AUTOIMMUNITY - PATHOGENESIS, CLINICAL ASPECTS AND THERAPY OF SPECIFIC AUTOIMMUNE DISEASES

Edited by **Katerina Chatzidionysiou**

Autoimmunity - Pathogenesis, Clinical Aspects and Therapy of Specific Autoimmune Diseases
http://dx.doi.org/10.5772/58718
Edited by Katerina Chatzidionysiou

Contributors

Ye Htun Oo, Nwe Ni Than, Mª Isabel Torres, Mitesh Kumar Dwivedi, Philippe Frachet, Pascale Tacnet-Delorme, Christine Gaboriaud, Nicole Thielens, Anna Pituch-Noworolska, Thomas Aune, Hiroshi Tanaka, Dilip Shah, Swapan Nath, Dheeraj Mohania, Nidhi Mahajan, Swapan K. Nath

Published by InTech

Janeza Trdine 9, 51000 Rijeka, Croatia

Publishing Process Manager Iva Lipovic

Technical Editor InTech DTP team

Cover InTech Design team

First published June, 2015

Printed in Croatia

Additional hard copies can be obtained from orders@intechopen.com

Autoimmunity - Pathogenesis, Clinical Aspects and Therapy of Specific Autoimmune Diseases, Edited by Katerina Chatzidionysiou

p. cm.

ISBN 978-953-51-2134-3

For EU product safety concerns:
IN TECH d.o.o., Prolaz Marije Krucifikse Kozulić 3, 51000 Rijeka, Croatia,
info@intechopen.com or visit our website at intechopen.com.

Meet the editor

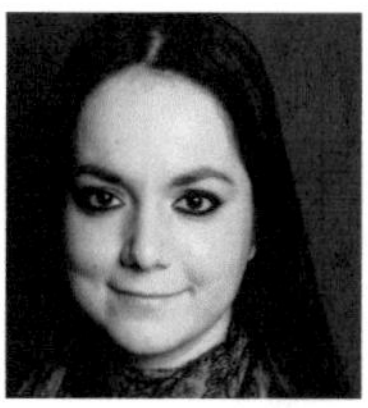

Katerina Chatzidionysiou, MD, PhD, is currently working at the Rheumatology Department at Karolinska University Hospital and at the Unit for Clinical Therapy Research, Inflammatory Diseases, at Karolinska Institute in Stockholm, Sweden. Her main research interest is therapy of Rheumatoid Arthritis and other inflammatory arthropathies. She has been involved in epidemiological studies based on large national and international registries, as well as translational research projects, which aim to optimize the use of biologic disease modifying antirheumatic drugs in clinical practice.

Contents

Preface

Autoimmune disorders represent a large group of disorders, from organ-specific to multi-system diseases. The understanding of the genetic background, immunopathogenesis, clinical presentation and therapeutic approach of these disorders is getting significantly deepened and broadened, as new evidence is arising. The aims of this book are:

• to provide insight into some pathogenic mechanisms with possible involvement in autoimmunity; the crosstalk between oxidative stress, autophagy and cell death; the role of C1Q in efferocytosis and self-tolerance; the implication of regional activation of toll-like receptor 3/interferon-β signaling in human mesangial cells.

• to describe clinical aspects of specific autoimmune diseases, like vitiligo, celiac disease and autoimmune liver disease, as well as the clinical spectrum of autoimmunity in primary immunodeficiency syndromes.

• to present new data regarding specific immunosuppressive therapies, such as methotrexate and triptolide. It is my hope that you will find the content of this book up-to-date, interesting and clinically relevant.

Katerina Chatzidionysiou, MD, PhD
Unit for Clinical Therapy Research, Inflammatory Diseases (ClinTRID), Karolinska Institute
Department of Rheumatology, Karolinska University Hospital
Stockholm, Sweden

Chapter 1

Crosstalk Between Oxidative Stress, Autophagy and Cell Death — Pathogenesis of Autoimmune Disease

Dilip Shah, Dheeraj Mohania, Nidhi Mahajan,
Sangita Sah, Bishnuhari Paudyal and
Swapan K. Nath

Additional information is available at the end of the chapter

http://dx.doi.org/10.5772/60696

1. Introduction

Increased free radical formation and altered redox state are fundamentally important in autoimmune diseases pathogenesis. Free radicals are mainly derived from oxygen (reactive oxygen species/ROS) and nitrogen (reactive nitrogen species/RNS) in mitochondria, cellular membranes, and the endoplasmic reticulum membrane as physiological responses to a variety of internal and external stress. These free radicals play both beneficial and deleterious roles in our body's defense system [1]. ROS/RNS are beneficial to our body at low/moderate concentrations via activation of redox-sensitive signaling pathways, phagocytosis of infected cells, induction of mitogenic responses for wound healing, and clearance of abnormal or aging cells as a part of an important surveillance mechanism [2-4].

Autophagy is a persistent homeostatic process in which certain cellular components are engulfed by autophagosomes, and are subsequently degraded in order to produce energy, or preserve viability and homeostasis. Autophagy breaks down compromised cellular components, such as damaged organelles and aggregated proteins, whose deposition within cells can lead to toxic effects resulting in destruction of tissues, organisms, and biological systems [5]. Alterations in autophagic cycle rate (flux), which initiates with formation of phagophore and terminates with degradation of autophagosome cargo after its fusion with lysosome, are generally observed in response to stress [6]. In most cases, autophagy primarily serves an adaptive role to protect organisms against diverse pathologies, including infections, cancer, neurodegeneration, aging, and heart disease. However, in certain experimental settings, autophagy may be deleterious [7]. Evidence from genetic, cell biology and lupus animal model studies suggests a pivotal role of autophagy in mediating the development of systemic lupus erythematosus (SLE) [8]. The current chapter will focus on the following areas: (i) molecular mechanism(s) by which ROS/RNS generate; (ii) redox signaling and altered autophagic flux rates; (iii) the role of autophagy as a cell death progression or survival mechanism in response to oxidative stress; and (iv) modulation of autophagy in antioxidant response relative to autoimmune disease. Attention is specifically focused on understanding the molecular basis of events by which autophagy is fine tuned by oxidation/reduction events in autoimmune disease, especially SLE. Understanding the intricate relationships between oxidative stress with both apoptosis and autophagy in SLE pathogenesis could be critical in elucidating key pathogenic mechanisms, possibly leading to novel interventions for clinical disease management.

2. Reactive Oxygen Species (ROS)

Reactive oxygen species (ROS) is a general term for chemical species which are generated from incomplete oxygen reduction. These are short lived molecules formed as a natural byproduct of normal cellular metabolism and have dual role; deleterious and beneficial effect in our body. ROS comprises several oxygen ion radicals such as superoxide anion radical ($O2^{\cdot-}$), peroxy radical ($ROO^{\cdot}$), extremely reactive hydroxyl radical ($^{\cdot}OH$), peroxide (hydrogen peroxide (H_2O_2), singlet oxygen ($^1O_2$), and perhydroxyl radical ($HO_2^{\cdot}$). Sources and modes of action of various reactive species are shown in Table 1 Beneficial role of ROS occur at low to moderate concentration that can be demonstrated by several important role of ROS in cell signaling and in defense against infectious agents and induction of a mitogenic response and immune functions.

When the ROS productions are not scavenged sufficiently by antioxidant system, it causes oxidative stress and shows harmful effect. These dangerous reactive species are formed by (1) enzymes such as nicotinamide adenine dinucleotide phosphate (NADPH) [9] or nitric oxide synthase [10], (2) non-enzymatic reactions through the mitochondrial electron transport chain [11], or (3) reduced transition metals [12]. ROS can also interact with nitric oxide (NO), whose expression is usually accompanied by inflammatory lesions. The product of NO synthases results in conversion of NO to various reactive nitrogen species (RNS.), including nitrosonium cation (NO^+), nitroxyl anion (NO^-), and peroxynitrite ($ONOO^{\cdot}$) (Table 1).

Reactive species	Sources	Modes of action
Super oxide (SO)	NADPH oxidase Xanthine oxidase Complex I/Complex III (mitochondria) 5-lipoxygenase, Cyclooxygenase Uncoupled nitric oxide synthase	Oxidative stress Redox signaling
Hydrogen peroxide (H_2O_2)	Peroxisomes	Redox signaling

Reactive species	Sources	Modes of action
	Super oxide dismutase	Oxidative stress
Hydroxyl radical (OH)	Fenton reaction Haber-Weiss reaction	Oxidative stress
Hypochlorous acid (HOCL)	Myeloperoxidase (MPO)	Chlorination Oxidative stress
Nitric oxide (NO)	Nitric oxide synthase	Nitrosylation of metal centers Redox signaling
Peroxynitrite (ONOO-)	Reaction between NO and SO	Nitration, oxidation Oxidative stress
Nitrogen dioxide radical (NO_2)	Reaction between NO and O_2	Nitration, oxidation Oxidative stress
Dinitrogen trioxide (N_2O_3)	Reaction between NO and NO_2	Nitrosation Nitrosative stress

Table 1. List of critical reactive oxygen and nitrogen species, their sources, and modes of action.

3. Sources of oxygen radicals and their scavengers

Reactive oxygen species mainly originate from mitochondria and blood compartment, including lymphocytes from SLE patients (Table 1). ROS show hyperpolarization of mitochondria and activated T lymphocytes [13, 14]. We and others have shown an increased production of ROS or diminished levels of intracellular reduced glutathione in various blood compartments (RBC, lymphocytes) from SLE patients [15, 16]. Beside these important source of ROS, these reactive oxygen species are also produced other sources such as NADPH oxidase (NOX enzyme) in activated phagocytes [9], and minor amount from endothelial cells, macrophage and polymononuclear cells [16-18], lysosome (myeloperoxidase undergoes a complex array of redox transformations and produces HOCl), and microsomes [19, 20]. Hydrogen peroxide is formed through the dismutation of $O_2^{\cdot -}$ catalyzed by enzyme superoxide dismutase, and is also produced via action of several other oxidase enzymes (e.g., amino acid oxidases) (Figure 1). Beside the role of ROS in cell damage, it is also involved in inflammation generation by activation of nuclear transcription factor NF-kB, a master pathway of inflammation generation. Once, the NF-kB is activated it leads to upregulation of pro-inflammatory cytokines and leukocyte adhesion molecules.

The most harmful ROS are hydroxyl radicals, $OH^{\cdot -}$ and $O_2^{\cdot -}$. Superoxide ion is converted into stable non-radical hydrogen peroxide by SOD enzyme which is then reduced by following 3 mechanisms. In a detoxification mechanism, catalase and glutathione peroxidase convert H_2O_2 to $H_2O + O_2$, this is considered as a detoxification mechanism. In the next mechanism, H_2O_2 is converted by myeloperoxidase (MPO) in neutrophils to hypochlorous acid (HOCl). This appears to be a mechanism for a physiological toxic agent, since HOCl is a strong oxidant that acts as a bactericidal agent in phagocytic cells. Reaction of HOCl with H_2O_2 yields singlet oxygen ($^1O_2$) and water. The biological significance of singlet oxygen is unclear. In the last mechanism, H_2O_2 is converted in a spontaneous reaction catalyzed by Fe^{2+} (Fenton reaction) to the highly reactive hydroxyl radical ($^{\cdot}OH$). As the hydroxyl radical cannot be removed without causing oxidative damage, it reacts rapidly with biological molecules such as lipid, protein and DNA, triggering severe consequences in SLE pathogenesis [21-24].

4. Mechanism of oxidative damage

Reactive oxygen species, specifically the hydroxyl radical, respond with lipid layers and produces receptive aldehydes, including malondialdehyde and 4-hydroxy-2-nonenal (HNE), in three phage responses. It can "spread" oxidative damage through flow in SLE patients [25]. In the start stage an essential receptive radical concentrates a hydrogen iota from a methylene gathering to begin peroxidation. These outcomes in the development of a conjugated diene, leaving an unpaired electron on the carbon. Carbon-focused unsaturated fat radicals consolidate with sub-atomic oxygen in the proliferation stage, yielding profoundly receptive peroxyl radicals that respond with an alternate lipid particle to structure hydroperoxides. Peroxyl radicals are fit for creating new unsaturated fat radicals, bringing about a radical chain response. The course of lipid peroxidation bring about a mixed bag of unsafe final items including conjugated dienes, isoprostanes, 4-hydroxy-2-nonenal (HNE), HNE-altered proteins, malondialdehyde (MDA), MDA-adjusted proteins, protein-bound acrolein and oxHDL,which are associated with SLE disease activity [26-28]. In addition to the involvement of ROS in lipid peroxidation, it can modify both structure and function of proteins in SLE patients [21, 29]. Metal-catalyzed protein oxidation brings about expansion of carbonyl gatherings, cross-connecting, or discontinuity of proteins. Lipid (peroxidation) aldehydes can respond with sulfhydryl (cysteine) or essential amino acids (histidine, lysine). Essentially, adjustment of individual nucleotide bases, single-strand breaks and cross-connecting are regular impacts of ROS on nucleic acids. All these communications of ROS with protein, lipid and nucleic corrosive prompts the development of adducts items which are exceedingly immunogenic and are perceived as an outside molecule to our body, which may be included in arrangement of pathogenic auto-immune response in SLE [30, 31].

5. Antioxidant defense system

The impact of ROS is restricted by the presence of various regulatory systems in aerobic organisms to maintain redox homeostasis. A comparatively large number of compounds possess some measurement of antioxidant activities. They keep up a harmony between the generation and scavenger of ROS, and shield the cell from oxidative damage [32, 33]. Antioxidant enzymes comprise SOD (superoxide dismutase), CAT (catalase) and glutathione related enzymes; GPx (glutathione peroxidase), GR (glutathione reductase) and GST (Glutathione S-transferase), while non-enzymatic scavengers include vitamins E, C and A and thiol containing compounds such as glutathione [34].

Reduced glutathione (L-γ-glutamyl-L-cysteinylglycine) is the most prevalent cellular thiol and the most abundant low molecular weight peptide present in all cells [35]. GSH has an amazingly essential role as a reductant in the very oxidizing environment of the erythrocyte. GSH levels in human tissues ordinarily run from 0.1 to 10 mM, and are most gathered in the liver (upto 10 mM), spleen, kidneys, lens, erythrocytes and leucocytes [36].]. In cell, more than 90% of the total glutathione pool is in the reduced form (GSH) and less than 10% exists in the oxidized form (GSSG). Reduced form of glutathione is required for many critical cellular processes and plays a cardinal role in cell maintenance and regulation of the thiol-redox [37]. Thus the ratio of GSH/GSSG is a significant marker for characterizing oxidative anxiety. Changes in this ratio relate with disease activity in SLE patients [15, 29]. Cellular GSH levels affect T helper cell maturation [38], T cell proliferation [39], and susceptibility to ROS secreted by inflammatory cells. Additionally, many correlations exist between immune system dysfunction and alterations in GSH levels in the cells of SLE patients. We and others have reported that GSH depletion in antigen presenting cells inhibits Th1-related cytokine production like IFN-γ and IL-12, which supports Th2- mediated humoral immune response in SLE patients [39]. Protection against oxidative damage is normally afforded by replenishing intracellular reduced glutathione through an antioxidant supplement of glutathione precursors N-acetylcysteine (NAC). Evidence from SLE patients and lupus prone mice supports the role of glutathione as antioxidant therapy to diminish oxidative stress and severity of disease. In (NZB × NZW) F1 lupus-prone mice NAC treatment prevented the decline of glutathione, including GSSG ratios, reduced autoantibody production, development of nephritis, and prolonged survival [40]. Two pilot studies of NAC treatment in SLE patients, Tewthanom (40 SLE patients) and Perl (36 SLE patients), showed that NAC treatment is effective in reversing glutathione depletion and improving disease activity and fatigue in SLE patients [16, 41]. These studies demonstrated that intracellular depletion displays an increased in oxidative stress and replenishment of intracellular glutathione may diminish disease activity in SLE patients.

Superoxide dismutase is a metalloprotein, thought to be the first line of resistance against free radicals. It catalyzes the dismutation of superoxide radical into oxygen and hydrogen peroxide [42]. If not rummaged successfully, superoxide radicals might specifically inactivate a few proteins like CAT and GPx, which are expected to take out hydrogen peroxide from intracellular medium [43]. This enzyme is found in 3 forms in human are: SOD1 located in the cytoplasm, SOD2 in the mitochondria, and extracellular SOD3 [44]. While SOD1 is dimeric [42], SOD2 and SOD3 are tetrameric [45, 46]. SOD1 and SOD3 contain copper and zinc, while SOD2 has manganese in its reactive center. Several groups reported decreased SOD activity and formation of auto-antibodies against SOD in SLE patients [47-49]. Antibodies against SOD are reported to have a role in the inactivation of SOD enzyme during increase oxidative state are responsible to deleterious effect in SLE patients.

Catalase is generally present in peroxisomes (80%) and cytosol (20%) of all oxygen consuming cells and responsible for managing harmful hydrogen peroxide produced inside cells. It catalyzes hydrogen peroxide to water and oxygen without production of free radicals [50, 51].

CAT is most elevated in the liver, kidney and erythrocytes and low in connective tissues [52]. In the most organs (e.g., liver, kidney), catalase is found as particle found (mitochondria and peroxisomes) where it exists in soluble state in erythrocytes. Under the physiological condition, H_2O_2 is catalyzed by glutathione peroxidase (high affinity for H_2O_2)while at high concentration H_2O_2 is removed by catalase enzyme [12]. The important of catalase enzyme in the SLE patients is well documented in SLE patients. The polymorphism catalase enzyme (-330CC genotype) showed remarkable association with several disease activities such as thrombocytopenia, renal manifestations, as well as production of anti-nRNP and anti-Scl-70 antibodies in SLE patients [53]. An elegant study by Mansour et al. reported that elevated levels of auto-antibodies against catalase in excessive oxidative stress state in SLE patients are associated with disease activity [54]. In two different studies they demonstrated that SLE patients have increased levels of IgG antibodies (Ab) against CAT in SLE patients compared to control subjects [54, 55].

Glutathione peroxidase belongs to the selenoprotein family and is one of the most important anti-oxidant enzymes in human. It catalyses hydroperoxides and protects biomembranes and cell structures from oxidative damage. [56]. This enzyme accomplishes these protections through utilization of glutathione as a reducing substrate and converting hydroperoxides to free hydrogen peroxide to water [57]. In animals studies the important of this enzyme can be illustrated by following evidences. Glutathione peroxidase knockout mice have abnormal cardiac mitochondria and associated with increase mitochondrial ROS production and oxidative mtDNA damage.

In SLE patients, decrease activity of glutathione peroxidase enzyme has been associated with increase in oxidized redox environment in cell [47]. Since, glutathione peroxidase enzyme is also required for maintaining intracellular glutathione levels, which is key antioxidant and control oxidative stress and involved in regulating several immune functions such as apoptosis [58]and cytokine network [38] in SLE pathogenesis.

6. Oxidative-stress and autophagy

Excessive oxidative stress and altered redox signaling are most commonly known to be involved in cell death signaling cascades. However, their role in regulation of autophagy is largely unknown in autoimmune diseases. Autophagy is a persistent homeostatic process in which certain cell components are engulfed by autophagosomes and, subsequently degraded in order to produce energy or preserve cellular viability and homeostasis [59]. Autophagy breaks down compromised cellular components, such as damaged organelles and aggregated proteins. Deposition of these components within cells can lead to toxicity, resulting in destruction of tissues, organisms, and biological systems [60]. Elevated ROS causing autophagy promotes either cell survival or cell death, the fate of which depends upon the severity of stress occurring with a particular disease.

Several studies have shown that ROS accumulation in the cell activates the autophagy process. For example, a mutation in an antioxidative superoxide dismutase (SOD1) gene modulates autophagy. Reports from different laboratories have described autophagy activation in transgenic mice expressing mutant SOD1 [61, 62]. In the first report, SOD1^{G93A} transgenic mice displayed inhibition of mTOR and accumulation of lipid-conjugated LC3, the mammalian homologue of Atg8 [62]. A recent report showed that mutant SOD1 interacts directly with p62 (also called SQSTM1), an LC3 binding partner known to target protein aggregates for autophagic degradation. Indeed, this interaction is proposed to mediate autophagic degradation of mutant SOD1 [63]. Ruth Scherz-Shouval's group has suggested two major ROS (H_2O_2 and $O_2^{\cdot-}$) as the main regulators of autophagy [64]. H_2O_2 is a striking contender for signaling because it is comparatively stable and long- lived as compared to other ROS species. Its neutral ionic state enables it to exit the mitochondria with ease. It has been implicated as a signaling molecule in various signal transduction pathways, including autophagy [65]. Indeed, ATG4, an essential protease in the autophagic pathway, has been identified as a direct target for oxidation by H_2O_2 during starvation [66]. Other studies report autophagy activation in response to exogenous H_2O_2 treatment [67] In most cases, this treatment leads to oxidative stress and mitochondrial damage, which induce autophagy. Taken together, this evidence supports the vital role of oxidative stress in the induction of autophagy.

7. Redox signaling and autophagy

Redox signaling involves targeted modification by reactive species through a chemically reversible reaction. The reaction of ROS/RNS with the target molecule acts as an on-off switch signal. Oxidative damage in response to oxidative stress leads to irreversible oxidation of proteins lipids and nucleic acids [68]. However, since amino-acid residues in proteins, fatty acids in lipids and nucleic acid bases have different susceptibility to oxidative stress. "Mild" oxidative stress appears to provide selectivity for a specifically targeted molecule and may constitute a signaling mechanism even when an irreversible modification is produced [69]. Oxidative damage can be repaired to a certain extent, as evident in the diverse array of DNA repair systems. In addition, oxidized proteins can be effectively degraded and recycled by both proteasome and autophagy systems. Proteasomal degradation of oxidatively modified proteins requires protein unfolding; thus, only mildly oxidized proteins are suitable proteasome substrates. During oxidative stress, the resulting cellular response and outcome is likely to involve both redox signaling and oxidative damage, whose contribution will depend on the concentration and nature of the ROS/RNS involved [70]. NAC decreased both cellular ROS production and autophagy, implicating redox thiol signaling as an important regulator of autophagy.

8. Autophagy as cell death progression or survival in response to oxidative stress

Similar to autophagy, ROS/RNS formation has been linked to the regulation of both pro-survival and cell death pathways (Figure 1). To generalize, basal levels of ROS/RNS formation and those induced by growth factor receptor activation are essential for maintaining appropriate cellular homeostasis and mediate cell proliferation by redox signaling [71]. ROS/RNS-mediated redox signaling also regulates survival-promoting adaptive responses to cellular stress. Redox signaling, generally occurs in the absence of an overall imbalance of pro-oxidants and antioxidants [71]. In contrast, when antioxidant defenses are surpassed by ROS/RNS formation, and oxidative damage is not repaired by endogenous mechanisms, oxidative stress leads to cell death. However, although oxidative damage to proteins, lipids, and nucleic acids is associated with activation of programmed cell death, both pro-apoptotic and pro-survival signaling proteins are modulated by specific reversible oxidative modifications [71, 72].

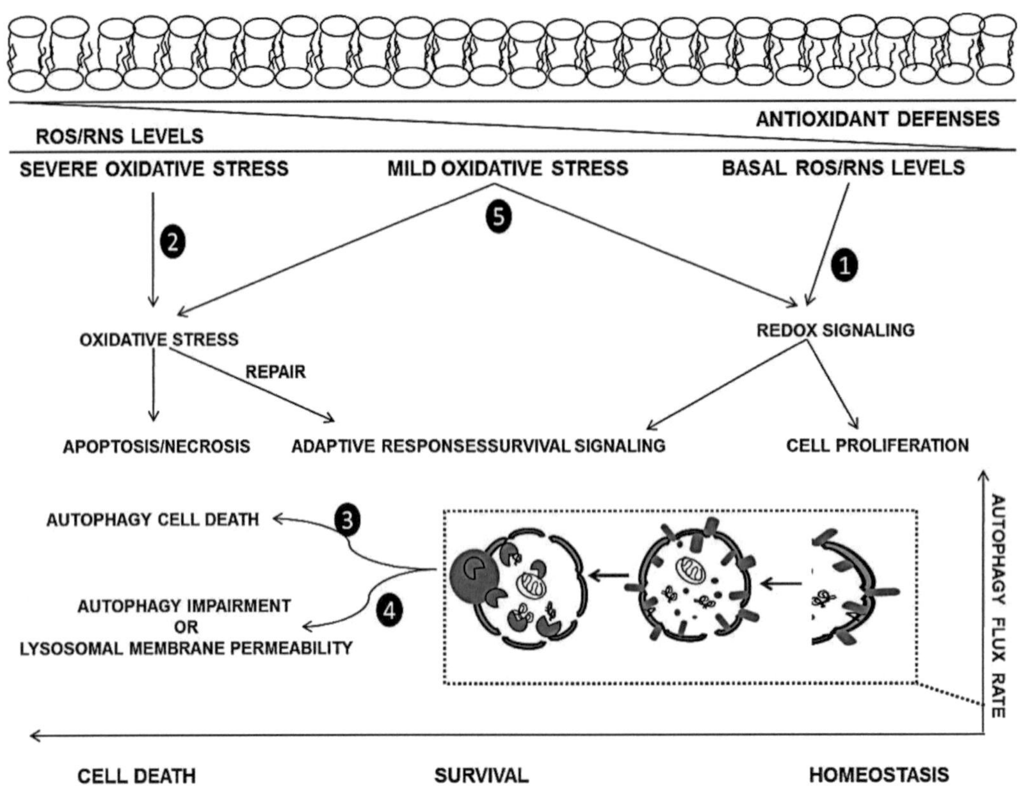

Figure 1. Oxidative stress, redox signaling, and autophagy: cell death versus survival. (1) Basal or physiological levels of ROS/RNS play an important homeostatic role regulating signal transduction involved in proliferation and survival. (2) In contrast, when antioxidant defenses are surpassed by ROS/RNS formation and oxidative damage is not repaired by endogenous mechanisms, oxidative stress leads to cell death. (3) Under these pathological conditions, "excessive" autophagy might promote cell death through degradation of important components within the cell. In addition, (4) lysosomal membrane permeabilization induced by stress can also contribute to cell death. However, (5) "mild" oxidative stress can act as a signaling mechanism leading to adaptive stress responses. Oxidative damage can be repaired to a certain extent and oxidized biomolecules, such as proteins, can be degraded and recycled by distinct processes, including autophagy. During oxidative stress the resulting cellular response and outcome is likely to involve both redox signaling and oxidative damage, whose contribution will depend on the concentration and nature of the ROS/RNS involved, the duration of the stress response, and cell type or gender. A clear distinction between both oxidative stress and redox signaling is hard to define.

9. Modulation of autophagy by antioxidant in autoimmune disease

There is a lack of literature on the role of redox signaling by oxidative cysteine modification in autophagy. Cysteines can act as post-translational modification sites which are utilized for targeting proteins to membranes and/or influence protein activity, localization, and/or protein–protein interactions [73]. In response to ROS or RNS, redox-sensitive cysteines undergo reversible and irreversible thiol modifications. Almost all physiological oxidants react with thiols [74]. $O_2^{\cdot -}$ and peroxides (H_2O_2, and $ONOO^-$) mediate one- and two-electron oxidation of protein cysteines respectively, leading to formation of reactive intermediates protein sulfenic acids (PSOH) and protein thiyl radicals (PS˙), respectively. PSOH can lead to formation of additional oxidative modifications that act as signaling events regulating protein function. The reaction of PSOH with either another protein cysteine or GSH will generate a disulfide bond or a glutathionylated residue (PSSG). PSSG is considered as a protective modification against irreversible cysteine oxidation. PSOH can undergo further reaction with H_2O_2 and irreversibly generate protein sulfinic (PSO_2H) and sulfonic (PSO_3H) acids. The reversible covalent adduction of a nitroso group (NO) to a protein cysteine is referred to as protein nitros(yl)ation (PSNO). PSNO occurs by endogenous NO-mediated nitros(yl)ating agents such as dinitrogen trioxide (N_2O_3) or by transition metal-catalyzed addition of NO. The transfer of NO groups between PSNO and GSNO (transnitros[yl]ation) is one of the major mechanisms mediating PSNO. GSNO is formed during oxidation of NO in the presence of GSH, or as a by-product from the oxidation of GSH by $ONOO^-$ [75].

Reversible conjugation of the Atg8 family of proteins to autophagosomal membrane is a hallmark event in the autophagic process. All Atg8 homologues (including LC3) are substrates for the Atg4 family of cysteine proteases. Atg4s cleave Atg8 near the C-terminus downstream of a conserved glycine, enabling its conjugation to PE. Atg4 further cleaves Atg8 (LC3)-PE, releasing it from the membrane. Thus, after initial cleavage of Atg8(LC3)-like proteins, Atg4 must be inactivated to ensure the conjugation of Atg8 (LC3) to the autophagosomal membrane. After the autophagosome fuses with the lysosome, Atg4 is re-activated in order to dilapidate and recycle Atg8 (LC3). Recently, it was revealed that upon starvation, increased generation of mitochondrial H_2O_2 oxidizes and inactivates Atg4 after the initial cleavage of LC3, ensuring structural integrity of the mature form [66]. A number of signaling molecules regulating apoptosis are reported to be regulated by oxidative cysteine modifications. For example, glutathionylation (PSSG) of nuclear factor-kappa B (NF-kB) and caspases, have been reported to regulate apoptotic cell death [76]. Similarly, caspases and the anti-apoptotic Bcl-2 protein have been shown to be nitros(yl)ated (PSNO) under basal conditions in human lung epithelial cancer cells, and their denitros(yl)ation is necessitated for their activation during apoptosis [77]. Both apoptosis and autophagy are simultaneously activated by the distinct stressors. Cross-talk between both the signaling pathways has been evidenced primarily by (1) interaction of Bcl-2 or Bcl-xl with Beclin-1, which inhibits autophagy; and (2) cleavage/degradation of Beclin-1 by caspases [78]. Thus, both glutathionylation and nitrosylation might exert regulatory roles in autophagy by indirect regulation of Bcl-2 and caspase activity [77]. Protein nitros(yl)ation exert inhibitory effects on autophagy. Nitros(yl)ation and inhibition of JNK1 and IKKb signaling pathways are also reported to inhibit autophagy by increased Bcl-2-Beclin-1 interaction and decreased AMPK phosphorylation [79].

AMPK is a key regulator of metabolism, particularly glycolysis. By regulation of ULK1 and mTORC1 complexes, AMPK has been demonstrated to regulate autophagy [80]. In HEK293 cells, H_2O_2 was recently demonstrated to oxidize cysteine residues of α-(Cys299 and Cys304) and β-subunits of AMPK via glutathionylation, with a concomitant increase in its kinase activity. Hypoxia is reported to activate AMPK via mitochondrial ROS formation independent from the AMP/ATP ratio in mitochondrial DNA-deficient cells [81]. Ataxia-telangiectasia mutated (ATM) protein kinase is activated by DNA double strand breaks (DSBs) to initiate DNA damage response. Cells lacking ATM are also hypersensitive to insults other than DSBs, particularly oxidative stress. Oxidation of ATM directly induces its activation in the absence of DNA damage via a disulfide-cross-linking dimerization [82]. Activation of ATM by oxidative stress or genotoxic damage was recently reported to activate AMPK and the tuberous sclerosis complex 2 (TSC2), which in turn participates in energy sensing and growth factor signaling to repress the kinase mTOR in the mTORC1 complex [83]. Studies regarding mechanisms by which ROS, redox signaling, and autophagy regulate autoimmune disease progression is a new research field that could provide pivotal information toward understanding and development of therapeutic to manage the disease.

10. Modulation of autophagy in systemic lupus erythematosus

SLE is an autoimmune disorder characterized by the auto-antibodies directed against self-antigens, immune complex formation and immune deregulation, resulting in damage to any organ, including kidneys, skin, blood cells, and nervous system [84]. It is a multifactorial disease and its etiology comprises hormonal, environmental and genetic background. While mechanisms underlying this systemic autoimmune response remain largely unknown, several vital studies show that uncontrolled reactive oxygen generation and defect in regulation of antioxidant system are, in part, crucial factors for the pathogenesis of SLE [85]. The uncontrolled oxidative species generations are speculated to be involved in the production, expansion of antibody flares [86] and various clinical features in SLE [87]. Oxidative damage mediated by ROS results in formation of deleterious byproducts, such as aldehydic products, and leads to development of adducts with proteins. The consequence of this effect makes them highly immunogenic, thus inducing pathogenic antibodies in SLE [88]. In the last 2 decades, there has been substantial progress in understanding the mechanism of oxidative stress in SLE pathogenesis (Figure 2) and the level of intracellular glutathione has been regarded as a checkpoint of oxidative stress [1]. Altered signal transduction pathways, mTOR is activated by relative depletion of glutathione and supplementation of N-acetyl cysteine (NAC), a precursor of glutathione. mTOR replenishes intracellular glutathione, inhibits mTOR signaling and diminished oxidative stress mediated damage in SLE [89]. Glutathione is a key cellular component, a small tri-peptide constructed from three amino acids (glycine, glutamic acid and cysteine), known to be a powerful antioxidant. The main function of glutathione is to protect the cell and mitochondria from oxidative damage, indicating its role in energy utilization.

Management of disease through supplement of NAC and rapamycin has shown promise as a therapy for SLE patients. Administration of rapamycin decreased production of autoantibodies, glomerular deposits of immunoglobulins, development of proteinuria, and prolonged survival in murine SLE. Interestingly, autophagy is regulated by mTOR pathway, and mTOR is activated by relative depletion of glutathione. Thus, redox signaling may provide a link between altered autophagy and depletion of glutathione and autophagy regulation by replenishment of intracellular glutathione may have a therapeutic intervention for disease management [90].

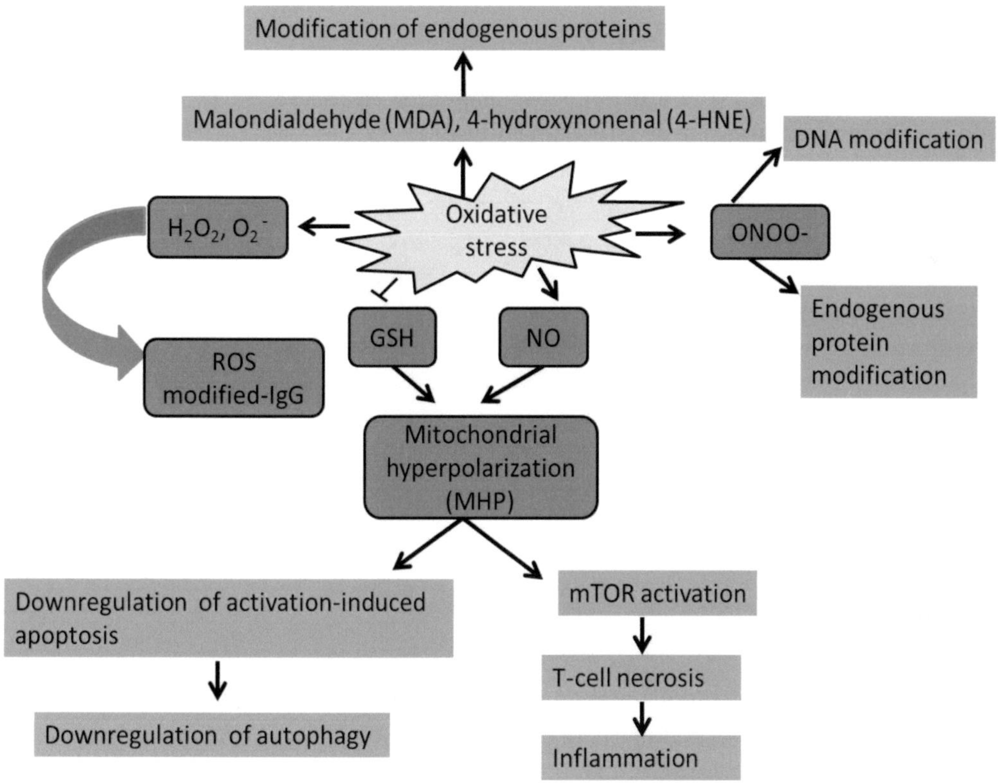

Figure 2. Oxidative stress involvement in the pathogenesis of SLE. MDA, malondialdehyde; 4-HNE, 4-hydroxynonenal; GSH, glutathione; MHP, mitochondrial hyperpolarization; NO, nitric oxide; $O_2^{\cdot -}$ superoxide; $ONOO^-$, peroxynitrite.

It has been shown that changes in the intracellular redox environment of in cells, through oxidative stress, have been reported to be critical for cellular immune dysfunction [48], activation of apoptotic enzymes, and apoptosis [15]. Decreased intracellular glutathione levels in the various blood components, including total lymphocytes and its subsets (CD4, CD8 T cell), are strongly associated with disease severity and linked to increase Th1/Th2 cytokine imbalance and lymphocyte apoptosis in SLE patients [49]. Similarly, Tewthanom et al. [41] reported that administration of NAC may be beneficial for patients with mild SLE in terms of decreasing lipid peroxidation. Lai et al. demonstrated that GSH regulates elevation of mitochondrial transmembrane potential ($\Delta\psi_m$) or mitochondrial hyperpolarization (MHP), which in turn activates mTOR in lupus T cells [91]. mTOR skews cell death signal processing, modulates T-cell differentiation, and, in particular, inhibits development of $CD4^+/CD25^+/$ $Foxp3^+$ regulatory T cells which are deficient in patients with active SLE. These studies are important as they suggest the blockade of mTOR with rapamycin and NAC improves lupus disease activity [89, 91].

In recent years, perturbation in autophagy has been implicated in a number of diseases, including SLE [8]. Towns et al. [92] found that serum factors, likely autoantibodies, purified from SLE patients were able to induce autophagy in neuroblastoma cell lines, providing a further link between autophagy and SLE. Several other groups have reported activated autophagy pathway in T and B lymphocytes as a mechanism for survival of autoreactive T and B lymphocytes. Inhibition of autophagy by blocking mTOR signaling has been suggested as a novel target for treatment in this disease. Importantly, Lai et. al. has shown that blockade of mTOR with supplementation of NAC reversing glutathione depletion and improving disease activity and fatigue in SLE patients [91]. NAC treatment promotes expansion of $CD4^+CD25^+FOXP3^+$ T cell subsets and inhibits anti-DNA antibody production. Indeed, NAC reversed expansion of $CD4^-CD8^-$ T cells, which exhibited the most prominent mTOR activation before treatment with NAC, and may be responsible for promoting anti-DNA autoantibody production by B cells. They showed that NAC acts as a sensor of $\Delta\Psi m$, mTOR governs T-cell signaling events implicated in pathogenesis [91]. Since, activation of autophagy has been considered to be principally regulated by the mTOR pathway, supplementation of NAC block mTOR signaling in SLE patients.

11. Conclusion

The autophagic process is highly regulated and is stimulated by several factors including oxidative stress. Cell death occurs when over production of ROS/NOS fails to be corrected by antioxidant machinery, activate autophagy, which in turn removes damaged components, or when damage exceeds a certain threshold. However, whether autophagy leads to a pro-survival response or cell death depends on the situation and severity of oxidative stress occurring in a particular pathologic setting. Evidence from genetics, cell biology and lupus animal model studies suggests a pivotal role of autophagy in mediating occurrence and development of SLE. Importantly, autophagy is regulated by the mTOR pathway, and mTOR is activated by relative depletion of glutathione. This suggests that redox signaling may provide a link between altered redox signaling and autophagy in SLE. Therefore it will be interesting to study the effect of therapeutic supplements of NAC on autophagy in animal models of lupus and in SLE patients. Such controlled clinical studies encourage exploration of the therapeutic potential of NAC, which might prove to provide an inexpensive and significant alternative therapy for SLE.

http://dx.doi.org/10.5772/60696

Acknowledgements

The authors thank Xana Kim-Howard for excellent assistance in editing and reviewing this manuscript. We also acknowledge the grant support from NIH (AI103399, AR060366) for this work. Some sections of this chapter were previously published in: Shah D and Nath SK. Glutathione: a possible link to autophagy in Systemic lupus erythematosus. *Am J Immunology.* 10 (3): 114-115, 2014; Shah D, Mahajan N, Sah S, Nath SK, Paudyal B. Oxidative stress and its biomarkers in systemic lupus erythematosus. *J Biomed Sci.* 2014 Mar 17;21:23; Shah D, Agawam A, Bhavnagar A, Koran R, Winch A. Association between T lymphocyte sub-set apoptosis and peripheral blood mononuclear cell oxidative stress in systemic lupus erythematosus. *Free Radic Res* 2011;45:559-567; Shah D, Wanchu A, Bhatnagar A. Interaction between oxidative stress and chemokines: possible pathogenic role in systemic lupus erythematosus and rheumatoid arthritis. *Immunobio.* 2011;216:1010-1017; Shah D, Kiran R, Wanchu A, Bhatnagar A. Oxidative stress in systemic lupus erythematosus: relationship to Th1 cytokine and disease activity. *Immunol Lett.* 2010;129:7-12; Shah D, Sah S, Nath SK. Interaction between glutathione and apoptosis in systemic lupus erythematosus. *Autoimmun Rev.* 2013 May;12(7):741-51; 4. Shah D, Sah S, Wanchu A, Wu MX, Bhatnagar A. Altered Redox State and Apoptosis in Systemic Lupus Erythematosus. *Immunobio.* 2013 Apr;218 (4):620-7.

Author details

Dilip Shah[1*], Dheeraj Mohania[2], Nidhi Mahajan[3], Sangita Sah[4], Bishnuhari Paudyal[5] and Swapan K. Nath[6]

*Address all correspondence to: Swapan-Nath@omrf.org; dilipkmc@gmail.com

1 Center for Translational Medicine, Thomas Jefferson University, Philadelphia, PA, USA

2 Department of Research, Sir Ganga Ram Hospital (S.G.R.H.), New Delhi, India

3 Department of Biochemistry, Panjab University, Chandigarh, India

4 Department of Biochemistry, JNMC, Karnataka, India

5 Department of Radiology, Thomas Jefferson University, Philadelphia, PA, USA

6 Arthritis and Clinical Immunology Research Program, Oklahoma Medical Research Foundation, Oklahoma City, OK, USA

The authors report no conflicts of interest.

References

[1] Shah, D., et al., *Oxidative stress and its biomarkers in systemic lupus erythematosus.* J Biomed Sci, 2014. 21: p. 23.

[2] D'Autreaux, B. and M.B. Toledano, *ROS as signalling molecules: mechanisms that generate specificity in ROS homeostasis.* Nat Rev Mol Cell Biol, 2007. 8(10): p. 813-24.

[3] Franco, R. and J.A. Cidlowski, *Apoptosis and glutathione: beyond an antioxidant.* Cell Death Differ, 2009. 16(10): p. 1303-14.

[4] Franco, R., M.I. Panayiotidis, and J.A. Cidlowski, *Glutathione depletion is necessary for apoptosis in lymphoid cells independent of reactive oxygen species formation.* J Biol Chem, 2007. 282(42): p. 30452-65.

[5] Choi, A.M., S.W. Ryter, and B. Levine, *Autophagy in human health and disease.* N Engl J Med, 2013. 368(7): p. 651-62.

[6] Kroemer, G., G. Marino, and B. Levine, *Autophagy and the integrated stress response.* Mol Cell, 2010. 40(2): p. 280-93.

[7] Levine, B. and G. Kroemer, *Autophagy in the pathogenesis of disease.* Cell, 2008. 132(1): p. 27-42.

[8] Alessandri, C., et al., *T lymphocytes from patients with systemic lupus erythematosus are resistant to induction of autophagy.* FASEB J, 2012. 26(11): p. 4722-32.

[9] Vignais, P.V., *The superoxide-generating NADPH oxidase: structural aspects and activation mechanism.* Cell Mol Life Sci, 2002. 59(9): p. 1428-59.

[10] Wei, C.C., et al., *The three nitric-oxide synthases differ in their kinetics of tetrahydrobiopterin radical formation, heme-dioxy reduction, and arginine hydroxylation.* J Biol Chem, 2005. 280(10): p. 8929-35.

[11] Turrens, J.F. and A. Boveris, *Generation of superoxide anion by the NADH dehydrogenase of bovine heart mitochondria.* Biochem J, 1980. 191(2): p. 421-7.

[12] Chance, B., H. Sies, and A. Boveris, *Hydroperoxide metabolism in mammalian organs.* Physiol Rev, 1979. 59(3): p. 527-605.

[13] Alam, K., Moinuddin, and S. Jabeen, *Immunogenicity of mitochondrial DNA modified by hydroxyl radical.* Cell Immunol, 2007. 247(1): p. 12-7.

[14] Perl, A., P. Gergely, Jr., and K. Banki, *Mitochondrial dysfunction in T cells of patients with systemic lupus erythematosus.* Int Rev Immunol, 2004. 23(3-4): p. 293-313.

[15] Shah, D., et al., *Altered redox state and apoptosis in the pathogenesis of systemic lupus erythematosus.* Immunobiology, 2013. 218(4): p. 620-7.

[16] Perl, A., *Oxidative stress in the pathology and treatment of systemic lupus erythematosus.* Nat Rev Rheumatol, 2013.

[17] Kim, J.Y., et al., *Osteoprotegerin causes apoptosis of endothelial progenitor cells by induction of oxidative stress.* Arthritis Rheum, 2013. 65(8): p. 2172-82.

[18] Li, K.J., et al., *Deranged bioenergetics and defective redox capacity in T lymphocytes and neutrophils are related to cellular dysfunction and increased oxidative stress in patients with active systemic lupus erythematosus.* Clin Dev Immunol, 2012. 2012: p. 548516.

[19] Ahmad, R., Z. Rasheed, and H. Ahsan, *Biochemical and cellular toxicology of peroxynitrite: implications in cell death and autoimmune phenomenon.* Immunopharmacol Immunotoxicol, 2009. 31(3): p. 388-96.

[20] Murphy, M.P., et al., *Peroxynitrite: a biologically significant oxidant.* Gen Pharmacol, 1998. 31(2): p. 179-86.

[21] Morgan, P.E., A.D. Sturgess, and M.J. Davies, *Evidence for chronically elevated serum protein oxidation in systemic lupus erythematosus patients.* Free Radic Res, 2009. 43(2): p. 117-27.

[22] Al-Shobaili, H.A., et al., *Hydroxyl radical modification of immunoglobulin g generated cross-reactive antibodies: its potential role in systemic lupus erythematosus.* Clin Med Insights Arthritis Musculoskelet Disord, 2011. 4: p. 11-9.

[23] Garg, D.K., Moinuddin, and R. Ali, *Hydroxyl radical modification of polyguanylic acid: role of modified guanine in circulating SLE anti-DNA autoantibodies.* Immunol Invest, 2003. 32(3): p. 187-99.

[24] Kurien, B.T. and R.H. Scofield, *Lipid peroxidation in systemic lupus erythematosus.* Indian J Exp Biol, 2006. 44(5): p. 349-56.

[25] Rimbach, G., et al., *Methods to assess free radicals and oxidative stress in biological systems.* Arch Tierernahr, 1999. 52(3): p. 203-22.

[26] Hartley, D.P., D.J. Kroll, and D.R. Petersen, *Prooxidant-initiated lipid peroxidation in isolated rat hepatocytes: detection of 4-hydroxynonenal- and malondialdehyde-protein adducts.* Chem Res Toxicol, 1997. 10(8): p. 895-905.

[27] Calingasan, N.Y., K. Uchida, and G.E. Gibson, *Protein-bound acrolein: a novel marker of oxidative stress in Alzheimer's disease.* J Neurochem, 1999. 72(2): p. 751-6.

[28] Levine, R.L., et al., *Determination of carbonyl content in oxidatively modified proteins.* Methods Enzymol, 1990. 186: p. 464-78.

[29] Shah, D., S. Sah, and S.K. Nath, *Interaction between glutathione and apoptosis in systemic lupus erythematosus.* Autoimmun Rev, 2013. 12(7): p. 741-51.

[30] Al-Shobaili, H.A., et al., *Antibodies against 4-hydroxy-2-nonenal modified epitopes recognized chromatin and its oxidized forms: role of chromatin, oxidized forms of chromatin and 4-*

hydroxy-2-nonenal modified epitopes in the etiopathogenesis of SLE. Dis Markers, 2012. 33(1): p. 19-34.

[31] Jovanovic, V., et al., *Lipid anti-lipid antibody responses correlate with disease activity in systemic lupus erythematosus.* PLoS One, 2013. 8(2): p. e55639.

[32] Halliwelly, B. and J. Gutteridge, M.,C., *Free Radical Biology and Medicine, 4ed (Oxford: Clarendon Press)* 2006.

[33] Halliwell, B., *Reactive oxygen species in living systems: source, biochemistry, and role in human disease.* Am J Med, 1991. 91(3C): p. 14S-22S.

[34] Sies, H., *Role of reactive oxygen species in biological processes.* Klin Wochenschr, 1991. 69(21-23): p. 965-8.

[35] Meister, A., *Glutathione metabolism and its selective modification.* J Biol Chem, 1988. 263(33): p. 17205-8.

[36] Bremer, H., J., M. Duran, and J. Kameling, P., *Glutathione. In: Bremer HJ, Duran M, Kamerling JP (eds) Disturbances of amino acid metabolism: clinical chemistry and diagnosis. Urban & Schwarzenberg, Baltimore-Munich.* 1981: p. 80-82.

[37] Schafer, F.Q. and G.R. Buettner, *Redox environment of the cell as viewed through the redox state of the glutathione disulfide/glutathione couple.* Free Radic Biol Med, 2001. 30(11): p. 1191-212.

[38] Peterson, J.D., et al., *Glutathione levels in antigen-presenting cells modulate Th1 versus Th2 response patterns.* Proc Natl Acad Sci U S A, 1998. 95(6): p. 3071-6.

[39] Messina, J.P. and D.A. Lawrence, *Cell cycle progression of glutathione-depleted human peripheral blood mononuclear cells is inhibited at S phase.* J Immunol, 1989. 143(6): p. 1974-81.

[40] Suwannaroj, S., et al., *Antioxidants suppress mortality in the female NZB x NZW F1 mouse model of systemic lupus erythematosus (SLE).* Lupus, 2001. 10(4): p. 258-65.

[41] Tewthanom, K., et al., *The effect of high dose of N-acetylcysteine in lupus nephritis: a case report and literature review.* Journal of Clinical Pharmacy and Therapeutics, 2009. 9999(9999).

[42] McCord, J.M. and I. Fridovich, *Superoxide dismutase. An enzymic function for erythrocuprein (hemocuprein).* J Biol Chem, 1969. 244(22): p. 6049-55.

[43] Blum, J. and I. Fridovich, *Inactivation of glutathione peroxidase by superoxide radical.* Arch Biochem Biophys, 1985. 240(2): p. 500-8.

[44] Johnson, F. and C. Giulivi, *Superoxide dismutases and their impact upon human health.* Mol Aspects Med, 2005. 26(4-5): p. 340-52.

[45] McCord, J.M., *Iron- and manganese-containing superoxide dismutases: structure, distribution, and evolutionary relationships.* Adv Exp Med Biol, 1976. 74: p. 540-50.

[46] Marklund, S.L., *Properties of extracellular superoxide dismutase from human lung*. Biochem J, 1984. 220(1): p. 269-72.

[47] Turgay, M., et al., *Oxidative stress and antioxidant parameters in a Turkish group of patients with active and inactive systemic lupus erythematosus*. APLAR Journal of Rheumatology, 2007. 10(2): p. 101-106.

[48] Shah, D., et al., *Oxidative stress in systemic lupus erythematosus: relationship to Th1 cytokine and disease activity*. Immunol Lett, 2010. 129(1): p. 7-12.

[49] Shah, D., et al., *Association between T lymphocyte sub-sets apoptosis and peripheral blood mononuclear cells oxidative stress in systemic lupus erythematosus*. Free Radic Res, 2011. 45(5): p. 559-67.

[50] Forman, H.J. and A.B. Fisher, *Antioxidant enzymes of rat granular pneumocytes. Constitutive levels and effect of hyperoxia*. Lab Invest, 1981. 45(1): p. 1-6.

[51] Jones, D.P., et al., *Metabolism of hydrogen peroxide in isolated hepatocytes: relative contributions of catalase and glutathione peroxidase in decomposition of endogenously generated H2O2*. Arch Biochem Biophys, 1981. 210(2): p. 505-16.

[52] Aebi, H., *Catalase in vitro*. Methods Enzymol, 1984. 105: p. 121-6.

[53] Warchol, T., et al., *Catalase -262C>T polymorphism in systemic lupus erythematosus in Poland*. Rheumatol Int, 2008. 28(10): p. 1035-9.

[54] Mansour, R.B., et al., *Increased levels of autoantibodies against catalase and superoxide dismutase associated with oxidative stress in patients with rheumatoid arthritis and systemic lupus erythematosus*. Scand J Rheumatol, 2008. 37(2): p. 103-8.

[55] Ben Mansour, R., et al., *Enhanced reactivity to malondialdehyde-modified proteins by systemic lupus erythematosus autoantibodies*. Scand J Rheumatol, 2010. 39(3): p. 247-53.

[56] Gamble, S.C., A. Wiseman, and P.S. Goldfarb, *Selenium-dependent glutathione peroxidase and other selenoproteins: their synthesis and biochemical roles*. J Chem Technol Biotech, 1999. 68(2): p. 123-134.

[57] Sen, C.K., *Cellular thiols and redox-regulated signal transduction*. Curr Top Cell Regul, 2000. 36: p. 1-30.

[58] Circu, M.L. and T.Y. Aw, *Reactive oxygen species, cellular redox systems, and apoptosis* Free Radic Biol Med, 2010. 48(6): p. 749-762.

[59] Zhou, X.J., F.J. Cheng, and H. Zhang, *Emerging View of Autophagy in Systemic Lupus Erythematosus*. Int Rev Immunol, 2014.

[60] Doria, A., M. Gatto, and L. Punzi, *Autophagy in human health and disease*. N Engl J Med, 2013. 368(19): p. 1845.

[61] Dobrowolny, G., et al., *Skeletal muscle is a primary target of SOD1G93A-mediated toxicity*. Cell Metab, 2008. 8(5): p. 425-36.

[62] Morimoto, N., et al., *Increased autophagy in transgenic mice with a G93A mutant SOD1 gene*. Brain Res, 2007. 1167: p. 112-7.

[63] Gal, J., et al., *Sequestosome 1/p62 links familial ALS mutant SOD1 to LC3 via an ubiquitin-independent mechanism*. J Neurochem, 2009. 111(4): p. 1062-73.

[64] Scherz-Shouval, R. and Z. Elazar, *Regulation of autophagy by ROS: physiology and pathology*. Trends Biochem Sci, 2010. 36(1): p. 30-8.

[65] Zhang, H., et al., *Oxidative stress induces parallel autophagy and mitochondria dysfunction in human glioma U251 cells*. Toxicol Sci, 2009. 110(2): p. 376-88.

[66] Scherz-Shouval, R., et al., *Reactive oxygen species are essential for autophagy and specifically regulate the activity of Atg4*. EMBO J, 2007. 26(7): p. 1749-60.

[67] Azad, M.B., Y. Chen, and S.B. Gibson, *Regulation of autophagy by reactive oxygen species (ROS): implications for cancer progression and treatment*. Antioxid Redox Signal, 2009. 11(4): p. 777-90.

[68] Forman, H.J., J.M. Fukuto, and M. Torres, *Redox signaling: thiol chemistry defines which reactive oxygen and nitrogen species can act as second messengers*. Am J Physiol Cell Physiol, 2004. 287(2): p. C246-56.

[69] Giordano, S., V. Darley-Usmar, and J. Zhang, *Autophagy as an essential cellular antioxidant pathway in neurodegenerative disease*. Redox Biol, 2013. 2: p. 82-90.

[70] Navarro-Yepes, J., et al., *Oxidative stress, redox signaling, and autophagy: cell death versus survival*. Antioxid Redox Signal, 2014. 21(1): p. 66-85.

[71] Nakamura, T. and S.A. Lipton, *Emerging role of protein-protein transnitrosylation in cell signaling pathways*. Antioxid Redox Signal, 2013. 18(3): p. 239-49.

[72] Allen, E.M. and J.J. Mieyal, *Protein-thiol oxidation and cell death: regulatory role of glutaredoxins*. Antioxid Redox Signal, 2012. 17(12): p. 1748-63.

[73] Fomenko, D.E., S.M. Marino, and V.N. Gladyshev, *Functional diversity of cysteine residues in proteins and unique features of catalytic redox-active cysteines in thiol oxidoreductases*. Mol Cells, 2008. 26(3): p. 228-35.

[74] Winterbourn, C.C. and M.B. Hampton, *Thiol chemistry and specificity in redox signaling*. Free Radic Biol Med, 2008. 45(5): p. 549-61.

[75] Foster, M.W., D.T. Hess, and J.S. Stamler, *Protein S-nitrosylation in health and disease: a current perspective*. Trends Mol Med, 2009. 15(9): p. 391-404.

[76] Qanungo, S., et al., *Glutathione supplementation potentiates hypoxic apoptosis by S-glutathionylation of p65-NFkappaB*. J Biol Chem, 2007. 282(25): p. 18427-36.

[77] Liu, Q., et al., *A Fenton reaction at the endoplasmic reticulum is involved in the redox control of hypoxia-inducible gene expression*. Proc Natl Acad Sci U S A, 2004. 101(12): p. 4302-7.

[78] Giansanti, V., A. Torriglia, and A.I. Scovassi, *Conversation between apoptosis and autophagy: "Is it your turn or mine?"* Apoptosis, 2011. 16(4): p. 321-33.

[79] Lista, P., et al., *On the role of autophagy in human diseases: a gender perspective*. J Cell Mol Med, 2011. 15(7): p. 1443-57.

[80] Han, D., et al., *LKB1/AMPK/mTOR signaling pathway in non-small-cell lung cancer.* Asian Pac J Cancer Prev, 2013. 14(7): p. 4033-9.

[81] Wu, W., P. Liu, and J. Li, *Necroptosis: an emerging form of programmed cell death.* Crit Rev Oncol Hematol, 2011. 82(3): p. 249-58.

[82] Guo, Z., et al., *ATM activation by oxidative stress*. Science, 2010. 330(6003): p. 517-21.

[83] Kubli, D.A. and A.B. Gustafsson, *Mitochondria and mitophagy: the yin and yang of cell death control.* Circ Res, 2012. 111(9): p. 1208-21.

[84] Wallace, D.J., *The clinical presentation of systemic lupus erythematosus. Dubois' lupus erythematosus. 7th ed. Baltimore (Maryland): Williams & Wilkins* 2007: p. 627–33..

[85] Graham, K.L. and P.J. Utz, *Sources of autoantigens in systemic lupus erythematosus.* Curr Opin Rheumatol, 2005. 17(5): p. 513-7.

[86] Kurien, B.T. and R.H. Scofield, *Free radical mediated peroxidative damage in systemic lupus erythematosus*. Life Sci, 2003. 73(13): p. 1655-66.

[87] Taysi, S., et al., *Serum oxidant/antioxidant status of patients with systemic lupus erythematosus*. Clin Chem Lab Med, 2002. 40(7): p. 684-8.

[88] Shah, D., et al., *Soluble granzyme B and cytotoxic T lymphocyte activity in the pathogenesis of systemic lupus erythematosus.* Cell Immunol, 2011. 269(1): p. 16-21.

[89] Fernandez, D. and A. Perl, *mTOR signaling: a central pathway to pathogenesis in systemic lupus erythematosus?* Discov Med, 2010. 9(46): p. 173-8.

[90] Shah, D. and S.K. Nath, *glutathione: a possible link to autophagy in systemic lupus erythematosus*. American Journal of Immunology, 2014. 10(3): p. 115.

[91] Lai, Z.W., et al., *N-acetylcysteine reduces disease activity by blocking mammalian target of rapamycin in T cells from systemic lupus erythematosus patients: a randomized, double-blind, placebo-controlled trial.* Arthritis Rheum, 2012. 64(9): p. 2937-46.

[92] Towns, R., et al., Sera from patients with type 2 diabetes and neuropathy induce autophagy and colocalization with mitochondria in SY5Y cells. Autophagy, 2005. 1(3): p. 163-70.

Chapter 2

Role of C1q in Efferocytosis and Self-Tolerance — Links With Autoimmunity

Philippe Frachet, Pascale Tacnet-Delorme,
Christine Gaboriaud and Nicole M. Thielens

Additional information is available at the end of the chapter

http://dx.doi.org/10.5772/60519

1. Introduction

C1q, the well-known initiator of the classical complement pathway, belongs to a family of soluble pattern recognition receptors (PRRs) called defense collagens comprised of a C-terminal globular region and an N–terminal collagen-like tail. The defense collagens include collectins (collagen containing lectins) such as mannan-binding lectin (MBL), lung surfactant protein A (SP-A), SP-D, CL-K1 CL-L1, conglutinin, collectin-43 and related proteins ficolins. They are capable of recognizing a wide range of microorganisms by binding to their pathogen-associated molecular patterns (PAMPs) [1-3].

C1q differs from the collectins and ficolins members of the defense collagens in that it does not contain a C-type lectin or fibrinogen like recognition domain [4]. Rather, it contains a "jellyroll" beta sandwich fold typical of tumor necrosis factor family [5]. Additionally, C1q is structurally related to some TNF-related proteins such as adiponectin, and the members of CTRP (C1q/TNF-related proteins) family [6], suggesting that C1q could share some "cytokine-like"functions with these molecules.

On the other hand, C1q is classically known for its ability to bind IgG-and IgM-containing immune complexes [7, 8] which initiates the classical complement cascade for microbial killing and phagocytosis.

The traditional view of the biological role of C1q as a first line of innate immunity against pathogens has been reconsidered over the past 15 years with evidences showing that C1q has the ability to sense many altered structures from self, including the pathological form of the prion protein [9, 10], β-amyloid fibrils [11], modified forms of low-density lipoprotein [12, 13] and apoptotic cells [14-16]. Unlike the other complement proteins that are expressed mostly, if not exclusively, in the liver, C1q is predominantly synthesized by myeloid cells such as macrophages and dendritic cells (DC) and also, in smaller quantities, by a wide range of cell types (reviewed in [17] and paragraph 3.2).

Importantly, C1q is one actor of efferocytosis, which is the mechanism of the clearance of altered self-cells and in particular of apoptotic cells, and is essential for development and to maintain tissue homeostasis [18]. C1q is involved in this process, at least as a physical bridge between the phagocyte and its prey. Numerous C1q-binding molecules at both sides of the phagocytic synapse have been characterized today (summarized in Tables 1 and 2), suggesting a multiligand-binding process even if the consequences of their molecular interplay are not deciphered yet.

Consistent with its importance in the fight against pathogens and as for the other complement proteins, genetic deficiency in C1q leads to a plethora of infections [19]. However, in the case of C1q, deficiency is also strongly correlated with autoimmune diseases, such as systemic lupus erythematosus (SLE) and glomerulonephritis, associated with compromised removal of apoptotic cells (as developed in paragraph 7).

A key element that highlights the non-traditional C1q functions, linking it to autoimmunity, is its capacity to regulate immune cells. This includes a wide range of effects such as regulation of dendritic cells and macrophage polarization, phagocytosis enhancement, stimulation of leukocytes, suppression of T and B cells proliferation. This chapter will provide an update of the C1q functions with an emphasis on its role in autoimmunity.

2. The C1q protein and its classical functions in complement activation

The association with a Ca^{2+}-dependent tetramer comprising two copies of two serine proteases, C1r and C1s [20, 21], allows C1q to trigger the classical complement pathway. C1q is a 460-kDa hexameric protein assembled from six heterotrimeric collagen-like fibers (Figure 1), each being prolonged by a C-terminal globular domain. One heterotrimeric fiber consists of 3 distinct but similar polypeptide chains, A, B, C encoded by 3 genes *C1QA*, *C1QB* and *C1QC* localized on human chromosome 1p, and aligned in the same orientation in the order A-C-B. From a structure-function point of view, the collagen-like domain (cC1q) and the globular heads (gC1q) define two well characterized functional domains. The gC1q domain has the ability to sense and engage an amazing variety of ligands that could be part of surface molecular patterns [20, 22] and is considered as the key to the versatility of C1q function [21, 23, 24]. Until even recently, cC1q specificity has been restricted to the interaction with the associated serine proteases C1r-C1s and with the phagocyte endocytic receptor CRT/CD91(LRP1). As the recognition molecule of the classical pathway, C1q is well known to recognize the IgG and IgM Fc fragments of membrane-bound antibodies, but also of aggregated immune complexes. In addition to this best known "classical" property, C1q recognizes C-reactive protein and other pentraxins bound to pathogens and other surfaces, as well as various molecular motifs on several Gram-negative bacteria and viruses (PAMPs), including gp41 or DNA [20, 25-27]. In most cases, recognition of these non-self ligands, as well as Ig and pentraxins, by C1q triggers activation of the classical complement pathway, thereby contributing to their elimination through enhanced phagocytosis, lysis, and inflammation (Figure 2).

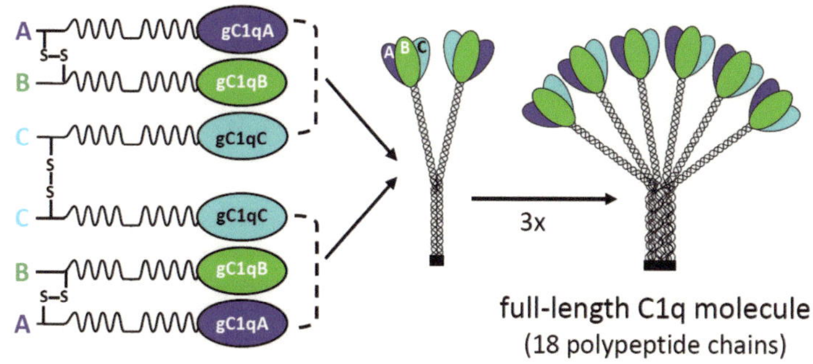

Figure 1. Schematic representation of the assembly of the C1q molecule. C1q is assembled from three polypeptide chains (A, B and C) encoded by 3 different genes (*C1QA, C1QB* and *C1QC*). Each chain comprises an N-terminal collagen-like sequence and a C-terminal globular gC1q module, with disulfide bridges linking the N-terminal ends of the A and B chains and two C chains. Each A-B dimer associates with a C chain, resulting in a basic subunit comprised of two disulphide-linked heterotrimeric collagen-like stalks prolonged by globular domains. The association of 3 subunits results in a full-length protein with a typical shape of a bouquet of six flowers, the stalks being held together in their N-terminal half through strong non-covalent interactions and then diverging to form six individual stems, each terminating in a globular head.

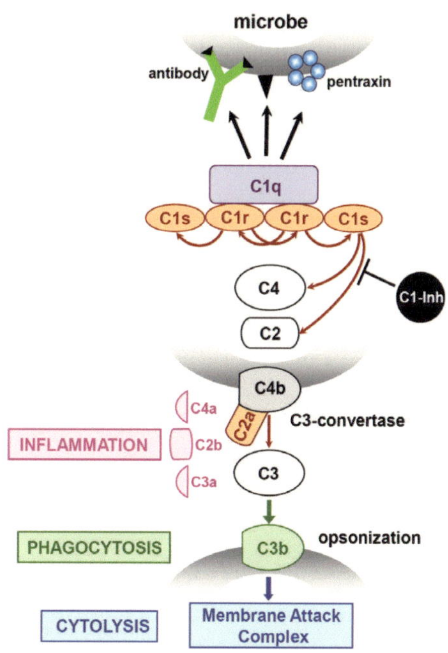

Figure 2. Activation of the classical pathway of complement. C1q binds to microbial surface motifs directly or via or other immune molecules (antibodies, pentraxins) through its globular heads. This multivalent binding triggers sequential activation of the C1r and C1s proteases associated to C1q collagen stalks. Activated C1s cleaves complement components C4 and C2, leading to the assembly of the C3 convertase responsible for C3 cleavage and opsonization of the target by C3b. Activation of the complement cascade generates fragments involved in inflammation, enhancement of phagocytosis and ends in target lysis by the membrane attack complex assembled from complement components C5b, C6, C7, C8 and C9. C1 inhibitor (C1-Inh), a member of the serine protease inhibitor (serpin) family, controls both C1 activation and C1s proteolytic activity.

3. New emerging C1q functions

3.1. A sensor of altered-self structure

One main starting point for revisiting C1q function was probably the work of Korb and Ahearn showing that gC1q binds specifically to apoptotic cells and that binding is important for prevention of autoimmunity in SLE [14]. Since then, numerous experimental proofs have established that C1q is an efficient sensor of self-modifications defined as ACAMPs and DAMPs (for Apoptotic Cells- and Danger-Associated Molecular Patterns, respectively). In contrast to PAMPs, DAMPs and ACAMPs are molecules that can initiate and perpetuate the immune response in a noninfectious inflammatory context. On one way, ACAMPs should be defined as a restricted class of DAMPs which is linked and/or restricted to apoptotic cell membrane modifications. Viewed from another angle, some DAMPs are ACAMPs when they are exposed at the surface of apoptotic cells, the best illustration being probably DNA: it is indeed a mainly intracellular molecule released upon cell damage, but DNA is also anchored at the cell surface in association with histone proteins as a consequence of apoptosis. C1q recognizes the deoxyribose moiety of DNA, through unexpected lectin-like property [28, 29].

At the surface of apoptotic cells, C1q also binds phosphatidylserine (PS), the canonical marker of apoptosis, and calreticulin (CRT) which was characterized as a strong "Eat–me" signal for phagocyte. Growing evidence emphasizes the role of **C1q as a sensor and integrator of the self-alteration** and the list of recognized molecules summed up in Table I (C1q ligands on apoptotic cells), is probably far from being closed. These interactions are mainly mediated by the globular region of C1q (gC1q) that were shown to contain the binding sites for self-molecules specifically exposed on altered-self cells surface. However, as the C1q collagenous tail (cC1q) is known to interact with several membrane receptors (see paragraph 6), widely distributed on various cell types, C1q can enter into a vast array of interactions by binding of its heads or/and its stalks depending of their accessibility in a particular situation. C1q binding to altered–self structures is not dependent on its associated serum proteases. Indeed, purified C1q freed of the $C1r_2$-$C1s_2$ tetramer, and the isolated gC1q domains retain its binding capacity [14, 28, 30, 31].

	Interaction with C1q domains	**Function(s)**	**Potential partners in complex(es)**	**References (first authors, years)**
DNA* on early and late ACs	gC1q through deoxy-D-ribose, interaction with C chain (Arg 98, Arg 111, and Asn 113)[1]	Promotion of phagocytosis, dependent on iC3b opsonin and on CD46 regulation[3]	Annexin II, factor H, histones	Jiang, H. 1992 [32] Tissot, B. 2003 [33] Palaniyar, N. 2004 [34] Elward, K. 2005 [35] Paidaissi. H, 2008 [28] Garlatti, V. 2010 [29]

	Interaction with C1q domains	Function(s)	Potential partners in complex(es)	References (first authors, years)
Ecto-Calreticulin (CRT)* isolated gC1q binds to CRT on early ACs (possibly preapoptotic)	gC1q and cC1q with CRT globular domain	Bridging AC and phagocyte, Modulation of cytokines release	PS	Paidaissi, H. 2011 [31] Verneret, M. 2014 [36] Donnelly, S. 2006 [37]
PS * characterized on early ACs[2]	gC1q through phosphoserine, interaction with C chain (Arg 98 and Arg 111)[1]	ACs recognition, Bridging AC and phagocyte(?) Modulation of PS-dependent signaling(?) Complement activation in the presence of serum	CRT, annexin(s)	Paidaissi, H. 2008 [30] Tan, L. 2010 [38]
Annexin V* most likely on late ACs	ND[4]	Modulation of ACs uptake(?) Modulation of complement activation(?)	PS, CRT	Martin, M. 2012 [39]
Annexin II* most likely on late ACs	ND[4]	Modulation of complement activation(?)	DNA, PS, Factor H, histones	Leffler, J. 2010[40] Martin, M. 2012[39]
GAPDH detected on early ACs[2]	gC1q	ND on ACs		Terrasse, R. 2012 [41]
CERT(L) most likely on late ACs	gC1q	Complement activation		Bode, G. 2014 [42]

*These ligands are autoantigens targeted in lupus erythematous. PS, phosphatidylserine; CERT(L), the longer splicing isoform of ceramide transporter protein (CERT); GAPDH, Glyceraldehyde-3-phosphate dehydrogenase;[1] determined by X-ray crystallography;[2] does not exclude a binding to late ACs;[3]CD46 was characterized as a "Don't Eat me" signal (Elward *et al*, 2005, [35]);[4] full length C1q was used in these studies; (?) probable function that remains to be further investigated; ND, not determined.

Table 1. C1q ligands characterized on apoptotic cells (ACs).

3.2. A modulator of the phagocyte functions

Other biological functions of C1q with particular emphasis on immune responses have been revealed. They include stimulation of leukocyte oxidative response, chemotaxis of monocytes derived cells, including neutrophils, modulation of lymphocytes proliferation, DC differentiation, cytokines expression by phagocytes (reviewed in [17]) and more recently macrophage

M1/M2 polarization [43]. The recent findings that C1q, together with its receptors, is directly involved in the safe removal of self-waste (paragraph 4), also provide strong evidence for a relationship between C1q activity, maintenance of immune tolerance and prevention of autoimmunity (developed in paragraph 7). Importantly, the monocyte lineage includes macrophages and dendritic cells which are key actors for phagocytosis, cytokines production and antigen presentation. This suggests a special place for C1q at the interface of both innate and acquired immunity. Indeed, recent observations by the group of Berhane Ghebrehiwet [44, 45] suggest that C1q functions as a molecular switch dictating the monocyte to dendritic cell transition and arresting DCs in an immature state, which influences the cell response, mainly in a "tolerogenic" way. Although not precisely known, this process seems supported by the oligo heterotrimeric nature of C1q which can bind to gC1q and cC1q receptors which are differentially expressed during monocytes maturation. It should also be mentioned that these interactions are likely differentially modulated by the pathogenic or altered-self nature of gC1q ligands (e. g, PAMPs or DAMPs).

In the same way, C1q influences the M1 pro-inflammatory / M2 pro-resolving macrophage polarization [46]. Specifically, the C1q-stimulated phagocyte is anti-inflammatory (M2-polarized) and this is also observed when C1q-opsonized apoptotic cells are engulfed. In blood, C3 complement component is another actor that, in the presence of C1 (C1q/C1r-C1s complex) helps the clearance of apoptotic debris in an anti-inflammatory manner, through its cleavage fragments C3b and iC3b generated by complement activation. Apoptotic blebs become opsonized by iC3b, which is recognized by complement receptor 3 (CR3, Mac-1) on phagocytes. This induces an immune suppression beneficial to the safe elimination of altered-self structures.

Interestingly, recent studies have also shown that T cell responses to apoptotic cells are regulated by complement in a C3-dependent manner [47, 48]. The group of Marina Botto has demonstrated that C3 bound to dying cells not only facilitates the uptake of apoptotic cells but also influences their intracellular processing, facilitating the MHC II/peptide presentation, and thus dedicates the T cell response to an "apoptotic cell" antigen [48]. This observation contributes to the understanding of how use of the same engulfing machinery yields different responses for a pathogen or an altered-self cell.

Whether C1q alone or C3b-derived opsonins are involved is certainly a key for understanding the cellular response mechanism. Therefore it must be dependent on the local delivery of C1q, i.e. in blood or in the surrounding tissues. Approximately 80% of C1q contained in the plasma is associated with the $C1r_2$–$C1s_2$ tetramer to form the C1 complex which is capable to trigger proteolytic processing of other serum complement components, including C3. Since monocyte-derived cells are the most abundant sources of C1q, local production of C1q in the absence of other complement proteins could induce a specific response, independently of the complement proteolytic cascade. The "phagocytic synapse", which organizes the information that will trigger a specific signaling event, is one of the micro environments where C1q produced by phagocytes may serve as an autocrine signal to induce specific responses. Interestingly, growing evidence is now in favor of C1q production in various tissues, such as endothelial cells [49], neurons [50], fibroblasts [51], osteoclasts [52], which reinforces the view that it may be involved in distinct functions in the absence of serum complement proteins.

3.3. A role in angiogenesis and development

C1q is produced by endothelial cells (ECs) and in the absence of other complement proteins such as the C1r and C1s proteases, C3 and C4, exerts a proangiogenic effect [49]. C1q is very efficient in inducing new vessel formation in wound healing. The globular region of C1q seems to be implicated in this function by binding specifically to the gC1q membrane receptor (gC1qR) expressed by ECs and mainly restricted to the skin ulcer. These observations provide significant insights in favor of a role of C1q in development, tissue repair and also tumor growth. Importantly, this is a new entry to apprehend the role of C1q in inflammatory processes. Angiogenesis is an essential component of inflammatory and it is related to inflammatory pathologies such as rheumatoid arthritis and other systemic autoimmune diseases [53, 54].

C1q produced by cells of the central nervous system (CNS) has been shown to play an important role in remodeling synaptic connections in the developing visual system by tagging unwanted synapses for elimination. These results suggest that complement-mediated synapse elimination may become aberrantly reactivated in neurodegenerative diseases [55]. In addition a dramatic increase of C1q level in the CNS (as much as 300-fold) during normal aging was demonstrated recently [56]. C1q has also been reported to activate Wnt signaling, a pathway involved in development of many organs and implicated in mammalian aging, thereby possibly promoting aging-associated decline in tissue regeneration [57].

4. Efferocytosis

Efferocytosis (from efferre, Latin for 'to take to the grave') is now the term admitted to name the mechanism of the clearance of apoptotic cells [58]. Apoptosis occurs throughout life as an essential process during development, tissue homeostasis but also in pathogenic events. Despite the billion of apoptotic cells produced per day in human [59], they were rarely observed in tissue excepted in pathological situations. Efficient removal of apoptotic cells before the onset of necrosis is considered as a pre-requisite for prevention of autoimmune and inflammatory diseases. This fundamental process, which appears to promote immune tolerance to self together with anti-inflammatory effects, is ongoingly studied since at least 15 years at the cellular and molecular levels and is increasingly better characterized. Such knowledge leads to discover signals that play together to modulate the way by which dead cells are recognized, engulfed by phagocytes and also determine the final immunological outcome. Of great interest, it was shown that drug-manipulating apoptosis of tumor cell for therapy could benefit to their elimination possibly in an immunogenic way [60, 61]. This also highlights that the balanced immune response to apoptotic cell death results from a fine regulation of "factors" promoting either immunity or tolerance. In brief, efferocytosis proceeds in successive steps, including (i) the contact between the damaged cell and the phagocyte, that could be affected by release of soluble "Find-me" signals by ACs, (ii) the specific recognition of the target with the organization of the phagocytic synapse, and (iii) the intracellular degradation and processing of the debris that impact the global "immune" response.

Because excellent reviews are available on this subject [18, 62-64], the next paragraphs will only summarize the pivotal steps of efferocytosis, with a particular emphasis on the role of C1q.

4.1. C1q recognizes apoptotic cells rapidly from death induction

If it is now clear that C1q binds to various molecules on "apoptotic surfaces" (see Table 1 and paragraph 3). The "age" of the apoptotic cells (young/early or rather aged/late) concerned by C1q-dependent clearance remains a subject of debate [65-67], essentially because extensive binding to necrotic cells is observed *in vitro*. Various elements must be taken into account to make up its mind on the question. At first, when does C1q bind to the cell? When does the recognized motif become accessible? An interesting element is the nature of the debris that is engulfed by the phagocyte and, importantly, this is clearly dependent on the type of phagocyte. Some phagocytes (mostly the professional phagocytes i.e. macrophages and DCs) are able to eat the apoptotic cell in whole [68, 69], whereas there are other instances where phagocytes engulf smaller cell fragments proceeding from membrane blebbing. This is one of the observations explaining why C1q has been involved in early or late apoptotic cells uptake, depending on the experimental setup. The efficiency of engulfment itself and the kinetics of the apoptosis process are two other factors that could impact the time course of the C1q effect. The presence of serum complement components (i.e. C3 and C4) is known to amplify the C1q effect. At last, an important point is certainly the nature of the ligands recognized by C1q that could impact its function. It is now known that C1q deficiency correlates with autoimmune diseases characterized by an increased number of non-engulfed apoptotic cells together with production of auto-antibodies (paragraph 7). It was also shown that in the case of patients with systemic lupus erythematosus who present auto-antibodies against C1q, anti-C1q specifically targeted C1q bound on early apoptotic cells [70]. These latter two observations strongly argue for an early action of C1q in the course of apoptosis development, nevertheless it does not preclude that C1q could also act on later stages of induced cell death and necrosis.

In favor of a rapid response during the elimination process of apoptotic cells, it was shown by our group and others that the C1q globular region binds cells with non-yet permeabilized plasma membrane. Among the C1q ligands on the outlet face of the plasma membrane, PS, CRT, DNA, annexins and GAPDH are molecules that become accessible or increase significantly at early stage of apoptosis [71]. In particular, we have observed by confocal microscopy and FRET (Fluorescence Resonance Energy Transfer) measurement that CRT/gC1q interaction occurs mainly on HeLa apoptotic cells without detectable membrane blebs and that this interaction decreases on developed blebs [71]. Additionally, in a study performed with Jurkat cells, gC1q binding was detected before the appearance of PS, which is a hallmark of very early stage of the morphologic changes of apoptosis. Importantly, Obeid and coworkers have shown a preapoptotic translocation of CRT to the plasma membrane [60].

4.2. C1q enhances phagocytosis

Despite numerous studies demonstrating the effect of C1q on phagocytosis, a clear understanding of the molecular events which support its functions is still lacking. Even if the enhancement of uptake was initially reported, it proved to be modest in most cases. Various factors that could modulate this effect have to be taken into account. First, efferocytosis is a very redundant process, involving a large number of molecules, which could partially compensate each other. Second, it depends on either the apoptotic cell or the phagocyte type and third it is conditioned by the cell microenvironment, i.e. the presence of serum proteins. In accordance with the observation that C1q by itself binds ACAMPs, the enhancement of uptake is observed independently from its ability to activate the classical complement pathway. However it was also clearly demonstrated that complement protein iC3b, a proteolytic inactive product of the cleavage of C3, could opsonize the target, resulting in enhanced phagocytosis due to iC3b recognition by phagocyte receptors (CR3) [35]. It cannot also be excluded that in some cases other complement opsonins such as C4b could also be involved.

4.2.1. C1q bridges the phagocyte and its prey

It was first proposed that C1q binds the prey through its globular regions and the phagocyte through its collagen stalks, essentially because CRT with its co-receptor CD91 (LRP1) at the phagocyte surface was characterized as a receptor for the collagen part of C1q, and because C1q binds directly to pathogens as well as damaged self–cells surface via its globular heads. This model is undoubtedly challenged by the increasing number of molecules and receptors known to recognize the globular and/or the collagen part of C1q, which could be exposed at both faces of the phagocytic synapse (reviewed in Tables 1 and 2).

4.2.2. C1q aggregates motifs and potentially helps synapse formation

By its capacity to recognize a large number of molecular motifs, mainly supported by the C1q globular region versatility (paragraph 5) but also by the collagen region, C1q has the potential to aggregate molecules in close proximity to help the phagocytic synapse formation in a way similar to the organization of the immunologic synapse. Beyond its role as a molecular bridge, a large number of studies demonstrate that C1q activates signals stimulating the cell responses, thereby providing evidence for its function as a "transmitter" molecule.

4.2.3. C1q induces cell signaling

An important primary observation was that C1q serves as an activation ligand for cells from the monocyte lineage. Indeed, it was shown that fluid phase or immobilized C1q binds to various membrane receptors, including β1 and β3 integrins and other not yet characterized molecules [72-74]. This binding correlates with various intracellular signaling events, such as integrin activation and platelet aggregation, cell migration and tissue remodeling, and also generation of NF-kappa B complexes, most obviously linked with anti–inflammatory effects and thus directly to efferocytosis. In addition, several independent investigators have analyzed the role of C1q on dendritic cells and proposed that C1q interaction with cC1qR(s), but also with gC1qR/p33 in cooperation with the DC-SIGN receptor, are responsible for the modulation of DC maturation and consequently for the "nonimmunogenic" presentation of self-antigens [75, 76]. Notably, DCs which express elevated levels of C1q co-localized with DC-SIGN-gC1qR are functionally immature, whereas inducing DC maturation with LPS and inflammatory cytokines decreases expression of both C1q and its receptors. A recent work has revealed a shared signaling pathway for C1q and adiponectin in murine macrophages, through the demonstration that C1q utilizes 5′ adenosine mono-phosphate-activated protein kinase (AMPK) to induce MER tyrosine kinase which is a receptor known to regulate efferocytosis [77]. Remarkably, various phagocyte receptors that are linked to efferocytosis have been shown to bind C1q, but so far the consequences of these interactions remain elusive. They include a scavenger receptor expressed by endothelial cell and also in some subsets of DCs (SREC-I/SCARF1), which binds C1q dependently of its interaction with PS on the apoptotic cell surface [51], the leukocyte-associated Ig-like receptor 1 (LAIR1) [78], but also the CD91(LRP1)-CRT complex (see paragraph 6).

4.2.4. C1q modulates cytokine production

It is now unambiguously demonstrated that C1q promotes an anti-inflammatory response and thus probably contributes to the global tolerogenic effect triggered by apoptotic cells. A major contribution was provided by Andrea Tenner and coworkers, who have analyzed the C1q effect on cytokine response during ingestion of apoptotic cells by the various monocyte derived-cells (monocytes, macrophages and DCs) [79]. This effect is mainly supported by increase of the IL-10 anti-inflammatory cytokine, inhibition of the pro-inflammatory NF-kappa B transcription factor [74] and modulation of interferon (IFN)-alpha [80, 81]. It however depends either on the maturation state of the phagocyte or on the nature of the apoptotic cell. In addition, the recent characterization of CRT as a major "Eat-me" signal that enhances phagocytosis of apoptotic cells [60, 82] had shed new light on the "signaling" potentiality of C1q, by showing that it could also trigger an immunogenic response in reaction to proapoptotic/anticancer drugs. CRT is a ligand of both the collagen stems and the heads of C1q and is present on each side of the phagocytic synapse. We have demonstrated the direct interaction between CRT and gC1q [71] on early apoptotic cells and also that decreasing CRT exposure impacts C1q binding [31], together with a modulation of cytokine released by macrophages that have engulfed these cells. We also showed that a deficiency of CRT induces contrasting effects on cytokine release by THP-1 macrophages, by increasing interleukin (IL)-6 and monocyte chemotactic protein 1/CCL2 and decreasing IL-8. Remarkably, these effects were greatly reduced when apoptotic cells were opsonized by C1q, which counterbalanced the effect of CRT deficiency. Most notably, these data emphasize the dual role of C1q on uptake and on signaling events during the elimination of apoptotic cells and highlight the crucial role of C1q in tissue homeostasis in controlling the inflammatory phagocyte status. However, the molecular mechanisms that control this effect remain to be fully elucidated. Interestingly, C1q and CRT share PS as a common ligand, itself characterized as a signal involved in the non-immunogenic handling of apoptotic cells. Other serum PS binding molecules have been shown to regulate C1q function such as factor H and beta 2-glycoprotein 1 [38, 83]. Annexins (II, V) which are PS binding molecules were also reported to interact with C1q [39]. All these observations suggest that these immunomodulatory proteins could interact inside complexes involving both faces of the phagocytic synapse.

5. How C1q interactions modulate its function

As stated above, both cC1q and gC1q can interact with different molecular partners, which modulate C1q function. For example, the C1q classical function is mediated by the cC1q-associated C1r and C1s proteases, whereas the cC1q interaction with the phagocyte endocytic receptor CRT-CD91(LRP1) is believed to occur only in the absence of the proteases. More intriguingly, the gC1q domain has the ability to recognize a wide variety of ligands, but the resulting gC1q-mediated C1 binding does not automatically activate the complement pathway as illustrated in figure 3 [21, 23, 24]. How can the nature of the ligand-binding surface modulate such an activation? We can very briefly sum up a current hypothesis as follows: the catalytic domain of the C1r protease lies inside the C1q cone in a 'resting dimeric' configuration preventing its spontaneous auto-activation, as strongly suggested by the combined use of electron microscopy and X-ray structural studies [84]. Therefore, a mechanical signal (or heating) is required to trigger C1 activation [23, 24, 85]). The mobile collagen stems of the C1q molecule can accommodate different positions and transmit molecular distortions to the proteases when binding to a target surface (Fig. 3). The magnitude of the corresponding mechanical stress will vary according to the nature and relative position of the molecular motifs on the surface; it will also be influenced by the position of its binding site on gC1q [29].

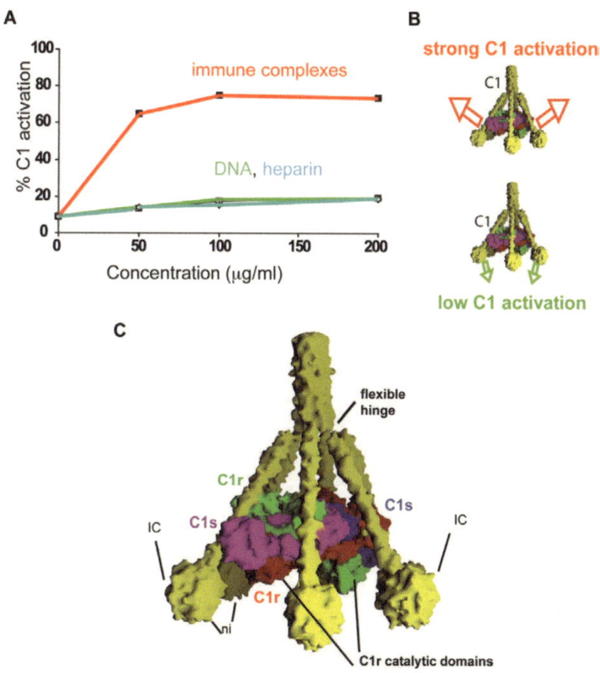

Figure 3. Differential C1 activation in response to various binding surfaces. A) Differential C1 activation by IgG-containing immune complexes, heparin and DNA (from Garlatti *et al.* 2010 [29]). The non-immune self-ligands DNA and heparin induce almost no complement activation in the presence of physiological concentrations of C1-inhibitor. B) Schematic molecular interpretation in terms of differential activating mechanical stress induced by C1q binding. C) Larger view of the C1 model showing the positions of C1q flexible hinges, of the inner C1r dimeric catalytic domains, and of the proposed immune complex binding site on the B chain (IC) and the non-immune self-ligand binding site on the C chain (ni).

6. C1q receptors on phagocytes

The identity of C1q receptors and their role in C1q-dependent efferocytosis have been a matter of controversy for many years and are still not fully elucidated. These receptors include cC1qR, gC1qR, C1qRp, CR1, the $\alpha 2\beta 1$ integrin and CD91, and several new receptors described during the past two years, including RAGE, CR3, DC-SIGN and LAIR-1. As will be seen below, certain of these receptors interact with each other and the interaction with C1q might involve ternary complexes.

Paradoxically, the first two receptors identified for C1q collagen-like and globular regions (**cC1qR**/collectin receptor and **gC1qR**, respectively) [86, 87] turned out to be multifunctional, multi-compartmental proteins normally present in the endoplasmic reticulum (cC1qR/ calreticulin/CRT) and in mitochondria (gC1qR/p33), but detected at the surface of a wide variety of cells. Since both proteins neither have transmembrane domain nor membrane anchor, they likely function as co-receptors in association with cell surface transmembrane proteins such as CD91/LRP1 (CRT) and DC-SIGN (gC1qR), which have recently been shown themselves to bind C1q [76, 88]. Both gC1qR and cC1qR have also been proposed to form a signaling complex with integrin $\beta 1$ on endothelial cells [89], but the possible binding of C1q to this complex was not investigated.

Two other receptors were described later, a receptor called **C1qRp** (C1q receptor that enhances phagocytosis) [90], further identified as the C-type lectin receptor CD93, and complement receptor 1 (CR1/CD35) [91]. It should be mentioned that CD93 is not considered any more as a C1q receptor due to the lack of direct interaction of the protein with C1q [92]. **CR1,** also called the immune adherence receptor, was initially identified as a receptor for complement fragments C4b and C3b, acting as a regulator of complement activation. CR1 is expressed on numerous cells, including erythrocytes, eosinophils, neutrophils, monocytes, macrophages, B-lymphocytes, some T cells subsets, follicular dendritic cells and glomerular podocytes (reviewed in [93]). CR1 on red blood cells (ECR1) has been shown to transport complement-tagged particles and immune complexes to the spleen and the liver for phagocytosis by resident macrophages. A marked decline in ECR1 has been observed in autoimmune diseases such as SLE [94]. CR1 was also identified as a receptor for C1q and other defense collagens such as MBL and ficolins [91, 95, 96]. However the involvement of C1q-CR1 interaction in phagocytosis has not been demonstrated so far. This receptor is a multi-modular type I membrane glycoprotein composed of an extracellular stretch of 30 complement control protein (CCP) modules, organized into four long homologous repeats (LHR-A, -B, -C and -D) of 7 CCPs each, a transmembrane domain and a short cytoplasmic tail (43 amino acids). The cytoplasmic tail of CR1 contains two PDZ (postsynaptic density protein, Drosophila disc large tumor suppressor and zonula occludens-1) motifs, allowing interaction of ECR1 with Fas-associated phosphatase 1, a scaffolding protein with tyrosine phosphatase activity [97]. LHR-A contains the major C4b binding site whereas LHR-B and LHR-C contain homologous C4b/C3b binding sites. C1q, MBL and ficolin-2 have been shown to bind LHR-D and their interaction with CR1 proposed to involve major ionic interactions between their collagen stalks and CCP24 and/or CCP25 of CR1 ([96] and unpublished data).

http://dx.doi.org/10.5772/60519

Integrin **α2β1** is known as a receptor for extracellular matrix components, including collagen, and is involved in inflammation and immunity (for a review on β1 integrins [98]. It is expressed on many cell types such as epithelial cells, endothelial cells, fibroblasts and hematopoietic cells, including platelets and specific subsets of leukocytes [99]. This integrin has been shown to interact with C1q and other members of the collectin family such as MBL and surfactant protein-A. The C1q-α2β1 interaction has been suggested to play a role in mast cell activation and cytokine secretion [99, 100]. However, its role on other cell types and its potential function in ACs clearance have not been investigated yet. Integrin α2β1 has been shown to interact with calreticulin at the surface of various cells, including platelets [101]. It has been proposed to interact with the collagen-like part of C1q and collectins through its α_2 inserted (I) domain, which is involved in collagen binding [100].

CD91/LRP1 (or α_2-macroglobulin receptor) is a multifunctional endocytic and cell-signaling receptor of the low density lipoprotein (LDL) receptor family, expressed on both professional (macrophages and dendritic cells) and non-professional phagocytes (epithelial, endothelial cells, fibroblasts, microglia...). It is composed of two non-covalently linked α (85 kDa, C-terminal, membrane-spanning) and β (515 kDa, N-terminal, extracellular) chains. The latter is involved in binding to a wide variety of ligands, including lipoproteins, extracellular matrix proteins or protease/inhibitor complexes [102]. The binding versatility is supported by the modular structure of LRP1 composed of four ligand-binding clusters of LDL receptor type A (LA, also called complement-like) repeats, β-propellers (YWTD repeats) and epidermal growth factor (EGF) modules. Binding of the various ligands was shown to involve mainly clusters II and IV. The cytoplasmic tail of LRP1 consists of 100 amino acids and exhibits diverse potential endocytosis and signaling motifs, including two NPXY motifs, one YXXL motif and two di-leucine motifs. It has been shown to interact with GULP, an adaptor protein involved in engulfment of apoptotic cells.

LRP1 was proposed to use CRT as a coreceptor for engulfment of C1q-opsonized targets, but also to serve as a docking platform for CRT-dependent recognition of dying cells by C1q. However, it has been reported that LRP1 is not always required for C1q-dependent enhancement of AC phagocytosis, suggesting involvement of other C1q receptors [103]. In addition, no direct interaction between isolated LRP1 and CRT has been reported yet while a direct interaction between the LRP1 and C1q molecules has been described, which involves both the collagen-like stalks and the globular heads of C1q [88]. This indicates that the role of LRP1 and CRT in C1q-dependent efferocytosis is more complex than anticipated and needs further clarification.

SREC-I (scavenger receptor (SR) expressed by endothelial cells I, also called **SCARF1** or **SR-F1**) is a class F type scavenger receptor expressed on endothelial cells, macrophages and dendritic cells, that binds various ligands including modified LDL, heat-shock proteins and fungal pathogens. It is characterized by an extracellular domain composed of 6-7 EGF/EGF-like modules, a transmembrane domain and a long (388 amino acids) C-terminal cytoplasmic tail containing serine/proline and glycine rich segments. SREC-I has been shown very recently to play a crucial role in the recognition and engulfment of ACs and in preventing autoimmunity. Most strikingly, this function is mediated through SREC-I interaction with C1q bound to PS exposed at the surface of AC [51]. This C1q-SREC-I efferocytosis pathway, although not fully non-redundant, contributed to AC clearance up to 70%, depending on the phagocyte type, again suggesting involvement of different pathways, depending on cell types and tissue environment. Interestingly, SREC-I has been described as an endocytic receptor for CRT [104], but no interaction was detected recently using isolated proteins [51]. SREC-I has also been shown to trans-interact through its ectodomain with SREC-II, a related type F SR [105], that however does not recognize typical SR ligands and is not involved in C1q-dependent efferocytosis [51]. Identification of protein domains and amino acid residues critical in C1q-SREC-I interaction, the potential existence of trimolecular complexes with CRT, and the signaling pathway triggered by SREC-I binding to C1q-opsonized ACs, remain to be investigated at both molecular and functional levels.

RAGE (receptor for advanced glycation end-products (AGEs) or **SR-J**) is a 45 kDa receptor of the immunoglobulin (Ig) superfamily comprising an extracellular domain of 3 Ig-like domains (V, C1 and C2 type), a transmembrane domain and a short C-terminal cytoplasmic tail (41 amino acids). RAGE oligomerization is believed to play a role in ligand recognition and signal transduction, which is mediated through association with cytoplasmic adaptor proteins [106]. RAGE is expressed on monocytes, macrophages and dendritic cells, and acts as a pattern recognition receptor for endogenous danger signals including AGEs, high mobility group box 1 (HMGB1), β–amyloid fibrils, S-100 protein and DNA, known to play a pathogenic role in chronic inflammatory diseases [107]. It has also been shown to participate in efferocytosis by acting as a PS receptor [108, 109] and proposed to contribute to the resolution of inflammation. This dual "friend or foe" role appears to depend on the cell context and environment [107]. Of note, soluble forms of RAGE (sRAGE), produced by alternative mRNA splicing or ectodomain shedding, were shown to act as decoys for RAGE ligands [110]. RAGE was shown recently to bind to the globular heads of C1q and to enhance C1q-mediated phagocytosis of ACs, a process suggested to involve formation of a receptor complex with **CR3** (see next paragraph) [111]. The RAGE domain and the amino acid residues of both partners participating in the receptor-C1q interaction remain to be determined. Interestingly, RAGE has been shown recently to bind collagen *in vitro* [112].

The phagocytic receptor **CR3** (alias Mac-1, integrin $\alpha_M\beta_2$, CD11bCD18) is an integrin expressed on most immune cells including neutrophils, dendritic cells and macrophages. It binds to a wide range of ligands including complement C3 fragments C3b/iC3b, extracellular matrix proteins, adhesion molecules (ICAM-1 and -2) and microbial motifs, most of them binding to the inserted (I) domain of the α chain. CR3 inside-out activation leads to a high affinity ligand binding state (extended conformation) allowing target uptake and triggering phagocytosis and signaling [113]. CR3 has been shown to interact extracellularly with other C1q receptors including LRP1 [114] and RAGE [111]. In addition, a direct interaction between CR3 and C1q was reported recently [111]. The receptor and C1q domains involved in the interaction are not known. Interestingly, CR3 has also been shown recently to bind collagens *in vitro* [115].

DC-SIGN (DC-specific intercellular adhesion molecule (ICAM)-3 grabbing non integrin/ CD209) is a C-type lectin receptor with a short N-terminal cytoplasmic tail (37 amino acids) containing recycling and internalization motifs, a transmembrane domain and a C-terminal extracellular domain comprising an extended tetrameric neck region surmounted by a cluster of 4 Ca^{2+}-dependent carbohydrate recognition domains (CRDs). It is expressed by DCs and specific macrophage populations and is a receptor involved in multiple functions including adhesion, pathogen recognition and antigen presentation [116]. Interactions between neutrophils and DCs are mediated through interaction of DC-SIGN with CR3 [117]. DC-SIGN was reported recently to bind C1q, and the interaction proposed to involve the IgG binding site of C1q globular heads and the Ca^{2+}-binding pocket of the lectin domain of DC-SIGN [76]. In addition, C1q and gC1qR were shown to associate with DC-SIGN on the surface of immature DCs and to regulate DC differentiation and function. Interestingly, SIGN-R1, a DC-SIGN homolog expressed on mouse splenic marginal zone macrophages, was shown recently to enhance ACs clearance through interaction with C1q and subsequent complement activation [118]. However, the potential capacity of DC-SIGN to activate the classical complement pathway remains to be investigated.

LAIR-1 (leukocyte-associated immunoglobulin-like receptor-1/CD305) is part of the family of inhibitory immune receptors and is expressed at the surface of both myeloid and lymphoid immune cells. LAIR-1 contains a single extracellular C2-type Ig-like domain, a transmembrane domain and a cytoplasmic tail of 101 amino acids with two immunoreceptor tyrosine-based inhibitory motifs (ITIMs) (reviewed in [119]). When phosphorylated, ITIM motifs can bind the SH2 domain of several SH2-containing phosphatases, leading to down-regulation of immune cell activation. LAIR-1 is a receptor for membrane and matrix collagens and its interaction with collagens is dependent on the presence of hydroxyproline residues [120]. LAIR-1 and its soluble homologue LAIR-2 have been shown to interact with several defense collagens, including C1q, MBL and surfactant protein D through their collagen-like regions [78, 121, 122]. LAIR-2 has been reported to inhibit the classical and MBL-dependent lectin complement pathways [121]. LAIR-1 engagement by C1q has been shown to trigger phosphorylation of LAIR-1 ITIMs in monocytes, which likely represents a mechanism involved in maintaining immunological tolerance [78, 123].

It has been classically considered that C1q binds to the apoptotic cell surface through its globular heads, which leaves the collagen-like stems available for interaction with the C1q receptor at the surface of phagocytes. As mentioned above, recently published results challenge this hypothesis since (i) LRP1 and CRT bind both functional C1q regions and may be present on both AC and phagocyte surfaces and, (ii) two recently identified C1q receptors, RAGE and DC-SIGN, bind the globular regions of C1q. Therefore alternative hypotheses about C1q orientation in the phagocytic synapse should be investigated, taking into account the hexameric structure of C1q, possibly allowing simultaneous interaction of the globular heads with both AC and phagocyte surfaces. Since many receptors seem to function as macromolecular complexes, simultaneous interaction of the C1q molecule with two receptors at the phagocyte surface may also be envisaged, as proposed for the globular heads of C1q within the gC1qR/C1q/DC-SIGN complex [76].

Another important feature of C1q receptors lies in the existence of soluble counterparts, that may arise from alternative gene splicing (soluble RAGE variants, DC-SIGN isoforms), as a result of gene duplication (LAIR-2), or after receptor proteolytic shedding from the membrane (as reported for LRP1 and CR1). These soluble proteins might act as decoy receptors by competing with membrane-bound receptors for ligand binding and preventing subsequent signal transmission, thereby playing a role in regulation of C1q-dependent clearance of altered self.

Names (CD number)	Receptor type	Ectodomain composition	C1q specificity	Main self ligands /partners	Functional relevance to autoimmunity
gC1qR, C1qBP, p33, p32	Mitochondrial protein	"doughnut-like" trimer	gC1q	DC-SIGN, CRT β1 integrin	Gene deletion in mouse: lethality
cC1qR, calreticulin, CRT	ER lectin-like chaperone	Lectin-like + "arm"	gC1q cC1q	MBL, ficolins, CD91	Gene deletion in mouse: lethality
CR1 (CD35)	Regulator of complement activation	4 long homologous repeats of CCP modules	?	C3b, C4b MBL, ficolins	Marked decline in CR1 observed on erythrocytes from SLE patients
LRP1 **α2M receptor** **(CD91)**	LDL receptor	4 clusters of LA, WTD and EGF-like modules	gC1q cC1q	Lipoproteins, ECM proteins, CRT, CR3, protease-inhibitor complexes	MΦ and DCs selective LRP1 KO mice: impaired efferocytosis
α2β1 **(CD49bCD29)**	β1 integrin	integrin	cC1q gC1q?	Collagen, laminin MBL, SP-A, CRT	KO mice: profound defect in the innate immune response
SREC-I, SCARF1, SR-F	Scavenger receptor	6/7 EGF-like modules	?	oxLDL, HSP CRT	KO mice: autoimmunity, deficient AC uptake
RAGE, SR-J	Scavenger receptor	3 IgG-like modules (V-C1-C2)	gC1q	HMGB1, AGE, PS, CR3	KO mice: deficient AC uptake
CR3, Mac1, αMβ2 **(CD11bCD18)**	β2 integrin	integrin	?	iC3b, sRAGE, LRP1, collagen	Reduced efferocytosis in CD11b-lupus associated variant
DC-SIGN (CD209)	C-type lectin receptor	Tetramer; neck + C-lectin domain	gC1q cC1q?	ICAM-3, gC1qR	SIGNR1 KO mice: delayed AC clearance
LAIR-1 (CD305)	Inhibitory immune receptor	Ig-like domain (C2)	cC1q gC1q?	MBL, SP-D, collagens	defective expression and function in B lymphocytes from SLE patients

Table 2. C1q receptors on phagocytes

7. C1q in autoimmune disease

Numerous studies suggest that C1q has a protective role in lupus erythematosus, an autoimmune disease resulting largely in dysregulation of the adaptive immunity, i.e; loss of tolerance and generation of autoreactive T-cells [124]. Other observations, however, argue in favor of a facilitating role of C1q in SLE (systemic lupus erythematosus) correlating with tissue damage due to complement activation. Indeed, the complement cascade generates pro-inflammatory products such as C3a and C5a but could also contribute to acquired-C1q deficiency. These two hypotheses are not exclusive and in any case this highlights the pivotal function of C1q at the interface of the innate and adaptive immunity.

It is well established that complete genetic deficiency of C1q is the strongest risk factor for development of SLE [125]. More than 90 % of individuals who are homozygous for a mutation impairing the expression of one of the *C1Q* genes (A, B or C) developed severe clinical manifestations common for SLE (cutaneous lupus and photosensibility, nephritis). It was also reported that partial genetic deficiency, subtle genetic variations (e.g. point mutations that could modify the assembly or function of the C1q molecule) or auto antibodies against C1q [126-128] and to the C1q receptor CRT are associated with SLE [129, 130]. Importantly, targeting genes for C1q in mice resulted in disease susceptibility similar to that observed in human, even if the mice genetic background was shown to contribute to the disease [125, 131, 132]. Of note, deficiencies of the early components of the classical complement pathway predispose to SLE in a hierarchical fashion (C1q>C1rs>C4->C2). In brief, this indicates that C1q deficiency is the most important factor whereas C3 is not critical. A feature that could link the C1q deficiency to the adaptive immune response is its role in prevention of immune precipitation. C1q is essential in keeping antigen–antibody complexes soluble and for their removal from the circulation through the CR1 receptor, thereby preventing inflammatory tissue injury [133]. Another C1q function of significance in autoimmune processes likely resides in its involvement in the removal of apoptotic cells. In agreement with this hypothesis, C1q-deficient mice developed a proliferative glomerulonephritis associated with the presence of multiple apoptotic cell bodies, and apoptotic cells are also observed in lymph node germinal centers in some SLE patients with severe disease [134]. Accordingly, most of the relevant autoantigens in SLE, which are nuclear and cytoplasmic molecules [135], are also found at the surface of apoptotic cells or blebs [136]. As previously mentioned, it is interesting to note that among the autoantigens in various forms of lupus are calreticulin, an "Eat–me" signal recognized by the gC1q domain also acting as a cC1q receptor on phagocyte, or C1q itself when bound to apoptotic surfaces.

The other major effect of C1q modulation of immune responses concerns its function in regulating cells from the immune system, independently from the binding to apoptotic bodies and the uptake mechanism. This includes the role of C1q on the function of the neutrophil. In particular, calreticulin is released from activated neutrophils [137] and, as it was previously shown that C1q-CRT interaction modulates the cytokine release by macrophages, it might be hypothesized that this could interfere with neutrophil-mediated inflammatory processes. Of interest, we have shown that CRT recognizes proteinase 3 (PR3), a member of the family of neutrophil-derived serine proteases, released from azurophilic granules but also present in secretory vesicles and membrane-exposed on viable and apoptotic neutrophils [138]. PR3 is a pro-inflammatory factor whose membrane expression can potentiate chronic inflammatory diseases such as anti-neutrophil cytoplasmic antibodies systemic vasculitis (AAV) or rheumatoid arthritis [139]. In addition, the role of C1q on the biology of the monocyte-derived cells and particularly DCs is probably of primary importance [140], because the presence of C1q influences the DC and macrophage responses mainly in a "tolerogenic" way [46, 141]. The interaction of C1q with B and T cells [142-144], which modulates cell proliferation, has also been shown to participate both in the activation and inhibition of T cells, and in the negative selection of B autoreactive-cells through mechanisms that remain to be elucidated.

8. How manipulating C1q could help autoimmune disease treatment, hopes and difficulties

Undoubtedly, the aforementioned observations strongly highlight that C1q has a central role in maintaining tissue homeostasis. In this respect, the fact that complement deficiencies, including C1q, are relatively rare according to national and supranational registries (1 to 10 % of all primary immunodeficiencies) [145] together with the observation that an abnormal C1q content generally induces autoimmunity, is one element that also argues for a critical role of this protein. In our opinion, its function in efferocytosis by helping the rapid elimination of cell debris together with its impact on the response developed by the phagocyte makes it a prime target for resolving autoimmune diseases. Indeed, it can be hypothesized that restoring an efficient engulfment of apoptotic cells would decrease the number of not properly cleared dead cells and thus diminish the release of intracellular autoantigens which are strongly correlated to chronic systemic autoimmune disease. Accordingly, apoptotic cell-based therapy has been developed to limit the graft rejection in transplantation [146]. Because all defects in apoptotic cell clearance are not systematically related to immune disease (CD14 or MBL deficiencies for example) [147, 148], this stresses the dual function of C1q in the uptake process and in modulating the phagocyte signaling response in a tolerogenic way, thus reinforcing its therapeutic potential.

However the fact that C1q reacts with a large spectrum of molecules and membrane receptors which will likely induce mutiple, possibly antagonist functions adds complexity for its potential use in therapy. A 2001 pilot study including 8 patients suggested that SLE might be treated successfully by immunoadsorption of plasma with a C1q column [149]. The parameters of SLE clinical disease activity improved upon removing from the circulation molecules that bind to and consume C1q, i. e. immune complexes, anti-C1q autoantibodies and inflammatory proteins such as pentraxins. More recently, administration of plasma in a SLE patient with complete C1q deficiency has been therapeutically successful [150] with reestablishment of complement haemolytic activity and absence of anti-C1q antibodies, suggesting that targeting C1q/C1q pathway could be a valid therapeutic option.

The fact remains that a better understanding of the molecular details that control the C1q interaction with its targets is a primary need. One major breakthrough for future strategies was clearly the recent success in production of a recombinant full length C1q molecule [151]. This now allows the production of mutated forms of the molecule to map the amino acid residues involved in the recognition of its different targets and receptors. Importantly, this opens the way to produce C1q variants devoid of a particular interaction or sensing property, as exemplified by the lysines B61 and C58 mutants of the collagen stalks which are both unable to trigger complement activation but retain other C1q binding functions. Recombinant C1q devoid of binding capacity for antibodies recognition motifs could represent an efficient tool to disconnect C1q binding to apoptotic bodies from pathways involved in pathogen recognition or in the clearance of immune complexes. Mutated forms targeting binding to specific receptors such as LRP1/CD91 and CRT, DC-SIGN, SCARF1, gC1qR present on various monocytes-derived cells and DCs would provide powerful tools to modulate their specific functions discussed previously. More than ever, producing engineered C1q paves the way to target efferocytosis in order to gain in or to restore a tolerogenic and efficient elimination of apoptotic cells.

9. Conclusion

Over the past 15 years, the status of the C1q molecule has changed from its classical primary role in the initiation of the classical complement pathway, acting in the first line of the immune defense against pathogens, to **an essential molecule for maintaining tissue homeostasis**, functioning at the crossroad between innate and adaptive immunity. This relatively new finding is undoubtedly one explanation why the primitive C1q status resisted over time. Thanks to an incredible number of studies, not all reported in this chapter, C1q is now known for its involvement in a multiplicity of immunologic functions and other tissue homeostasis-related mechanisms that, when defective, could induce autoimmune and inflammatory diseases as well as cancer. This was emphasized by the discovery of its roles in several steps of the safe clearance of altered-self cells which elicits a global tolerogenic immune response. In our opinion, these properties of C1q arise from its multivalent heterotrimeric structure which supports its amazing ability to recognize and to interpret multiple molecular motifs that, taken individually, would possibly not be sufficient to yield a comprehensive signal. C1q appears to act either as a sensor or a transmitter of subtle changes that must be considered for a balanced appropriate response in numerous physiological processes, including immunity and inflammation.

This remarkable property to interact which a very large number of targets and receptors, involved in various biological processes, is also the major difficulty for its use in therapy. In this respect the recent success in the production of functional full-length recombinant C1q opens new avenues. Indeed, it paves the way for its engineering, first to decipher its molecular mechanisms of action, and second for developing new strategies by specifically targeting one C1q pathway, without undesirable side effects associated with other pathways. **We are only at the beginning of what is possible to imagine or of imagining what is possible.**

Author details

Philippe Frachet*, Pascale Tacnet-Delorme, Christine Gaboriaud and Nicole M. Thielens

*Address all correspondence to: philippe.frachet@ibs.fr

Immune Response to Pathogens and Altered Self (IRPAS) Group, Université Grenoble Alpes, CNRS and CEA, Institut de Biologie Structurale (IBS), Grenoble, France

References

[1] Holmskov U, Malhotra R, Sim RB, Jensenius JC: Collectins: collagenous C-type lectins of the innate immune defense system. *Immunol Today* 1994, 15:67-74.

[2] Holmskov U, Thiel S, Jensenius JC: Collections and ficolins: humoral lectins of the innate immune defense. *Annu Rev Immunol* 2003, 21:547-578.

[3] Selman L, Hansen S: Structure and function of collectin liver 1 (CL-L1) and collectin 11 (CL-11, CL-K1). *Immunobiology* 2012, 217:851-863.

[4] Hoppe HJ, Reid KB: Collectins--soluble proteins containing collagenous regions and lectin domains--and their roles in innate immunity. *Protein Sci* 1994, 3:1143-1158.

[5] Shapiro L, Scherer PE: The crystal structure of a complement-1q family protein suggests an evolutionary link to tumor necrosis factor. *Curr Biol* 1998, 8:335-338.

[6] Schaffler A, Buechler C: CTRP family: linking immunity to metabolism. *Trends Endocrinol Metab* 2012, 23:194-204.

[7] Lu J, Wiedemann H, Timpl R, Reid KB: Similarity in structure between C1q and the collectins as judged by electron microscopy. *Behring Inst Mitt* 1993:6-16.

[8] Gadjeva MG, Rouseva MM, Zlatarova AS, Reid KB, Kishore U, Kojouharova MS: Interaction of human C1q with IgG and IgM: revisited. *Biochemistry* 2008, 47:13093-13102.

[9] Klein MA, Kaeser PS, Schwarz P, Weyd H, Xenarios I, Zinkernagel RM, Carroll MC, Verbeek JS, Botto M, Walport MJ, et al.: Complement facilitates early prion pathogenesis. *Nat Med* 2001, 7:488-492.

[10] Erlich P, Dumestre-Perard C, Ling WL, Lemaire-Vieille C, Schoehn G, Arlaud GJ, Thielens NM, Gagnon J, Cesbron JY: Complement protein C1q forms a complex with cytotoxic prion protein oligomers. *J Biol Chem* 2010, 285:19267-19276.

[11] Tacnet-Delorme P, Chevallier S, Arlaud GJ: Beta-amyloid fibrils activate the C1 complex of complement under physiological conditions: evidence for a binding site for A beta on the C1q globular regions. *J Immunol* 2001, 167:6374-6381.

[12] Biro A, Ling WL, Arlaud GJ: Complement protein C1q recognizes enzymatically modified low-density lipoprotein through unesterified fatty acids generated by cholesterol esterase. *Biochemistry* 2010, 49:2167-2176.

[13] Biro A, Thielens NM, Cervenak L, Prohaszka Z, Fust G, Arlaud GJ: Modified low density lipoproteins differentially bind and activate the C1 complex of complement. *Mol Immunol* 2007, 44:1169-1177.

[14] Korb LC, Ahearn JM: C1q binds directly and specifically to surface blebs of apoptotic human keratinocytes: complement deficiency and systemic lupus erythematosus revisited. *J Immunol* 1997, 158:4525-4528.

[15] Taylor PR, Carugati A, Fadok VA, Cook HT, Andrews M, Carroll MC, Savill JS, Henson PM, Botto M, Walport MJ: A hierarchical role for classical pathway complement proteins in the clearance of apoptotic cells in vivo. *J Exp Med* 2000, 192:359-366.

[16] Navratil JS, Watkins SC, Wisnieski JJ, Ahearn JM: The globular heads of C1q specifically recognize surface blebs of apoptotic vascular endothelial cells. *J Immunol* 2001, 166:3231-3239.

[17] Ghebrehiwet B, Hosszu KK, Valentino A, Peerschke EI: The C1q family of proteins: insights into the emerging non-traditional functions. *Front Immunol* 2012, 3.

[18] Hochreiter-Hufford A, Ravichandran KS: Clearing the dead: apoptotic cell sensing, recognition, engulfment, and digestion. *Cold Spring Harb Perspect Biol* 2013, 5:a008748.

[19] Nishino H, Shibuya K, Nishida Y, Mushimoto M: Lupus erythematosus-like syndrome with selective complete deficiency of C1q. *Ann Intern Med* 1981, 95:322-324.

[20] Cooper NR: The classical complement pathway: activation and regulation of the first complement component. *Adv Immunol* 1985, 37:151-216.

[21] Gaboriaud C, Thielens NM, Gregory LA, Rossi V, Fontecilla-Camps JC, Arlaud GJ: Structure and activation of the C1 complex of complement: unraveling the puzzle. *Trends Immunol* 2004, 25:368-373.

[22] Kishore U, Gaboriaud C, Waters P, Shrive AK, Greenhough TJ, Reid KB, Sim RB, Arlaud GJ: C1q and tumor necrosis factor superfamily: modularity and versatility. *Trends Immunol* 2004, 25:551-561.

[23] Gaboriaud C, Juanhuix J, Gruez A, Lacroix M, Darnault C, Pignol D, Verger D, Fontecilla-Camps JC, Arlaud GJ: The crystal structure of the globular head of complement protein C1q provides a basis for its versatile recognition properties. *J Biol Chem* 2003, 278:46974-46982.

[24] Gaboriaud C, Frachet P, Thielens NM, Arlaud GJ: The human c1q globular domain: structure and recognition of non-immune self ligands. *Front Immunol* 2011, 2:92.

[25] Ebenbichler CF, Thielens NM, Vornhagen R, Marschang P, Arlaud GJ, Dierich MP: Human immunodeficiency virus type 1 activates the classical pathway of comple-

ment by direct C1 binding through specific sites in the transmembrane glycoprotein gp41. *J Exp Med* 1991, 174:1417-1424.

[26] Szalai AJ, Agrawal A, Greenhough TJ, Volanakis JE: C-reactive protein: structural biology and host defense function. *Clin Chem Lab Med* 1999, 37:265-270.

[27] Thielens NM, Tacnet-Delorme P, Arlaud GJ: Interaction of C1q and mannan-binding lectin with viruses. *Immunobiology* 2002, 205:563-574.

[28] Paidassi H, Tacnet-Delorme P, Lunardi T, Arlaud GJ, Thielens NM, Frachet P: The lectin-like activity of human C1q and its implication in DNA and apoptotic cell recognition. *FEBS Lett* 2008, 582:3111-3116.

[29] Garlatti V, Chouquet A, Lunardi T, Vives R, Paidassi H, Lortat-Jacob H, Thielens NM, Arlaud GJ, Gaboriaud C: Cutting edge: C1q binds deoxyribose and heparan sulfate through neighboring sites of its recognition domain. *J Immunol* 2010, 185:808-812.

[30] Paidassi H, Tacnet-Delorme P, Garlatti V, Darnault C, Ghebrehiwet B, Gaboriaud C, Arlaud GJ, Frachet P: C1q binds phosphatidylserine and likely acts as a multiligand-bridging molecule in apoptotic cell recognition. *J Immunol* 2008, 180:2329-2338.

[31] Paidassi H, Tacnet-Delorme P, Verneret M, Gaboriaud C, Houen G, Duus K, Ling WL, Arlaud GJ, Frachet P: Investigations on the C1q-calreticulin-phosphatidylserine interactions yield new insights into apoptotic cell recognition. *J Mol Biol* 2011, 408:277-290.

[32] Jiang H, Cooper B, Robey FA, Gewurz H: DNA binds and activates complement via residues 14-26 of the human C1q A chain. *J Biol Chem* 1992, 267:25597-25601.

[33] Tissot B, Daniel R, Place C: Interaction of the C1 complex of complement with sulfated polysaccharide and DNA probed by single molecule fluorescence microscopy. *Eur J Biochem* 2003, 270:4714-4720.

[34] Palaniyar N, Nadesalingam J, Clark H, Shih MJ, Dodds AW, Reid KB: Nucleic acid is a novel ligand for innate, immune pattern recognition collectins surfactant proteins A and D and mannose-binding lectin. *J Biol Chem* 2004, 279:32728-32736.

[35] Elward K, Griffiths M, Mizuno M, Harris CL, Neal JW, Morgan BP, Gasque P: CD46 plays a key role in tailoring innate immune recognition of apoptotic and necrotic cells. *J Biol Chem* 2005, 280:36342-36354.

[36] Verneret M, Tacnet-Delorme P, Laurin D, Aspord C, Thielens N, Kleman JP, Frachet P: Investigations on the cell surface calreticulin-C1q interactions and their involvement in the uptake of apoptotic cells. *Mol Immunol* 2011, 48:1706-1706.

[37] Donnelly S, Roake W, Brown S, Young P, Naik H, Wordsworth P, Isenberg DA, Reid KB, Eggleton P: Impaired recognition of apoptotic neutrophils by the C1q/calreticulin and CD91 pathway in systemic lupus erythematosus. *Arthritis Rheum* 2006, 54:1543-1556.

[38] Tan LA, Yu B, Sim FC, Kishore U, Sim RB: Complement activation by phospholipids: the interplay of factor H and C1q. *Protein Cell* 2010, 1:1033-1049.

[39] Martin M, Leffler J, Blom AM: Annexin A2 and A5 serve as new ligands for C1q on apoptotic cells. *J Biol Chem* 2012, 287:33733-33744.

[40] Leffler J, Herbert AP, Norstrom E, Schmidt CQ, Barlow PN, Blom AM, Martin M: Annexin-II, DNA, and histones serve as factor H ligands on the surface of apoptotic cells. *J Biol Chem* 2010, 285:3766-3776.

[41] Terrasse R, Tacnet-Delorme P, Moriscot C, Perard J, Schoehn G, Vernet T, Thielens NM, Di Guilmi AM, Frachet P: Human and pneumococcal cell surface glyceraldehyde-3-phosphate dehydrogenase (GAPDH) proteins are both ligands of human C1q protein. *J Biol Chem* 2012, 287:42620-42633.

[42] Bode GH, Losen M, Buurman WA, Veerhuis R, Molenaar PC, Steinbusch HW, De Baets MH, Daha MR, Martinez-Martinez P: Complement activation by ceramide transporter proteins. *J Immunol* 2014, 192:1154-1161.

[43] Benoit ME, Clarke EV, Morgado P, Fraser DA, Tenner AJ: Complement protein C1q directs macrophage polarization and limits inflammasome activity during the uptake of apoptotic cells. *J Immunol* 2012, 188:5682-5693.

[44] Hosszu KK, Santiago-Schwarz F, Peerschke EI, Ghebrehiwet B: Evidence that a C1q/C1qR system regulates monocyte-derived dendritic cell differentiation at the interface of innate and acquired immunity. *Innate Immun* 2010, 16:115-127.

[45] Hosszu KK, Valentino A, Ji Y, Matkovic M, Pednekar L, Rehage N, Tumma N, Peerschke EI, Ghebrehiwet B: Cell surface expression and function of the macromolecular c1 complex on the surface of human monocytes. *Front Immunol* 2012, 3:38.

[46] Bohlson SS, O'Conner SD, Hulsebus HJ, Ho MM, Fraser DA: Complement, c1q, and c1q-related molecules regulate macrophage polarization. *Front Immunol* 2014, 5:402.

[47] Kemper C, Atkinson JP: T-cell regulation: with complements from innate immunity. *Nat Rev Immunol* 2007, 7:9-18.

[48] Baudino L, Sardini A, Ruseva MM, Fossati-Jimack L, Cook HT, Scott D, Simpson E, Botto M: C3 opsonization regulates endocytic handling of apoptotic cells resulting in enhanced T-cell responses to cargo-derived antigens. *Proc Natl Acad Sci U S A* 2014, 111:1503-1508.

[49] Bossi F, Tripodo C, Rizzi L, Bulla R, Agostinis C, Guarnotta C, Munaut C, Baldassarre G, Papa G, Zorzet S, et al.: C1q as a unique player in angiogenesis with therapeutic implication in wound healing. *Proc Natl Acad Sci U S A* 2014, 111:4209-4214.

[50] Bialas AR, Stevens B: TGF-beta signaling regulates neuronal C1q expression and developmental synaptic refinement. *Nat Neurosci* 2013, 16:1773-1782.

[51] Ramirez-Ortiz ZG, Pendergraft WF, 3rd, Prasad A, Byrne MH, Iram T, Blanchette CJ, Luster AD, Hacohen N, El Khoury J, Means TK: The scavenger receptor SCARF1 me-

diates the clearance of apoptotic cells and prevents autoimmunity. *Nat Immunol* 2013, 14:917-926.

[52] Teo BH, Bobryshev YV, Teh BK, Wong SH, Lu J: Complement C1q production by osteoclasts and its regulation of osteoclast development. *Biochem J* 2012, 447:229-237.

[53] Szekanecz Z, Koch AE: Mechanisms of Disease: angiogenesis in inflammatory diseases. *Nat Clin Pract Rheumatol* 2007, 3:635-643.

[54] Imhof BA, Aurrand-Lions M: Angiogenesis and inflammation face off. *Nat Med* 2006, 12:171-172.

[55] Stevens B, Allen NJ, Vazquez LE, Howell GR, Christopherson KS, Nouri N, Micheva KD, Mehalow AK, Huberman AD, Stafford B, et al.: The classical complement cascade mediates CNS synapse elimination. *Cell* 2007, 131:1164-1178.

[56] Stephan AH, Madison DV, Mateos JM, Fraser DA, Lovelett EA, Coutellier L, Kim L, Tsai HH, Huang EJ, Rowitch DH, et al.: A dramatic increase of C1q protein in the CNS during normal aging. *J Neurosci* 2013, 33:13460-13474.

[57] Naito AT, Sumida T, Nomura S, Liu ML, Higo T, Nakagawa A, Okada K, Sakai T, Hashimoto A, Hara Y, et al.: Complement C1q activates canonical Wnt signaling and promotes aging-related phenotypes. *Cell* 2012, 149:1298-1313.

[58] deCathelineau AM, Henson PM: The final step in programmed cell death: phagocytes carry apoptotic cells to the grave. *Essays Biochem* 2003, 39:105-117.

[59] Ravichandran KS: Find-me and eat-me signals in apoptotic cell clearance: progress and conundrums. *J Exp Med* 2010, 207:1807-1817.

[60] Obeid M, Tesniere A, Ghiringhelli F, Fimia GM, Apetoh L, Perfettini JL, Castedo M, Mignot G, Panaretakis T, Casares N, et al.: Calreticulin exposure dictates the immunogenicity of cancer cell death. *Nat Med* 2007, 13:54-61.

[61] Kroemer G, Galluzzi L, Kepp O, Zitvogel L: Immunogenic cell death in cancer therapy. *Annu Rev Immunol* 2013, 31:51-72.

[62] Savill J, Dransfield I, Gregory C, Haslett C: A blast from the past: clearance of apoptotic cells regulates immune responses. *Nat Rev Immunol* 2002, 2:965-975.

[63] Paidassi H, Tacnet-Delorme P, Arlaud GJ, Frachet P: How Phagocytes Track Down and Respond to Apoptotic Cells. *Crit Rev Immunol* 2009, 29:111-130.

[64] Poon IK, Lucas CD, Rossi AG, Ravichandran KS: Apoptotic cell clearance: basic biology and therapeutic potential. *Nat Rev Immunol* 2014, 14:166-180.

[65] Liang YY, Arnold T, Michlmayr A, Rainprecht D, Perticevic B, Spittler A, Oehler R: Serum-dependent processing of late apoptotic cells for enhanced efferocytosis. *Cell Death Dis* 2014, 5:e1264.

[66] Gaipl US, Kuenkele S, Voll RE, Beyer TD, Kolowos W, Heyder P, Kalden JR, Herrmann M: Complement binding is an early feature of necrotic and a rather late event during apoptotic cell death. *Cell Death Differ* 2001, 8:327-334.

[67] Nauta AJ, Trouw LA, Daha MR, Tijsma O, Nieuwland R, Schwaeble WJ, Gingras AR, Mantovani A, Hack EC, Roos A: Direct binding of C1q to apoptotic cells and cell blebs induces complement activation. *Eur J Immunol* 2002, 32:1726-1736.

[68] Wood W, Turmaine M, Weber R, Camp V, Maki RA, McKercher SR, Martin P: Mesenchymal cells engulf and clear apoptotic footplate cells in macrophageless PU.1 null mouse embryos. *Development* 2000, 127:5245-5252.

[69] Parnaik R, Raff MC, Scholes J: Differences between the clearance of apoptotic cells by professional and non-professional phagocytes. *Curr Biol* 2000, 10:857-860.

[70] Bigler C, Schaller M, Perahud I, Osthoff M, Trendelenburg M: Autoantibodies against complement C1q specifically target C1q bound on early apoptotic cells. *J Immunol* 2009, 183:3512-3521.

[71] Verneret M, Tacnet-Delorme P, Osman R, Awad R, Grichine A, Kleman JP, Frachet P: Relative contribution of c1q and apoptotic cell-surface calreticulin to macrophage phagocytosis. *J Innate Immun* 2014, 6:426-434.

[72] Peerschke EI, Reid KB, Ghebrehiwet B: Platelet activation by C1q results in the induction of alpha IIb/beta 3 integrins (GPIIb-IIIa) and the expression of P-selectin and procoagulant activity. *J Exp Med* 1993, 178:579-587.

[73] Agostinis C, Bulla R, Tripodo C, Gismondi A, Stabile H, Bossi F, Guarnotta C, Garlanda C, De Seta F, Spessotto P, et al.: An alternative role of C1q in cell migration and tissue remodeling: contribution to trophoblast invasion and placental development. *J Immunol* 2010, 185:4420-4429.

[74] Fraser DA, Arora M, Bohlson SS, Lozano E, Tenner AJ: Generation of inhibitory NFkappaB complexes and phosphorylated cAMP response element-binding protein correlates with the anti-inflammatory activity of complement protein C1q in human monocytes. *J Biol Chem* 2007, 282:7360-7367.

[75] Castellano G, Woltman AM, Nauta AJ, Roos A, Trouw LA, Seelen MA, Schena FP, Daha MR, van Kooten C: Maturation of dendritic cells abrogates C1q production in vivo and in vitro. *Blood* 2004, 103:3813-3820.

[76] Hosszu KK, Valentino A, Vinayagasundaram U, Vinayagasundaram R, Joyce MG, Ji Y, Peerschke EI, Ghebrehiwet B: DC-SIGN, C1q, and gC1qR form a trimolecular receptor complex on the surface of monocyte-derived immature dendritic cells. *Blood* 2012, 120:1228-1236.

[77] Galvan MD, Hulsebus H, Heitker T, Zeng E, Bohlson SS: Complement Protein C1q and Adiponectin Stimulate Mer Tyrosine Kinase-Dependent Engulfment of Apoptotic Cells through a Shared Pathway. *J Innate Immun* 2014, 6:780-792.

[78] Son M, Santiago-Schwarz F, Al-Abed Y, Diamond B: C1q limits dendritic cell differentiation and activation by engaging LAIR-1. *Proc Natl Acad Sci U S A* 2012, 109:E3160-3167.

[79] Fraser DA, Laust AK, Nelson EL, Tenner AJ: C1q differentially modulates phagocytosis and cytokine responses during ingestion of apoptotic cells by human monocytes, macrophages, and dendritic cells. *J Immunol* 2009, 183:6175-6185.

[80] Santer DM, Hall BE, George TC, Tangsombatvisit S, Liu CL, Arkwright PD, Elkon KB: C1q deficiency leads to the defective suppression of IFN-alpha in response to nucleoprotein containing immune complexes. *J Immunol* 2010, 185:4738-4749.

[81] Lood C, Gullstrand B, Truedsson L, Olin AI, Alm GV, Ronnblom L, Sturfelt G, Eloranta ML, Bengtsson AA: C1q inhibits immune complex-induced interferon-alpha production in plasmacytoid dendritic cells: a novel link between C1q deficiency and systemic lupus erythematosus pathogenesis. *Arthritis Rheum* 2009, 60:3081-3090.

[82] Gardai SJ, McPhillips KA, Frasch SC, Janssen WJ, Starefeldt A, Murphy-Ullrich JE, Bratton DL, Oldenborg PA, Michalak M, Henson PM: Cell-surface calreticulin initiates clearance of viable or apoptotic cells through trans-activation of LRP on the phagocyte. *Cell* 2005, 123:321-334.

[83] Tan LA, Yang AC, Kishore U, Sim RB: Interactions of complement proteins C1q and factor H with lipid A and Escherichia coli: further evidence that factor H regulates the classical complement pathway. *Protein Cell* 2011, 2:320-332.

[84] Budayova-Spano M, Lacroix M, Thielens NM, Arlaud GJ, Fontecilla-Camps JC, Gaboriaud C: The crystal structure of the zymogen catalytic domain of complement protease C1r reveals that a disruptive mechanical stress is required to trigger activation of the C1 complex. *Embo J* 2002, 21:231-239.

[85] Gaboriaud C, Ling, W, Thielens, N. M., Bally, I, and Rossi, V Deciphering the fine details of C1 assembly and activation mechanisms: 'mission impossible'? *Front. Immunol* 2014. doi: 10.3389

[86] Malhotra R, Willis AC, Jensenius JC, Jackson J, Sim RB: Structure and homology of human C1q receptor (collectin receptor). *Immunology* 1993, 78:341-348.

[87] Ghebrehiwet B, Lim BL, Peerschke EI, Willis AC, Reid KB: Isolation, cDNA cloning, and overexpression of a 33-kD cell surface glycoprotein that binds to the globular "heads" of C1q. *J Exp Med* 1994, 179:1809-1821.

[88] Duus K, Hansen EW, Tacnet P, Frachet P, Arlaud GJ, Thielens NM, Houen G: Direct interaction between CD91 and C1q. *FEBS J* 2010, 277:3526-3537.

[89] Feng X, Tonnesen MG, Peerschke EI, Ghebrehiwet B: Cooperation of C1q receptors and integrins in C1q-mediated endothelial cell adhesion and spreading. *J Immunol* 2002, 168:2441-2448.

[90] Nepomuceno RR, Henschen-Edman AH, Burgess WH, Tenner AJ: cDNA cloning and primary structure analysis of C1qR(P), the human C1q/MBL/SPA receptor that mediates enhanced phagocytosis in vitro. *Immunity* 1997, 6:119-129.

[91] Klickstein LB, Barbashov SF, Liu T, Jack RM, Nicholson-Weller A: Complement receptor type 1 (CR1, CD35) is a receptor for C1q. *Immunity* 1997, 7:345-355.

[92] McGreal EP, Ikewaki N, Akatsu H, Morgan BP, Gasque P: Human C1qRp is identical with CD93 and the mNI-11 antigen but does not bind C1q. *J Immunol* 2002, 168:5222-5232.

[93] Liu D, Niu ZX: The structure, genetic polymorphisms, expression and biological functions of complement receptor type 1 (CR1/CD35). *Immunopharmacol Immunotoxicol* 2009, 31:524-535.

[94] Khera R, Das N: Complement Receptor 1: disease associations and therapeutic implications. *Mol Immunol* 2009, 46:761-772.

[95] Ghiran I, Barbashov SF, Klickstein LB, Tas SW, Jensenius JC, Nicholson-Weller A: Complement receptor 1/CD35 is a receptor for mannan-binding lectin. *J Exp Med* 2000, 192:1797-1808.

[96] Jacquet M, Lacroix M, Ancelet S, Gout E, Gaboriaud C, Thielens NM, Rossi V: Deciphering complement receptor type 1 interactions with recognition proteins of the lectin complement pathway. *J Immunol* 2013, 190:3721-3731.

[97] Ghiran I, Glodek AM, Weaver G, Klickstein LB, Nicholson-Weller A: Ligation of erythrocyte CR1 induces its clustering in complex with scaffolding protein FAP-1. *Blood* 2008, 112:3465-3473.

[98] Margadant C, Monsuur HN, Norman JC, Sonnenberg A: Mechanisms of integrin activation and trafficking. *Curr Opin Cell Biol* 2011, 23:607-614.

[99] Zutter MM, Edelson BT: The alpha2beta1 integrin: a novel collectin/C1q receptor. *Immunobiology* 2007, 212:343-353.

[100] Edelson BT, Stricker TP, Li Z, Dickeson SK, Shepherd VL, Santoro SA, Zutter MM: Novel collectin/C1q receptor mediates mast cell activation and innate immunity. *Blood* 2006, 107:143-150.

[101] Elton CM, Smethurst PA, Eggleton P, Farndale RW: Physical and functional interaction between cell-surface calreticulin and the collagen receptors integrin alpha2beta1 and glycoprotein VI in human platelets. *Thromb Haemost* 2002, 88:648-654.

[102] Herz J, Strickland DK: LRP: a multifunctional scavenger and signaling receptor. *J Clin Invest* 2001, 108:779-784.

[103] Lillis AP, Greenlee MC, Mikhailenko I, Pizzo SV, Tenner AJ, Strickland DK, Bohlson SS: Murine low-density lipoprotein receptor-related protein 1 (LRP) is required for

phagocytosis of targets bearing LRP ligands but is not required for C1q-triggered enhancement of phagocytosis. *J Immunol* 2008, 181:364-373.

[104] Berwin B, Delneste Y, Lovingood RV, Post SR, Pizzo SV: SREC-I, a type F scavenger receptor, is an endocytic receptor for calreticulin. *J Biol Chem* 2004, 279:51250-51257.

[105] Ishii J, Adachi H, Aoki J, Koizumi H, Tomita S, Suzuki T, Tsujimoto M, Inoue K, Arai H: SREC-II, a new member of the scavenger receptor type F family, trans-interacts with SREC-I through its extracellular domain. *J Biol Chem* 2002, 277:39696-39702.

[106] Fritz G: RAGE: a single receptor fits multiple ligands. *Trends Biochem Sci* 2011, 36:625-632.

[107] Sorci G, Riuzzi F, Giambanco I, Donato R: RAGE in tissue homeostasis, repair and regeneration. *Biochim Biophys Acta* 2013, 1833:101-109.

[108] Friggeri A, Banerjee S, Biswas S, de Freitas A, Liu G, Bierhaus A, Abraham E: Participation of the receptor for advanced glycation end products in efferocytosis. *J Immunol* 2011, 186:6191-6198.

[109] He M, Kubo H, Morimoto K, Fujino N, Suzuki T, Takahasi T, Yamada M, Yamaya M, Maekawa T, Yamamoto Y, et al.: Receptor for advanced glycation end products binds to phosphatidylserine and assists in the clearance of apoptotic cells. *EMBO Rep* 2011, 12:358-364.

[110] Santilli F, Vazzana N, Bucciarelli LG, Davi G: Soluble forms of RAGE in human diseases: clinical and therapeutical implications. *Curr Med Chem* 2009, 16:940-952.

[111] Ma W, Rai V, Hudson BI, Song F, Schmidt AM, Barile GR: RAGE binds C1q and enhances C1q-mediated phagocytosis. *Cell Immunol* 2012, 274:72-82.

[112] Milutinovic PS, Englert JM, Crum LT, Mason NS, Ramsgaard L, Enghild JJ, Sparvero LJ, Lotze MT, Oury TD: Clearance kinetics and matrix binding partners of the receptor for advanced glycation end products. *PLoS One* 2014, 9:e88259.

[113] Dupuy AG, Caron E: Integrin-dependent phagocytosis: spreading from microadhesion to new concepts. *J Cell Sci* 2008, 121:1773-1783.

[114] Ranganathan S, Cao C, Catania J, Migliorini M, Zhang L, Strickland DK: Molecular basis for the interaction of low density lipoprotein receptor-related protein 1 (LRP1) with integrin alphaMbeta2: identification of binding sites within alphaMbeta2 for LRP1. *J Biol Chem* 2011, 286:30535-30541.

[115] Lahti M, Heino J, Kapyla J: Leukocyte integrins alphaLbeta2, alphaMbeta2 and alphaXbeta2 as collagen receptors--receptor activation and recognition of GFOGER motif. *Int J Biochem Cell Biol* 2013, 45:1204-1211.

[116] Garcia-Vallejo JJ, van Kooyk Y: The physiological role of DC-SIGN: a tale of mice and men. *Trends Immunol* 2013, 34:482-486.

[117] Ludwig IS, Geijtenbeek TB, van Kooyk Y: Two way communication between neutrophils and dendritic cells. *Curr Opin Pharmacol* 2006, 6:408-413.

[118] Prabagar MG, Do Y, Ryu S, Park JY, Choi HJ, Choi WS, Yun TJ, Moon J, Choi IS, Ko K, et al.: SIGN-R1, a C-type lectin, enhances apoptotic cell clearance through the complement deposition pathway by interacting with C1q in the spleen. *Cell Death Differ* 2013, 20:535-545.

[119] Meyaard L: The inhibitory collagen receptor LAIR-1 (CD305). *J Leukoc Biol* 2008, 83:799-803.

[120] Lebbink RJ, de Ruiter T, Adelmeijer J, Brenkman AB, van Helvoort JM, Koch M, Farndale RW, Lisman T, Sonnenberg A, Lenting PJ, et al.: Collagens are functional, high affinity ligands for the inhibitory immune receptor LAIR-1. *J Exp Med* 2006, 203:1419-1425.

[121] Olde Nordkamp MJ, Boross P, Yildiz C, Jansen JH, Leusen JH, Wouters D, Urbanus RT, Hack CE, Meyaard L: Inhibition of the classical and lectin pathway of the complement system by recombinant LAIR-2. *J Innate Immun* 2014, 6:284-292.

[122] Olde Nordkamp MJ, van Eijk M, Urbanus RT, Bont L, Haagsman HP, Meyaard L: Leukocyte-associated Ig-like receptor-1 is a novel inhibitory receptor for surfactant protein D. *J Leukoc Biol* 2014, 96:105-111.

[123] Son M, Diamond B: C1q-mediated repression of human monocytes is regulated by LAIR-1. *Mol Med* 2014.

[124] Morgan BP, Walport MJ: Complement deficiency and disease. *Immunol Today* 1991, 12:301-306.

[125] Manderson AP, Botto M, Walport MJ: The role of complement in the development of systemic lupus erythematosus. *Annu Rev Immunol* 2004, 22:431-456.

[126] Trendelenburg M, Lopez-Trascasa M, Potlukova E, Moll S, Regenass S, Fremeaux-Bacchi V, Martinez-Ara J, Jancova E, Picazo ML, Honsova E, et al.: High prevalence of anti-C1q antibodies in biopsy-proven active lupus nephritis. *Nephrol Dial Transplant* 2006, 21:3115-3121.

[127] Siegert C, Daha M, Westedt ML, van der Voort E, Breedveld F: IgG autoantibodies against C1q are correlated with nephritis, hypocomplementemia, and dsDNA antibodies in systemic lupus erythematosus. *J Rheumatol* 1991, 18:230-234.

[128] Schaller M, Bigler C, Danner D, Ditzel HJ, Trendelenburg M: Autoantibodies against C1q in systemic lupus erythematosus are antigen-driven. *J Immunol* 2009, 183:8225-8231.

[129] van den Berg RH, Siegert CE, Faber-Krol MC, Huizinga TW, van Es LA, Daha MR: Anti-C1q receptor/calreticulin autoantibodies in patients with systemic lupus erythematosus (SLE). *Clin Exp Immunol* 1998, 111:359-364.

[130] Roumenina LT, Sene D, Radanova M, Blouin J, Halbwachs-Mecarelli L, Dragon-Durey MA, Fridman WH, Fremeaux-Bacchi V: Functional complement C1q abnormality leads to impaired immune complexes and apoptotic cell clearance. *J Immunol* 2011, 187:4369-4373.

[131] Botto M: C1q knock-out mice for the study of complement deficiency in autoimmune disease. *Exp Clin Immunogenet* 1998, 15:231-234.

[132] Botto M, Walport MJ: C1q, autoimmunity and apoptosis. *Immunobiology* 2002, 205:395-406.

[133] Nash JT, Taylor PR, Botto M, Norsworthy PJ, Davies KA, Walport MJ: Immune complex processing in C1q-deficient mice. *Clin Exp Immunol* 2001, 123:196-202.

[134] Baumann I, Kolowos W, Voll RE, Manger B, Gaipl U, Neuhuber WL, Kirchner T, Kalden JR, Herrmann M: Impaired uptake of apoptotic cells into tingible body macrophages in germinal centers of patients with systemic lupus erythematosus. *Arthritis Rheum* 2002, 46:191-201.

[135] Ippolito A, Wallace DJ, Gladman D, Fortin PR, Urowitz M, Werth V, Costner M, Gordon C, Alarcon GS, Ramsey-Goldman R, et al.: Autoantibodies in systemic lupus erythematosus: comparison of historical and current assessment of seropositivity. *Lupus* 2011, 20:250-255.

[136] Eggleton P, Ukoumunne OC, Cottrell I, Khan A, Maqsood S, Thornes J, Perry E, Isenberg D: Autoantibodies against C1q as a Diagnostic Measure of Lupus Nephritis: Systematic Review and Meta-analysis. *J Clin Cell Immunol* 2014, 5:210.

[137] Kishore U, Sontheimer RD, Sastry KN, Zappi EG, Hughes GR, Khamashta MA, Reid KB, Eggleton P: The systemic lupus erythematosus (SLE) disease autoantigen-calreticulin can inhibit C1q association with immune complexes. *Clin Exp Immunol* 1997, 108:181-190.

[138] Gabillet J, Millet A, Pederzoli-Ribeil M, Tacnet-Delorme P, Guillevin L, Mouthon L, Frachet P, Witko-Sarsat V: Proteinase 3, the autoantigen in granulomatosis with polyangiitis, associates with calreticulin on apoptotic neutrophils, impairs macrophage phagocytosis, and promotes inflammation. *J Immunol* 2012, 189:2574-2583.

[139] Witko-Sarsat V, Reuter N, Mouthon L: Interaction of proteinase 3 with its associated partners: implications in the pathogenesis of Wegener's granulomatosis. *Curr Opin Rheumatol* 2010, 22:1-7.

[140] Ghebrehiwet B, Hosszu KK, Valentino A, Ji Y, Peerschke EI: Monocyte Expressed Macromolecular C1 and C1q Receptors as Molecular Sensors of Danger: Implications in SLE. *Front Immunol* 2014, 5:278.

[141] Castellano G, Woltman AM, Schlagwein N, Xu W, Schena FP, Daha MR, van Kooten C: Immune modulation of human dendritic cells by complement. *Eur J Immunol* 2007, 37:2803-2811.

[142] Peerschke EI, Ghebrehiwet B: Modulation of platelet responses to collagen by Clq receptors. *J Immunol* 1990, 144:221-225.

[143] Jiang K, Chen Y, Xu CS, Jarvis JN: T cell activation by soluble C1q-bearing immune complexes: implications for the pathogenesis of rheumatoid arthritis. *Clin Exp Immunol* 2003, 131:61-67.

[144] Barilla-LaBarca ML, Atkinson JP: Rheumatic syndromes associated with complement deficiency. *Curr Opin Rheumatol* 2003, 15:55-60.

[145] Grumach AS, Kirschfink M: Are complement deficiencies really rare? Overview on prevalence, clinical importance and modern diagnostic approach. *Mol Immunol* 2014, 61:110-117.

[146] Morelli AE, Larregina AT: Apoptotic cell-based therapies against transplant rejection: role of recipient's dendritic cells. *Apoptosis* 2010, 15:1083-1097.

[147] Devitt A, Parker KG, Ogden CA, Oldreive C, Clay MF, Melville LA, Bellamy CO, Lacy-Hulbert A, Gangloff SC, Goyert SM, et al.: Persistence of apoptotic cells without autoimmune disease or inflammation in CD14-/- mice. *J Cell Biol* 2004, 167:1161-1170.

[148] Stuart LM, Takahashi K, Shi L, Savill J, Ezekowitz RA: Mannose-binding lectin-deficient mice display defective apoptotic cell clearance but no autoimmune phenotype. *J Immunol* 2005, 174:3220-3226.

[149] Pfueller B, Wolbart K, Bruns A, Burmester GR, Hiepe F: Successful treatment of patients with systemic lupus erythematosus by immunoadsorption with a C1q column: a pilot study. *Arthritis Rheum* 2001, 44:1962-1963.

[150] Mehta P, Norsworthy PJ, Hall AE, Kelly SJ, Walport MJ, Botto M, Pickering MC: SLE with C1q deficiency treated with fresh frozen plasma: a 10-year experience. Rheumatology (Oxford) 2010, 49:823-824.

[151] Bally I, Ancelet S, Moriscot C, Gonnet F, Mantovani A, Daniel R, Schoehn G, Arlaud GJ, Thielens NM: Expression of recombinant human complement C1q allows identification of the C1r/C1s-binding sites. Proc Natl Acad Sci U S A 2013, 110:8650-8655.

Chapter 3

Implication of Regional Activation of Toll-Like Receptor 3/Interferon-β Signaling in Human Mesangial Cells — Possible Involvement in the Pathogenesis of Lupus Nephritis

Hiroshi Tanaka, Kazushi Tsuruga and
Tadaatsu Imaizumi

Additional information is available at the end of the chapter

http://dx.doi.org/10.5772/59756

1. Introduction

It has been reported that toll-like receptors (TLRs) play a central role in the response of both the innate and adaptive immune systems to microbial ligands [1]. The activation of transcriptional factors, such as interferon regulatory factors (IRF) and nuclear factor kappa B (NF-κB) is induced by intracellular signaling cascades after recognition of presumptive antigenic ligands by TLRs. These signaling pathways result in the release of proinflammatory cytokines and chemokines which play a pivotal role in the innate and adaptive immune responses [1]. Both innate and adaptive immune systems reportedly play important roles in the pathogenesis of systemic lupus erythematosus (SLE) and lupus nephritis (LN) [2-4]. Given the pivotal roles for type I interferons (IFNs) in the pathogenesis of SLE and LN [2-5], the involvement of renal TLRs and their signaling pathways have recently been studied [4, 6, 7]. Since activation of TLRs and their downstream signaling pathways can be induced by non-infectious stimuli, endogenous ligands, this mechanism may be possibly involved in the pathogenesis of autoimmune renal diseases [1-6]. Indeed, recent studies have revealed the expressions of TLRs in resident renal cells, suggesting the involvement of the activations of TLRs and their downstream signaling pathway in the pathogenesis of glomerular diseases [4, 6].

It has been reported that glomerular mesangial cells (MCs) produce a wide variety of proinflammatory molecules that play an important role in both immune and inflammatory reactions in the kidney [7]. Thus, MCs themselves also have a pivotal role in the pathogenesis of renal diseases [8]. Given the implication of "pseudoviral" immunity in the pathogenesis of

LN, we examined the TLR3 signaling cascades triggered by polyinosinic-polycytidylic acid (poly IC), a synthetic analogue of viral dsRNA, that mimics "pseudoviral" infection in cultured human MCs, and found that activation of mesangial TLR3 signaling resulted in increased expressions of functional molecules acting as monocyte/macrophage and lymphocyte chemoattractants: CC chemokine ligand (CCL) 2 [monocyte chemoattractant protein-1 (MCP-1)], CCL5 [regulated on activation, normal T-cell expression and secretion (RANTES)], C-X-C motif ligand 10 (CXCL10) [interferon (IFN)-γ-induced protein 10 (IP-10)], and CX3CL1/fractalkine, in cultured human MCs [5, 6, 9-13]. And we found that poly IC-induced signaling in MCs via TLR3 results in induction of IFN-β, but not IFN-α, in the experimental setting we employed [5, 6, 9, 10, 13], and that newly synthesized IFN-β induces the expression of proinflammatory chemokines and cytokines [6, 9, 10, 13]. With respect to glomerular expression of TLRs, TLR 3, TLR 4, TLR 7 and TLR 9 may play roles in the modulation of inflammatory processes in glomerulonephritis, including LN and IgA nephropathy (IgAN) [2, 3, 6, 14-16]. Interestingly, TLR 7 and TLR 9 recognize mammalian nucleic acids as well as bacterial DNA or viral RNA. Thus, the generation of some autoantibodies may be attributable to possible roles of TLR 7 and TLR 9 in selected patients with LN [3, 6]. However, in this paper, we do not discuss the in-depth roles of TLR4, TLR 7 and TLR 9 in mesangial inflammation. Other general reviews of TLRs should be referred to regarding these issues. In the present paper, we summarize mesangial expressions of proinflammatory chemokines via TLR3/IFN-β signaling pathways [5, 9-13].

2. Expressions of retinoic acid-inducible gene-I (RIG-I) and melanoma differentiation-associated gene-5 (MDA5), and TLR3/IFN-β signaling in MCs

During hepatitis C virus (HCV) infection, the activation of mesangial TLR3-mediated proinflammatory chemokine/cytokine releases are reportedly involved in the pathogenesis of HCV glomerulonephritis [18]. In an experimental setting also, it has been reported that the expressions of matrix alteration-associated functional molecules, such as matrix metalloproteinase 9, plasminogen activator inhibitor type 1, and tissue plasminogen activator in human MCs induced by mesangial TLR3 activation [19, 20]. These findings suggest that viral RNA can influence subsequent glomerulosclerosis through the generation and degradation of the extracelluar matrix in the MCs except for direct viral stimulation [19, 20]. Viral double-stranded RNA (dsRNA) can activate not only TLR3 located in intracellular endosomes, but also retinoic acid-inducible gene-I (RIG-I)-like helicases receptors located in the cytosol, such as RIG-I and melanoma differentiation-associated gene-5 (MDA5) [21, 22]. Therefore, RIG-I and MDA5 may also be involved in the pathogenesis of LN [6, 7, 9, 11]. It has previously been reported that RIG-I, and not TLR3, mediated the secretion of type I IFN in poly IC/cationic lipid complex-treated glomerular endothelial cells [23]. In an experiment study using TLR3 signaling-deficient mice, it has been reported that MDA5, but not RIG-I, was required for signaling induced by poly IC/cationic lipid complex in murine MCs [7]. The cells transfected with poly IC/cationic lipid complex is thought to be a model of entry of RNA virus into the cytoplasm.

However, the precise role of RIG-I and the interaction between TLR3, MDA5 and RIG-I in mesangial inflammation remains to be elucidated.

We previously found significant expression of RIG-I in the glomeruli of biopsy specimens from patients with proliferative LN, and the level of expression correlated with the severity of the acute inflammatory lesions (Figure 1.) [24].

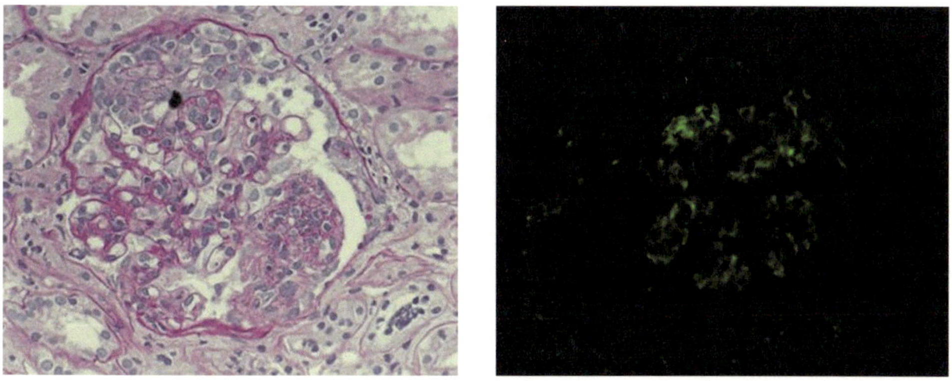

Figure 1. Glomerular immunoreactivity for RIG-I in patients with proliferative LN. The histological picture by light microscopy was classified as class IV according to the ISN/RPS criteria (left), and significant increase in the immunostaining intensity for RIG-I was observed (right) (quoted and modified from Ref. no. 24).

In addition, we found that the levels of RIG-I mRNA in the urinary sediment of patients with LN were higher than those in patients with IgAN and controls [25]. Further, repeated measurements of the mRNA expression of RIG-I in the urinary sediment of lupus patients revealed a reduction in the expression following immunosuppressive treatment [25]. These findings suggest that RIG-I may be involved in the acute inflammatory process in human LN. To examine the effect of TLR3 activation on the expression of RIG-I, human MCs were simply treated with poly IC. Treatment with poly IC is a model of cells exposed to viral dsRNA released from dying cells. Stimulation with poly IC resulted in an increase in the expression of both RIG-I mRNA and protein in a concentration- and time-dependent manner, and this was accompanied with CCL5 expression [9]. Also, we found that poly IC-induced signaling in MCs via TLR3 results in induction of IFN-β, but not IFN-α, in the experimental setting we employed (the results of our recent papers, Ref no. 9, 10, 13, should be referred to regarding this issue). Furthermore, knockdown of RIG-I expression by small interfering RNA (siRNA) significantly lowered poly IC-induced CCL5 expression. In contrast, the poly IC-induced expression of CCL2 mRNA was not affected by RIG-I siRNA. Interestingly, the poly IC-induced RIG-I expression was suppressed in response to treatment with siRNA against TLR3. Furthermore, TLR3 siRNA decreased the poly IC-induced expressions of TLR3 and IFN-β. On the other hand, RIG-I siRNA did not affect the expression of either TLR3 or IFN-β. To confirm the role of IFN-β acting as a potential mediator of poly IC-induced RIG-I expression, IFN-β siRNA results in markedly decreases in the expressions of poly IC-induced IFN-β and RIG-I. Pretreatment of the cells with an anti-type I IFN receptor antibody also reduced the poly IC-induced expression of RIG-I. Moreover, pretreatment of the cells with dexamethasone reduced the poly IC-induced expression of both RIG-I and IFN-β, but this treatment had no effect on IFN-β-induced RIG-I expression [9]. Our recent study showed that siRNA-mediated knock-down of TLR3 inhibited the poly IC-induced expression of both IFN-β and RIG-I, whereas RIG-I knockdown had no effect on poly IC-induced IFN-β expression. Thus, RIG-I may function downstream to TLR3 in the signaling cascade activated by poly IC-induced expression of CCL5 in MCs [9]. In this signaling pathway in MCs, TLR3 and newly synthesized IFN-β are involved in poly IC-induced CCL5 expression (TLR3/IFN-β/RIG-I/CCL5 pathway).

It has been reported a pivotal role of IFN-α, rather than IFN-β, in the pathogenesis of LN [2]. In an interesting experiment using murine lupus model, early IFN receptor blockade with anti-IFN-α receptor antibody attenuated the development of glomerular inflammation [26]. However, apart from its physiological antiviral activity, IFN-β has also been reported to play a pivotal role in the inflammatory reactions in GN [2]. With respect to this issue, we think that *de novo* synthesized IFN-β from MCs acts, at least in part, as a "autocrine" mediator in residual renal cells in our experimental setting employing "human" MCs, whereas IFN-α, generally, may be released from infiltrating proinflammatory cells and acts as a "paracrine" mediator in selected clinical and experimental settings, although this theory remains speculative. Recently, it has been reported an interesting case of so-called IFN-β nephropathy which developed after long-term IFN-β treatment for relapsing multiple sclerosis [27]. Thus, regional role of IFN-β, especially in case of sustained activation, in human MCs remains to be examined in the future.

Since implications for the expression of MDA5 in human MCs have not been clarified, we next examined the role of MDA5 in CXCL10 expression in cultured human MCs [11]. Poly IC, either simply applied to the cells or transfected as a complex with a cationic lipid, induced MDA5 expression in concentration- and time-dependent manners. Transfection of the cells with siRNA against TLR3 suppressed the poly IC-induced expression of MDA5 mRNA and protein, while siRNA against TLR3 did not suppress the poly IC/cationic lipid complex-induced expression of MDA5. On the other hand, siRNA against RIG-I significantly inhibited the MDA5 expression induced by poly IC/cationic lipid complex, whereas knockdown of MDA5 had no effects on the expression of RIG-I induced by poly IC or poly IC/cationic lipid complex, suggesting that MDA5 may be located in the downstream of RIG-I in this signaling pathway in MCs [11]. These results are inconsistent with a previous report dealing with MDA5 expression in murine MCs [7]. The molecular mechanisms of pathogen recognition may vary between species, although this remains to be determined in future studies. In this experiment also, TLR3 knockdown suppressed IFN-β induction in the poly IC-treated cells, while RIG-I knockdown suppressed the induction in the cells transfected with poly IC/cationic lipid. Transfection of the cells with IFN-β siRNA markedly inhibited production of MDA5 and CXCL10 induced by poly IC treatment or poly IC/cationic lipid transfection. On the other hand, MDA5 was markedly induced by the transfection with an IFN-β expression plasmid. Thus, it is considered that newly synthesized IFN-β mediates poly IC-induced MDA5 expression. In our previous studies, poly IC treatment of MCs induced the expression of IFN-β and *de novo* synthesized IFN-β mediated the expressions of RIG-I and IFN stimulated gene (ISG) 20 [9,

10]. In the present study, we observed that IFN-β is induced either by poly IC or a poly IC/cationic lipid complex, and *de novo* synthesized IFN-β may mediate the expression of MDA5 [11]. RIG-I is involved in IFN-β expression induced by poly IC/cationic lipid complex, but not in the MDA expression by IFN-β. Taking together, we concluded that the TLR3/IFN-β/MDA5/CXCL10 pathway activates by poly IC treatment, while RIG-I/IFN-β/MDA5/CXCL10 pathway activates by poly IC/cationic lipid complex treatment in anti-viral and inflammatory reactions in MCs [11]. Furthermore, we observed mesangial MDA5 immunoreactivity in biopsy specimens from patients with both severe LN and proteinuric IgAN but no MDA5 expression in patients with non-inflammatory renal diseases. Interestingly, there was no mesangial expression of RIG-I in the specimens from patients with IgAN despite positive MDA5 staining. These observations suggested that the expression of MDA5 in severe LN is associated with signaling pathway activation via RIG-I [6, 11], whereas MDA5 expression in IgAN may be RIG-I-independent. The differential roles of MDA5 and RIG-I in severe LN and proteinuric IgAN may predict the specific molecular mechanisms of these glomerulonephritis forms [6].

3. Expression of myxovirus resistance protein 1 (Mx1) and TLR3/IFN-β signaling in MCs

It has been reported that human myxovirus resistance protein 1 (Mx1), a type I IFN-dependent transcript, which belongs to the class of dynamin-like large guanosine triphosphatases, play a role against a wide range of RNA viruses by interfering with viral replication [28]. Although its precise role in the pathogenesis of SLE remains speculative, *Mx1* gene expression in peripheral blood cells has been reported as a possible biomarker for LN therapy [29]. However, the regional implication of Mx1 for innate immune response in MCs remains to be elucidated [30].

We recently examined the expression of Mx1 in response to poly IC in cultured human MCs. Both poly IC alone and poly IC/cationic acid complex-induced Mx1 expressions in MCs are shown both time- and dose-dependently, and siRNA against IFN-β inhibited both poly IC treatment and transfection with a poly IC/cationic lipid complex-induced Mx1 expression [4]. Further, intense glomerular Mx1 expression was observed in biopsy specimens from patients with LN, whereas negative staining occurred in specimens from patients with IgAN or purpura nephritis (PN), even though both showed moderately to severe mesangial proliferation (Figure 2.).

Based on our experimental and clinical observations, both TLR3/IFN-β and RIG-I/IFN-β signaling pathways are responsible for poly IC-induced Mx1 expression in MCs. Regarding the detailed function of Mx1, we previously found that neither cell viability nor the expression of various IFN-stimulated genes was altered by Mx1 knockdown [31]. Thus, mesangial expression of Mx1 in LN patients may be a sequel of marked regional innate immune system activation [4]. We previously reported significant expression of both RIG-I and MDA5 in the glomeruli of biopsy specimens from patients with proliferative LN [11, 24]. Taking together, glomerular expressions of Mx1 as well as RIG-I and MDA5 in biopsy specimens from patients

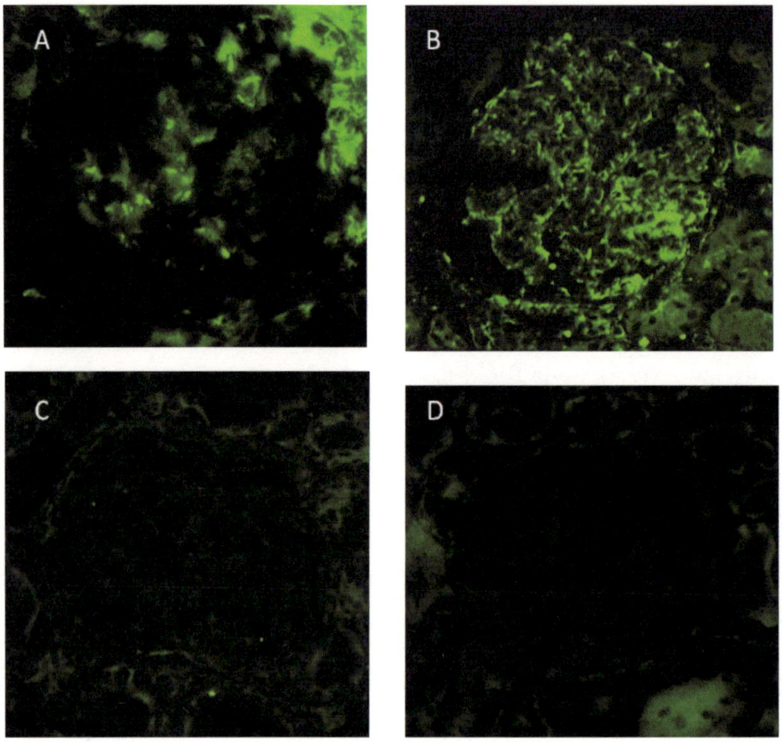

Figure 2. Immunofluorescence staining of Mx1 in renal biopsy specimens obtained from patients with proliferative LN (A, Class IV-G (A), and B, Class III (A) LN), proteinuric IgAN (C, diffuse proliferative mesangial proliferation6), and orthostatic proteinuria (D, served as a non-inflammatory control), respectively. A significant increase in Mx1 immunoreactivity was observed LN specimens (A and B), whereas immunoreactivity was negligible in the other specimens (C and D) (quoted and modified from Ref. no. 4).

with proliferative LN may further support the theory of innate immunity activation in the pathogenesis of LN [4].

4. Local activation of tumor necrosis factor (TNF)-α and TLR3/IFN-β signaling in MCs

It has been reported that patients with active SLE have local as well as systemic activation of proinflammatory cytokines [32, 33]. Among the increased serum proinflammatory cytokines in SLE, Koenig et al. recently reported that only serum soluble receptor of tumor necrosis factor (TNF)-α is actually and significantly increased, thereby possible local activation of TNF-α exists in active lupus patients [32]. However, mainly based on the observation murine LN models, it has been reported that TNF-α have both protective and deleterious effects in the pathogenesis of LN [33]. Therefore, precise role of regional TNF-α activation of in the pathogenesis of human LN remains to be determined.

Pretreatment of cultured normal human MCs with 1 ng/ml TNF-α markedly enhanced the poly IC-induced expression of CCL5 mRNA and protein, in a concentration-dependent manner. TNF-α pretreatment also enhanced the expression of protein and mRNA for IFN-β and RIG-I induced by poly IC, whereas treatment of MCs with 1 ng/ml TNF-α alone did not induce the expression of IFN-β. Transfection of siRNA against IFN-β partially but significantly inhibited the expression of CCL5 and RIG-I mRNA and protein induced by TNF-α followed by poly IC [13]. We found that the combination of pretreatment of cells with TNF-α, even at low dose (?) and subsequent treatment with poly IC resulted in the synergistic induction of CCL5 expression in MCs. Therefore, this experimental observation suggests that over production of CCL5 due to pre-existing regional activation of TNF-α may be involved in the development of LN in patients with active SLE. Increased IFN-β due to pre-existing regional activation of TNF-α may be a key mediator of CCL5 expression in MCs in this experimental setting. In a clinical setting, long-term beneficial effect of early induction regimen including TNF-α blockade has been reported in some patients with refractory LN [34], suggesting potential deleterious effects of regional TNF-α activation. Both pre-existing TNF-α activation and IFN-β/RIG-I/CCL5 axis may be involved in the pathogenesis of LN in patients with active SLE [13].

5. Expression of fractalkine/CX3CL1 and TLR3 signaling in MCs

Fractalkine/CX3CL1 (Fkn) is a chemokine that induces the chemotaxis and activation of inflammatory cells expressing its receptor, CX3CR1, and primarily regulated by proinflammatory cytokines such as TNF-α and IL-1 [35]. Fkn expression in mesangial lesions has been reported to be significantly correlated with histopathological disease activity in a rat model of human and mouse models of LN [36]. Moreover, mesangial Fkn expression may play an important role in the development of prolonged glomerular inflammation [37], and an antagonist of Fkn ameliorates the progression of this condition in a mouse model of LN [38]. However, the role of Fkn in innate immunity in human MCs remains to be elucidated.

We previously found that poly IC treatment of MCs induced both Fkn mRNA and protein expressions in a time-dependent manner. In contrast, induction of Fkn mRNA expression by poly IC/cationic lipid complex treatment was minimal, while RIG-I mRNA and protein were significantly induced. Poly IC-induced Fkn mRNA and protein expression was suppressed in response to treatment with siRNA against TLR3, while siRNAs against RIG-I and MDA5 did not affect poly IC-induced Fkn mRNA expression [12]. Transfection of MCs with siRNA against IRF3 suppressed the expression of Fkn mRNA and protein, whereas siRNA against NF-κB p65 did not affect Fkn protein expression. Interestingly, pre-treatment of cells using a blocking antibody against type I IFN receptor did not affect poly IC-induced Fkn mRNA expression, although this treatment clearly suppressed mRNA expression of poly IC-induced ISG 15. These results suggest that poly IC-induced expression of Fkn in MCs does not depend on cytosolic RNA recognition sensors RIG-I but may depend on the extracellular sensor TLR3. We then observed that knockdown of IRF3, but not NF-κB p65, inhibited poly IC-induced Fkn expression in MCs, and retreatment of cells using a blocking antibody against type I IFN receptor did not affect poly IC-induced mesangial Fkn expression, although it clearly inhibited poly IC-induced ISG15 expression, suggesting that poly IC-induced Fkn expression in MCs primarily depends on the TLR3/IRF3 signaling pathway, but not TLR3/IFN-β signaling [12]. Recently, it has been reported that Fkn is not a target of IRF3-dependent direct response genes in "embryo" fibroblast from virally-infected mice [39]. This discrepancy may attributable to cell maturity, types, or species. Future detailed studies focused on this issue using Fkn-deficient mice are needed.

6. Conclusions

We believe that involvement of the novel TLR3/IFN-β signaling pathways, those are TLR3/IFN-β/RIG-I/CCL5 and TLR3/IFN-β/MDA5/CXCL10 pathways, and type I IFNs-independent TLR3/IRF3/Fkn pathway in MCs may contribute to mesangial inflammation (Figure 3). Cross-talk of between these signaling pathways may be involved in the pathogenesis of human LN. Since the inhibitory effect of dexamethasone may depend on the suppression of IFN-β production and not on IFN-β induced RIG-I and MDA5 expressions [9, 10], effective treatment strategies for the intervening in these signaling pathways are needed. We believe that intervention within these signaling pathways may lead to the development of future therapeutic strategies for LN.

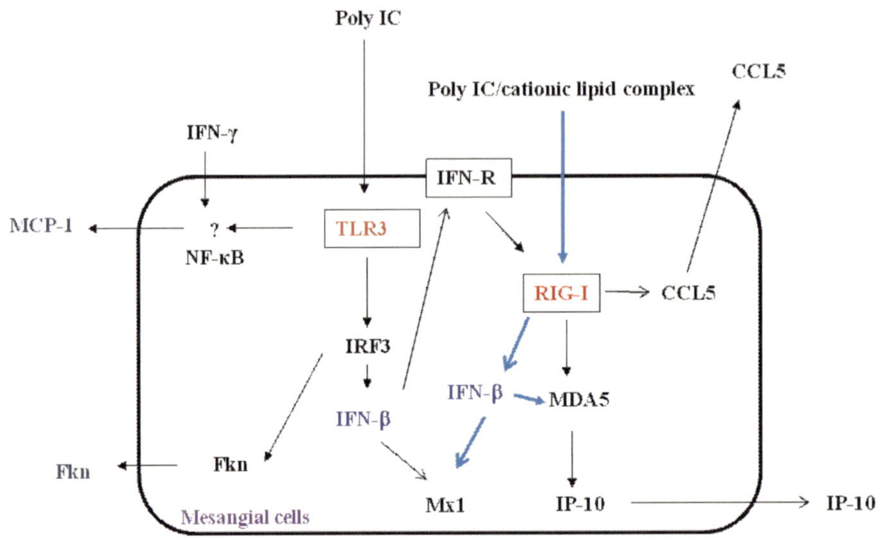

Figure 3. Proposed inflammatory signaling pathways via TLR3 induced by poly IC (black arrows) and RIG-I induced by poly IC/cationic lipid complex (blue arrows) in human mesangial cells (MCP-1, monocyte chemoattractant prorein-1; Fkn, fractalkine; IFN, interferon; NF-κB, nuclear factor kappa B; TLR, toll-like receptor; IRF3, interferon regulatory factor 3; Mx1, human myxovirus resistance protein 1; RIG-I, retinoic acid-inducible gene-1; MDA5, melanoma differentiation-associated gene-5; IP-10, interferon (IFN)-γ-induced protein 10; CCL5, CC chemokine ligand 5).

http://dx.doi.org/10.5772/59756

Acknowledgements

These studies were supported by Grants-in-Aid for Japan Society for Promotion of Science.

Author details

Hiroshi Tanaka[1,2], Kazushi Tsuruga[2] and Tadaatsu Imaizumi[3]

1 Department of School Health Science, Faculty of Education, Hirosaki University, Japan

2 Department of Pediatrics, Hirosaki University Hospital, Japan

3 Department of Vascular Biology, Hirosaki University Graduate School of Medicine, Hirosaki, Japan

We have no conflict of interest to be declared.

References

[1] Robson MG. Toll-like receptors and renal disease. Nephron Exp Nephrol 2009; 113: e1-7.

[2] Anders HJ, Lichtnekert J, Allam R. Interferon-α and -β in kidney inflammation. Kidney Int 2010; 77: 848-54.

[3] Karageorgas TP, Tseronis DD, Mavragani CP. Activation of type I interferon pathway in systemic lupus erythematosus: Association with distinct clinical phenotypes. J Biomed Biotechnol 2011; 2011: 273907.

[4] Migliorini A, Anders HJ. A novel pathogenetic concept - antiviral immunity in lupus nephritis. Nat Rev Nephrol 2012; 8: 183-9.

[5] Watanabe S, Imaizumi T, Tsuruga K, et al. Glomerular expression of myxovirus resistance protein 1 (Mx1) in human mesangial cells: possible activation of innate immunity in the pathogenesis of lupus nephritis. Nephrology (Carlton) 2013; 18: 833-7.

[6] Tanaka H, Imaizumi T. Inflammatory chemokine expression via toll-like receptor 3 signaling in normal human mesangial cells. Clin Dev Immunol 2013; 2013: 984708.

[7] Flur K, Allam R, Zecher D, et al. Viral RNA induces type I interferon-dependent cytokine release and cell death in mesangial cells via melanoma-differentiation-associated gene-5. Implications for viral infection-associated glomerulonephritis. Am J Pathol 2009; 175: 2014-22.

[8] Migliorini A, Ebid R, Scherbaum CR, Anders HJ. The danger control concept in kidney disease: mesangial cells. J Nephrol 2013; 26: 437-9.

[9] Imaizumi T, Tanaka H, Matsumiya T, et al. Retinoic acid-inducible gene-I is induced by double-stranded RNA and regulates the expression of CC chemokine ligand (CCL) 5 in human mesangial cells. Nephrol Dial Transplant 2010; 25: 3534-9.

[10] Imaizumi T, Tanaka H, Mechti N, et al. Polyinosinic-polycytidylic acid induces the expression of interferon-stimulated gene 20 in mesangial cells. Nephron Exp Nephrol 2011; 119: e40-8.

[11] Imaizumi T, Aizawa-Yashiro T, Tsuruga K, et al. "Melanoma differentiation-associated gene 5 regulates the expression of a chemokine CXCL10 in human mesangial cells: implications for chronic inflammatory renal diseases. Tohoku J Exp Med 2012; 228: 17-26.

[12] Aizawa-Yashiro T, Imaizumi T, Tsuruga K, et al. Glomerular expression of fractalkine is induced by polyinosinic-polycytidylic acid in human mesangial cells: possible involvement of fractalkine after viral infection. Pediatr Res 2013; 73: 180-6.

[13] Imaizumi T, Aizawa T, Hayakari R, et al. Tumor necrosis factor-α synergistically enhances polyinosinic-polycytidylic acid-induced toll-like receptor 3 signaling in cultured normal human mesangial cells: possible involvement in the pathogenesis of lupus nephritis. Clin Exp Nephrol 2015; 19: 75-81.

[14] Coppo R, Amore A, Peruzzi L, Vergano L, Camilla R. Innate immunity and IgA nephropathy. J Nephrol 2010; 23: 626-32.

[15] Papadimitraki ED, Tzardi M, Bertsias G, Sotsiou E, Boumpas DT. Glomerular expression of toll-like receptor-9 in lupus nephritis but not in normal kidney: implications for the amplification of the inflammatory response. Lupus 2009; 18: 831-5.

[16] Imaizumi T, Aizawa-Yashiro T, Watanabe S et al. TLR4 signaling induces retinoic acid inducible gene-I and melanoma differentiation-associated gene 5 in mesangial cells. J Nephrol 2013; 26: 886-93.

[17] Patole PS, Pawar RD, Lechet M al. Expression and regulation of Toll-like receptors in lupus-like immune complex glomerulomephritis of MRL-Fas (lpr) mice. Nephrol Dial Transplant 2006; 21: 3062-73.

[18] Wörnle M, Schmid H, Banas B et al. Novel role of Toll-like receptor 3 in hepatitis C-associated glomerulonephritis. Am J Pathol 2006 ; 168: 370-85.

[19] Wörnle M, Roeder M, Sauter M, Riberio A. Role of matrix mettalloproteinases in viral-associated glomerulonephritis. Nephrol Dial Transplant 2009; 24: 1113-21.

[20] Wörnle M, Roeder M, Sauter M, Merkle M, Ribeiro A. Effect of dsRNA on mesangial cell synthesis of plasminnogen activator inhibitor type 1 and tissue plasminogen activator. Nephron Exp Nephrol 2009; 113: e57-65.

[21] Takeuchi O, Akira S. MDA5/RIG-I and virus recognition. Current Opin Immunol 2008; 20: 17-22.

[22] Yoneyama M, Kikuchi M, Natsukawa T, et al. The RNA helicase RIG-I has an essential function in double-stranded RNA-induced innate antiviral responses. Nat Immunol 2004; 5: 730-7.

[23] Hagele H, Allam R, Pawar RD, Anders HJ. Double-stranded RNA activates type I interferon secretion in glomerular endothelial cells via retinoic acid-inducible gene (RIG)-I. Nephrol Dial Transplant 2009; 24: 3312-8.

[24] Suzuki K, Imaizumi T, Tsugawa K, Ito E, Tanaka H. Expression of retinoic acid-inducible gene-I in lupus nephritis. Nephrol Dial Transplant 2007; 22: 2407-9.

[25] Tsugawa K, Suzuki K, Oki E, Imaizumi T, Ito E, Tanaka H. Expression of mRNA for functional molecules in urinary sediment in glomerulonephritis. Pediatr Nephrol 2008; 23: 395-401.

[26] Baccalo R, Gonzalez-Quintial R, Schreiber RD, Lawson BR, Kono DW, Theofilopoulos AN. Anti-IFN-α/β receptor antibody treatment ameliorates disease in lupus-predisposed mice. J Immunol 2012; 189: 5976-84.

[27] Capobianco M, Piccoli G, Vigotti FN, et al. Interferon beta-related nephropathy and interstitial lung disease: a new association and a long-term warning. Mult Scler 2014; 20: 889-91.

[28] Haller O, Staeheli P. Kochs G. Interferon-induced Mx proteins in antiviral host defense. Biochemie 2007; 89: 812-8.

[29] Feng X, Wu H, Grossman JM, et al. Association of increased interferon-inducible gene expression with disease activity and lupus nephritis in patients with systemic lupus erythematosus. Arthritis Rheum 2006; 54: 2951-62.

[30] Floege J, Burg M, Al Masri AN, Gröne HJ, von Wussow P. Expression of interferon-inducible Mx-proteins in patients with IgA nephropathy or Henoch-Schönlein purpura. Am J Kidney Dis 1999; 33: 434-40.

[31] Dempoya J, Matsumiya T, Imaizumi T, et al. Double-stranded RNA induces biphasic STAT1 phosphorylation by both type I IFN-dependent and type I IFN-independent pathways. J Virol 2012; 86: 12760-9.

[32] Koenig KF, Groeschl I, Pesickova SS, Tesar V, Eisenberger U, Trendelenburg M. Serum cytokine profile in patients with active lupus nephritis. Cytokine 2012; 60: 410-6.

[33] Yung S, Cheung KF, Zhang Q, Chan TM. Mediators of inflammation and their effect on resident renal cells: Implications in lupus nephritis. Clin DevImmunol 2013; 2013: 317682.

[34] Aringer M, Houssiau F, Gordon C, et al. Adverse events and efficacy of TNF-α blockade with infliximab in patients with systemic lupus erythematosus: long-term follow-up of 13 patients. Rheumatology (Oxford) 2009; 48: 1451-4.

[35] Bazan JF, Bacon KB, Hardiman G, et al. A new class of membrane-bound chemokine with a CX3C motif. Nature 1997; 385: 640-7.

[36] Nakatani K, Yoshimoto S, Iwano M, et al. Fractalkine expression and $CD16^+$ monocyte accumulation in glomerular lesions: association with their severity and diversity in lupus models. Am J Physiol Ren Physiol 2010; 299: F207-16.

[37] Ito Y, Kawachi H, Morioka Y, et al. Fractalkine expression and the recruitment of CX_3CR1^+ cells in the prolonged mesangial proliferative glomerulonephritis. Kidney Int 2002; 61: 2044-57.

[38] Inoue A, Hasegawa H, Kohno M, et al. Antagonist of fractalkine (CX3CL1) delays the initiation and ameliorates the progression of lupus nephritis in MRL/lpr mice. Arthritis Rheum 2005; 52: 1522-33.

[39] Anderson J, VanScoy S, Cheng TF, Gomez D, Reich NC. IRF-3-dependent and augmented target genes during viral infection. Genes Immunity 2008; 9: 168-75.

Chapter 4

Autoimmunity in Children with Primary Immunodeficiency – Diagnosis, Management and Therapy

Anna Pituch-Noworolska

Additional information is available at the end of the chapter

http://dx.doi.org/10.5772/60882

1. Introduction

The list of primary immunodeficiencies (PID) includes now more than 200 different diseases and syndromes characterised by dysfunction of immune system with different epidemiology ranging from common, like selected IgA deficiency, to very rare, diagnosed in singular patients. The deficiencies of humoral immunity are frequent including transient hypogammaglobulinemia of infants (THI), common variable immunodeficiency (CVID), selected IgA deficiency (IgAD), hyper IgM syndrome (hyperIgM) or agammaglobulinemia (XLA). The hypogammaglobulinemia of selected immunoglobulins' class (IgG or IgA) or all classes (e.g. CVID) are associated with allergy and autoimmunity in significant percentage of patients. The hypothesis explaining autoimmune diseases in humoral immunodeficiency includes presence of autoreactive T and B lymphocytes, deregulation of immune response associated with number and function of T regulatory cells and other mechanisms. The typical clinical symptoms of autoimmune process in patients with humoral deficiency (CVID, IgAD, hyper IgM) include cytopenias, gastrointestinal tract diseases like celiac or inflammatory bowel diseases, endocrine system autoimmunity, rheumatoid arthritis and systemic autoimmune diseases. The diagnosis of autoimmunity in humoral immunodeficiency is difficult, due to low production of antibodies, overlapping of clinical symptoms of immunodeficiency and autoimmunity. Autoimmunity is noted also in group of well defined immunodeficiency or immunodysregulation syndromes with autoimmune symptoms as criteria of given immunodeficiency, e.g., autoimmune lymphoproliferative syndrome (ALSP) and Wiskott-Aldrich syndrome (WAS). Therapy of autoimmunity in immunodeficient patients includes steroids, immunosuppression, similar to patients without PID. However, if, in some patients with PID, the standard therapy of autoimmune disease is not effective, the immunoglobulins in high dose and/or, monoclonal antibodies are used. Progress and severity of autoimmune process, resistance to therapy, life-threatening symptoms are now the indications for haematopoietic stem cells transplantation for these patients.

2. Introduction to primary immunodeficiency associated with autoimmunity

The primary immunodeficiencies (PID) consist of more than 200 diseases with one common background – dysfunction of immune system as effect of T, B lymphocytes, NK cells and neutrophils' disturbances in ontogeny and function. The first, most extreme group of PIDs are severe combined immunodeficiencies (SCID) characterised by the lack of immunocompetent cell populations. In these deficiencies, the different patterns of lack of cells are noted- without T lymphocytes and/or NK cells (SCID T-B+NK-, SCID T-B+NK+), and/or B lymphocytes (SCID T-B-NK-, SCID T-B-NK+). The one way to safe life of newborn babies and infants with SCID is haematopoietic stem cells transplantation (HSCT) from matched related or unrelated donor (Table 1). In SCID, the autoimmunity is rare, practically seen only in Omenn's syndrome (Rag1/ Rag2 deficiency). In this type of SCID, besides antibacterial, antifungal, antiviral therapy, substitution of immunoglobulins as standard therapy for SCID, the use of steroids and/or cyclosporine A is indicated to resolve the erythrodermia and eosinophilia. This symptomatic therapy is effective in majority of patients. Thrombocytopenia, neutropenia and leukopenia are often due to hyperactivity of spleen.

Type of deficiency	Laboratory data	Genetic background	Clinical features	Effective therapy
T-B+ Gamma chain deficiency	T, NK decreased, B normal, low IgG	Defect of receptors for: IL-2, -4, -7, -9, -15, -21, X-linked	Severe infections (bacterial, viral, fungal), failure to thrive	Antibiotics, antimycotics, IVIG substitution, HSCT as curative
Other deficiency with known genetic background	like above	JAK3, IL-7R alfa chain, CD45 deficiency Autosomal recessive	Like above	Like above
T-B-(NK-) Omenn's syndrome	T, B, NK decreased, IgG low, IgE high	RAG1/RAG2	Erythrodermia, eosinophilia, autoimmunity, CMV infection, splenomegaly	Steroids and/or cyclosporine A, IVIG, antibacterial, antiviral therapy, HSCT
Reticular dysgenesis	T, B, NK decreased, low IgG	Adenylate kinase (AK2) deficiency	Neutropenia, deafness	Antibiotics, antimycotics, Antiviral therapy, IVIG, HSCT

http://dx.doi.org/10.5772/60882

Type of deficiency	Laboratory data	Genetic background	Clinical features	Effective therapy
Adenosine deaminase deficiency (ADA)	may be progressive decrease of T, B, NK cells number	ADA deficiency	Costochondral junction flaring, neurological features, hearing impairment, lung and liver involvement	Like above
MHC class I	decreased CD8, normal B and NK cells	TAP, TAP2 or TAPBP mutation	Severe infections, vasculitis	Like above
MHC class II	decreased CD4, normal B and NK cells number	Transcription factors mutation (CIITA, RFX5, RFXAP, RFXANK)	Infections, failure to thrive, chronic diarrhoea	Like above

Table 1. Selected types of severe combined immunodeficiencies (SCID) [acc. 1]

In general consensus, the primary immunodeficiencies are divided into groups depending on the basic defect: humoral immunodeficiency -- common deficiency with prevalence of disorders in immunoglobulins and antibodies production, cellular immunodeficiency and well-defined syndromes of immunodeficiency with prevalence of cellular mechanisms leading to functional deficiency. The bacterial, viral infections with severe clinical course and poor response to therapy are common and typical symptoms of immune deficiency, due to lack of proper reaction of immune system. In patients with SCID, these infections are life-threatening and together with failure to thrive and weight gaining, they lead to death within first year of life. The autoimmunity process and symptoms are noted as associated disease or complications in different types of immune deficiency. The autoimmunity, in particular types of PID (e.g. hyper IgM syndrome, autoimmune lymphoproliferative syndrome (ALPS), Wiskott-Aldrich syndrome (WAS), is one of criteria of these immunodeficiencies (Table 2). In CVID, one of common immune deficiency of immunoglobulin and specific antibodies synthesis, the autoimmune co-existent process and diseases are noted in more than 30% of patients (up to 60% in different groups). The similar frequency of autoimmunity is observed within IgA deficiency patients.

Type of deficiency	Laboratory data	Genetic background	Clinical features	Effective therapy
WAS Wiskott-Aldrich syndrome	Decreasing T number, B normal, IgA, IgE increased	Mutation in WAS X-linked	Microthrombocytopenia, eczema, autoimmunity, IgA nephropathy, infections, lymphoma	Antibiotics, antiviral therapy, IVIG, HSCT
ALPS (defects of apoptosis) 1.Fas defect (CD95) 2.FasL (CD95L)	Increased DNT (CD3/CD4-/CD8-), normal B and NK cells	Mutation of TNFRSF6 (surface apoptosis receptor)	Lymphadenopathy, splenomegaly, cytopenias, high or normal IgG level	Steroids (often resistance), high-dose IgG, MMF, sirolimus, HSCT

Type of deficiency	Laboratory data	Genetic background	Clinical features	Effective therapy
3.Caspase 10 4. Caspase 8		Mutation TNFSF6 (Fas ligand) Mutation of Casp10 (intracellular apoptosis pathway) Mutation of Casp8	Lymphadenopathy, splenomegaly, cytopenias, recurrent bacterial and viral infections, low IgG	
APECED, Polyendo-crinopathy, candidiasis, enctodermal dystrophy	T, B and NK cells normal, IgG normal	Mutation of AIRE	Autoimmunity of endocrinal glands, chronic candidiasis, hypoplasia of dental enamel	Symptomatic supplementary therapy, steroids
IPEX polyendocrino pathy, enteropathy	Impaired function of T regulatory, B and NK cells normal, high IgA, IgE	Mutation of FOXP3 X-linked	Autoimmune enteropathy, diabetes, thyroiditis, eczema, haemolytic anaemia, thrombocytopenia	Symptomatic therapy
CD25 deficiency	T, B and NK cells normal	Mutation of IL-2 receptor alfa chain	Lymphoproliferation, autoimmunity	Symptomatic therapy

Table 2. Diseases of immunodysregulation with autoimmunity [acc.1]

The primary immunodeficiency described below are selected from a list of known PIDs, based on high frequency or obligatory occurrence of autoimmunity, before or during the course of basic immunodeficiency disease [1-11].

2.1. Humoral immunodeficiency

X-linked agammaglobulinaemia (XLA, former name – Bruton's disease) with *Btk* mutation (Bruton's tyrosinae kinase) is typical example of B lymphocyte ontogeny disturbances. The inhibition of maturation between proB and preB cell stage, results in lack of mature B lymphocytes in the periphery. The first symptoms, typically severe bacterial infections, are noted after 4 months of life, when maternal IgG immunoglobulins have been used, without replacement by immunoglobulins produced by immune system of the affected patient. In serum, the level of IgG, IgA and IgM is often below detection; B cells are below 1% of lymphocyte population; T lymphocytes are normal in all aspects – total number, subpopulations' ratio and function. In part of XLA patients, the activation and function of NK cells are impaired. Sometimes, the number of NK cells is very low, due to particular mutation of *Btk*, essential to normal ontogeny of NK cells. In physical examination, the lack of B cell in periphery is seen as small or absent tonsils and lymph nodes. Autoimmunity is very rare in XLA, but in singular patients, rheumatoid arthritis or myositis symptoms were noted [12-15]. Within our group of 10 boys with XLA, the Shulman disease (eosinophilic fasciitis) was diagnosed in a 14-year-old patient [case report in preparation].

Hyper IgM syndrome (HIGM) is the name for a family of 5 different types of this immunodeficiency, with X-linked form as the most severe. This X-linked type of hyper IgM syndrome (HIGM1) is associated with T lymphocytes defect – lack of expression or function of CD40 ligand (*CD40LG*). The other forms of hyper IgM syndrome are results of mutation of genes encoding: CD40 expression on B cells (HIGM3), activation-induced cytidine deaminase (*AICDA*) (HIGM2), uracyl-N-glucosylase (*UNG*) (HIGM5). The signal transduction between T and B lymphocytes are critical for proper response to pathogens, so the disturbances in this function of lymphocytes explain the severe and recurrent bacterial infections in HIGM patients. In laboratory, very low or undetectable levels of IgG, IgA, normal or increased level of IgM, normal number of B and T lymphocytes are found. The other symptoms typical for hyper IgM syndrome include leukopenia, mainly due to severe neutropenia, high sensitivity to infection with *Cryptosporidium parvum* leading to sclerosing cholangitis and liver cirrhosis. In X-linked type of hyper IgM syndrome, HSCT is suggested as curable procedure, especially for patients with neutropenia refractory to G-CSF therapy, patients with cryptosporidiosis and severe bacterial infections, e.g., osteomyelitis [16-19].

Selected IgA deficiency (IgAD) is the most common immunodeficiency of humoral immunity (the mean frequency in Europe is 1/600 people). Diagnosis of IgAD is based on low level (often below detection) of IgA, normal or compensatory high level of IgG, normal level of IgM. IgAD is observed in small children (below 4 years of age), but the stable, definite selected IgA deficiency is diagnosed in children older than 4 years. This time is enough, like in transient hypogammaglobulinemia of infancy (THI), for development of the immune system and correction of immunoglobulin deficiency including IgA. In IgAD, the majority of affected children (70–80%) are asymptomatic. The remaining (20–30%) IgAD patients suffer from recurrent infections, mainly of the respiratory tract. In both subgroups of IgAD patients (with and without symptoms of immunodeficiency), allergic and autoimmune diseases are noted. The respiratory and gastrointestinal tract is involved in majority of patients. Recurrent upper respiratory tract infections caused by different bacteria, often encapsulated, are noted in younger children; prolonged sinusitis is typical for older children, teenagers and adults. The incidence of allergy in IgAD patients is 20 times higher than in healthy population with asthma, allergic rhinitis, conjunctivitis, food allergy, atopic dermatitis and urticaria as typical features [5, 11, 20-23].

The pathogenesis of IgAD is based on the defective terminal maturation of B cells into IgA secreting plasma cells, resulting in reduced levels of serum and secretory (mucosal) IgA (sIgA) [5, 22]. The IgA circulating in serum consists of IgA1 and IgA2 subclasses. Depending on the localisation of IgA production', the monomeric and dimeric forms of IgA (with joining (J)-chain in structure) are noted – monomeric circulating in serum, dimeric seen on surface of mucous membranes of small and large intestine, respiratory and urinary tract. The sIgA is produced by cells present within lymphoid tissue under the mucous membranes (MALT) [22, 24]. sIgA composed of IgA2 molecules characterise high resistance to enzymatic digestion by bacterial proteases. This secretory IgA immunoglobulin plays an important role in protection of mucous membranes from pathogens present within the lumen by agglutinating activity and facilitating the clearance of pathogens in the gastrointestinal, respiratory and urinary tracts [25]. Functions of sIgA include direct neutralization of pathogens, intracellular neutralization of viruses during transepithelial transport and inhibition of receptors-mediated activation of immune system. The role of sIgA in selection of antigens entering through the mucous membrane is also postulated. The lack of sIgA on surface of mucous membranes is compensated by IgG and IgM [22, 25].

Common variable immunodeficiency (CVID) presents variety of symptoms and heterogeneous clinical profiles. CVID has a frequency of 1:25000 to 1:66000 people; however, the delay of diagnosis is serious and estimated as years. Historically, the first description of CVID came from adults with typical clinical symptoms noted in these patients. CVID is diagnosed in adults and children older than 4 years of age (THI) after exclusion of all other known causes of hypogammaglobulinemia. The criteria of CVID include hypogammaglobulinemia in one or more classes of immunoglobulins (IgG only or IgG and IgA, and/or IgM), disturbances of cellular immunity noted in majority of patients. The consequence of disorders in cellular immunity (low number of T lymphocytes, reverse CD4:CD8 ratio, low response to stimulation *in vitro*) and low production of immunoglobulins are poor responses to pathogens and vaccines antigens [6, 8, 21, 25-31]. The hypogammaglobulinemia is a result of deregulation of B-cell differentiation process and disturbances of T-cell regulatory function, including signalling process and function of T-cell receptor. Number of B lymphocytes in peripheral blood and in lymph nodes is usually within normal range, but the disturbances in maturation resulted in decreased number of plasma cells and B memory cells. However, the low number of B cells, even below 1%, is noted in minority of CVID patients (about 10%) [28], suggesting the differential diagnosis of XLA if the patient is a boy with the level of immunoglobulins below detection. The clinical severity of course of CVID (e.g. splenomegaly, bronchiectases, autoimmunity) is associated with the reduction of memory B cells number (CD19+CD27+IgD-) observed in majority of CVID patients. To date, it is the one parameter with predictive value for the clinical course of CVID [32, 33]. The search for genetic background of CVID resulted in description of mutation in TACI gene (transmembrane activator and calcium-modulator) in about 10% of patients. The role of TACI, as member of TNF-like receptor family, is transduction of signals imported for cell survival, apoptosis and isotype switching. The ligands for TACI are BAFF (B-cell activating factor) and APRIL (a proliferation-inducing ligand), both associated with survival of autoreactive B-cell clones and overt autoimmunity. The mechanisms of BAFF and APRIL activity include induction of isotype switching of B cells. The absence of TACI (their receptor) resulted in inhibition of plasma cell maturation and inhibition of immunoglobulin production [34]. Defects like TACI deficiency, BAFF deficiency, APRIL deficiency, loss of inducible co-stimulator and others, led to heterogeneity of clinical features that were observed in CVID patients. This genetic and clinical heterogeneity was the cause of named "variable" this type of humoral deficiency and proposition of CVID subclassifications [5, 11, 35, 36].

The observations of CVID in children showed heterogeneity of clinical symptoms like in adults, but the course of disease is often different. In a large study of 248 CVID patients (children and adults), majority of them (90%) showed severe and recurrent infections, mostly in the respiratory tract [26]. Chronic lung disease developed in a reasonable number (27%) of adult patients. Recurrent infections of lower respiratory tract may lead to the development of bronchiectases. However, the bronchiectases may also be the result of few but severe and prolonged lung infections. In young children, chronic lung disease and bronchiectases are rare. Observations in a group of teenagers suggest that the time of CVID onset and duration are important for the occurrence of these complications. Moreover, in children with CVID, lymphoid interstitial pneumonia (LIP), an unusual and rare type of lung disease, is observed [37]. In our group of 52 children with CVID, the histology of lung biopsy showed LIP in 3 patients (2 boys and a girl). Chronic sinusitis, LIP or bronchiectases develop and progress independently of regular substitution of IgG, even in higher doses [38, 39].

2.2. Cellular immunodeficiency with autoimmunity

Wiskott-Aldrich syndrome (WAS) is an X-linked immunodeficiency and platelets disease caused by mutation of gene WASP (WAS protein) (Table 2). The disease is characterised by microthrombocytopenia (reduced platelets volume); eczema; high susceptibility to bacterial, viral infections; autoimmunity and high frequency of lymphomas (mainly B cell origin) [40-43]. The defects of T lymphocytes include cytoskeletal disorders leading to paucity of surface microvilli, defective polymerisation of actin, defective internalisation of CD3 after cross-linking of T-cell receptor (TCR) resulting in poor response of T cell to stimulation [40, 41]. Typical clinical symptoms of WAS are: thrombocytopenia with poor response to immunoglobulins and/or steroids, infections with severe clinical course and eczema from mild to very severe form, progressing with time. The other WASP gene mutations are associated with thrombocytopenia or agranulocytosis resistant to therapy with steroids or G-CSF. For these clinical syndromes, like for typical X-linked Wiskott-Aldrich syndrome, HSCT is suggested as curative therapy [4, 5, 40, 42, 43].

Autoimmune lymphoproliferative syndrome (ALPS) belongs to a group of diseases associated with immunoregulation and apoptosis disturbances (Table 2). The mutation of genes regulating production of proteins responsible for apoptosis process induced by FAS is the basis of this syndrome. Apoptosis disorders lead to polyclonal proliferation of T lymphocytes, accumulation of these cells in lymph nodes and spleen, and severe autoimmune symptoms. Clinical forms ALPS include: type Ia – mutation of FAS gene (CD95), autosomal dominating type of heredity with typical symptoms and high risk of lymphomas; type Ib – mutation of FAS ligand gene (CD95L), autosomal dominating or recessive heredity, often SLE and other autoimmune diseases; type IIa – mutation of Caspase-10 gene, autosomal dominating showing wide spectrum of autoimmune diseases; type IIb – mutation of Caspase-8 gene, autosomal dominating, in clinic – bacterial and viral infections; type III – mutation of NRAS (neuroblastoma ras viral oncogene homolog) activation gene coding protein binding GTP, autosomal dominating with high risk of leukaemias and lymphomas [4, 5, 44-46]. In the laboratory, increased percentage (and number) of double-negative T lymphocytes (DNT) with phenotype CD3+/CD4-/CD8-, TCR α/β chains and decreased number of T regulatory cells are seen. These DNT T lymphocytes showed high expression of HLA-DR as activation marker, weak response to stimulation, expression of CD45 isoform. It is believed, that the low number of T regulatory cells (Treg) is associated with autoimmune symptoms observed in patients. The B lymphocytes showed low production of specific antibodies to pathogens, but high production of autoantibodies against platelets, neutrophils, erythrocytes, and less frequent, antibodies against cell nuclei, phospholipids and rheumatoid factor. Production of autoantibodies is noted despite lower number of B cells in peripheral blood [44-46]. Clinical manifestation of symptoms and severity of disease course depend on type of ALPS and age of onset. The episodes of acute thrombocytopenia, haemolytic anaemia, splenomegaly (megaspleen) and chronic thrombocytopenia are severe, even life-threatening [44, 45, 47]. Steroids are first-line therapy in ALPS, but, in almost half of patients, the results are transient with progress of lymphadenopathy and splenomegaly. The ALPS patients resistant to steroids are treated with second-line therapy, consisting of infusion of immunoglobulins in high doses (1.0–2.0 g/kg b.w.), mofetil mycophenolate (MMF) and sirolimus. Good response is noted in about 40% of patients; for the remaining, traditional suppression (vincristine, methotrexate, mercaptopurine), rituximab, splenectomy and stem cells transplantation are proposed [44, 45, 48]. Among our 3 infants with ALPS, the resistance to steroid was noted in all; moreover, effect of MMF was partial and short lasting. The best clinical results were obtained with sirolimus, used in children under one year of age. All our patients were transplanted successfully with matched HSC from unrelated donors (in 2 infants) and related donor (father) in one boy. The clinical course and therapy results in these infants with severe symptoms of ALPS are shown in Table 3 [47].

Symptom/patients	D.G. Boy	Z.A. Girl	W.S. Boy
Family history of ALPS Age of	No 20 months	Father – mild form	No
diagnosis Lymphadenopathy	Present	12 days of life	12 months
Splenomegaly	megaspleen	Present	Present
		Present	megaspleen
Autoimmunity:	Severe	Severe	Mild
Thrombocytopenia	Mild	Severe	No
Haemolytic anaemia	Bronchial asthma	No	No
Allergy:			
Therapy:	Transient effect	Resistance	Transient effect
Steroids	Good effect	No effect	Good effect
High dose IVIG	Related	Good effect	Unrelated
Other – sirolimus	Without complications	Unrelated	Loss of chimerism
HSCT:		Loss of chimerism	Second transplant
Donor		Second transplant	
Course of transplant			
Laboratory data:	53 000	67 000	86 000
Platelets (/ul) before and	145 000	159 000	314 000
after sirolimus	2 900	22 100	11 100
Leukocytes (/ul) before	10 500	7 200	5 600
after sirolimus	97	67	73
Hemoglobin (g/l) before	111	96	123
after sirolimus	31	26	22
DNT (CD3+/CD4-/CD8-)	9	8	2
(%) before			
after sirolimus			

Table 3. Infants with ALPS – clinical course and therapy results of our patients [acc.47]

http://dx.doi.org/10.5772/60882

3. Pathogenesis of autoimmunity in humoral immunodeficiency

3.1. Role of autoantibodies

Autoantibodies are produced in the same way, like antibodies to pathogens and vaccine antigens, by B-1 subpopulation of B lymphocytes and plasma cells. The main production is localised in lymph nodes and bone marrow. Autoantigens originate from cells and tissues, so the structure of cell surface (e.g. determinants, receptors present on cell), products of cell (enzymes, hormones, pro-hormones, cytokines and other) and particles released after cell death have become recognised antigens. Autoantibodies against DNA result from circulation of nucleosomes containing DNA. The persistence of small population of self-reacting T and B lymphocytes in thymus and bone marrow in physiology is responsible for physiological presence of autoantibodies at low level. The increased occurrence and increasing amount of autoantibodies with age, suggest the presence of this small population of self-reactive lymphocytes during the entire lives of healthy people [49].

The inducing factor of autoantibodies production is not known to date, so different views are postulated, e.g. chronic inflammation, molecular mimicry with microbial antigens, aberrant expression of HLA-DR on cell surface (facilitating factor for immune response) as triggering signal. However, in diseases like lupus with intracellular autoantigen, this hypothesis is not very suitable. Perhaps the release of cytoplasmic organelles by dying cells and formation of nucleosomes containing pure DNA, induce production of antibodies against them. The antibodies' pattern (e.g. against histones, centromers, centriols, nucleoli, Golgi apparatus, mitochondria, peroxidase, specific proteins: Scl-70, RNP) is typical for particular diseases, but the association between autoantibodies' pattern and clinical features is far from explained [49]. The high level of autoantibodies present in serum is, in general view, associated with damage of target cells, tissues or organs, followed by occurrence of clinical symptoms. The reaction of antibodies with antigen forms immune complexes which circulate in serum and/or produce deposits in capillary vessels, in the tissue expressing the autoantigen. With time, injury of tissue is enough for clinical onset of disease. These immune complexes bind the complement and activate its cascade, stimulating the production of pro-inflammatory cytokines, chemotactic factors for infiltrating cells. This stimulation and hyper activation of immunocompetent cells support the permanent synthesis of autoantibodies and amplification of chronic inflammation (self-perpetuating inflammatory process). The antibodies play important role in the pathomechanism of clinical symptoms in autoimmune diseases, though, not in all of them. Although, the precise role of autoantibodies is unknown, their persistent production suggests the participation in pathomechanism of disease. For example, the anti-transglutaminase antibodies present in celiac disease are associated with reduction of intestinal epithelial cells endocytosis, differentiation and proliferation, which results in decreased function of intestinal/epithelial barrier. In histology of mucous membrane in untreated celiac disease, the epithelium tends to blister or totally detach from the basement membrane, possibly the effect of inhibition of epithelial cells adhesion caused by antibodies [50]. On the other hand, the role of autoantibodies in pathomechanisms of tissue damage in inflammatory bowel diseases (IBD – Leśniowski-Crohn's disease and ulcerative colitis) is not fully described [51-53].

3.2. Production of autoantibodies in immunodeficiency

The serological diagnosis of autoimmune diseases is based on autoantibodies circulating in the serum, as a marker of this process and presence of tissue deposits containing autoantibodies and complement. In CVID, the production of specific antibodies including autoantibodies is low, due to immune system dysfunction. Moreover, in CVID the deficiency of IgA is frequent, so there is lack of antibodies in this immunoglobulin class. The histology of affected tissues, in patients without PIDs, is typical and well known. In this group of patients, as an effect of immunoglobulins and cells deficiency, the histology of affected tissue by autoimmune process is different. B-cell deficiency and disturbances in maturation (e.g. memory cell decrease, low number of plasma cells) are probable causes of different histology of intestine in IBD present in CVID patients [8, 54]. In biopsy of jejunum mucous in celiac or Leśniowski-Crohn's disease in CVID patients, the infiltrates contain T lymphocytes, almost exclusively, with low number of B and plasma cells. To differentiate atypical histological pattern of intestine infiltrates in CVID from typical histology of affected intestine in otherwise healthy patients, the celiac disease and Leśniowski-Crohn's disease are termed "celiac-like, " and "Crohn-like" for CVID patients [8, 55-57].

In IgAD patients with celiac disease, the production of antibodies to gliadin, endomysium and tissue transglutaminase are preserved, but in IgG class. However, in some IgAD patients, the presence and high level of anti-transglutaminase antibodies may be shown in IgA, despite lack of IgA in serum (assayed with nephelometry). In these cases, the trace level of IgA in serum is enough to show antibodies to tissue transglutaminase, but with high sensitivity technique (e.g. ELISA). The histology of jejunum in IgAD patients is typical for celiac disease and similar to observed in children without IgAD. In some IgAD patients, serological diagnosis of celiac disease is suggested by other symptoms then directly associated with digestive tract (e.g. underweight, inhibition of growth, afts, low iron level). Moreover, in these patients, the typical changes of structure of jejunum villi may be absent (Marsh type 0). The time of introduction of restricted gluten-free diet (GFD) is a matter of discussion, depending on clinical symptoms from digestive tract, occurrence or progress of other symptoms, e.g. growth inhibition, loss of weight. It is obvious that in IgAD, plasma cells producing IgA are missing, although, total number of plasma cells is normal within infiltrates in jejunum. The GFD is effective in resolving the clinical symptoms of celiac disease in majority of IgAD patients [25, 55].

In CVID, the serological diagnosis of celiac disease is more difficult and doubtful, due to low production of antibodies both in IgG and IgA due to IgA deficiency in CVID [7-8, 55]. However, the permanent stimulation with autoantigens and antigens (e.g. gliadin) is enough to induce and to support the synthesis of antibodies/autoantibodies, overcoming the impaired function of immune system. The level of autoantibodies in serum is often lower than in patients without immune deficiency [54, 56-58]. In our observations, these antibodies present in low level were clinically significant, so, they should be considered in CVID patients as marker of celiac disease.

3.3. Role of T regulatory cells

The T regulatory subpopulation of T lymphocytes (Treg, CD4+/CD25+/FoxP3+) consists of the natural Treg from thymus and inducible Treg (iTreg), both involved in regulation of autoimmune reaction of immune system. Extensive studies have shown the role of Treg in monitoring the immune response, especially, in control of hyperactivity leading to imbalance of immune response to pathogens and self-perpetuating inflammation process. Treg cells are important for regulation of the activity of mucous membrane associated lymphoid tissue of gastrointestinal and respiratory tracts [59-61]. The population of Treg lymphocytes in peripheral blood is assayed with flow cytometry; Treg lymphocytes localised in the tissue and in inflammatory infiltrates are detected with immunohistochemistry. The immunohistochemistry is a sensitive method commonly used for analysis of the presence, proportion and characteristics of different – not only Treg – cells, within inflammatory focuses in tissues, e.g. macrophages, T and B lymphocytes, plasma cells. The data from many indicated the central role of this T lymphocytes subpopulation in regulation of prolonged inflammatory process within mucous membrane of gastrointestinal and respiratory tracts, joints and other tissues. The analysis of Treg lymphocytes number in Leśniowski-Crohn's disease and ulcerative colitis (UC) showed increased amount of these cells within lamina propria; whereas, the number of Treg in peripheral blood was decreased as compared to healthy people. This study of Treg cells in biopsy of intestine helped to classify the IBD patients into subgroups, based on relations between Treg number within infiltrates, clinical symptoms and course of disease. It will create specific "biological signature, " unique to each patient, leading to individualisation of therapy ("patient tailored") with hope for more rational therapy targeting the specific intestinal inflammatory pathway recognised in this patient [59, 62].

4. Autoimmune haematological syndromes

4.1. Thrombocytopenia acute and chronic

Thrombocytopenia associated with immunodeficiency presents two clinical forms – episodes of acute thrombocytopenia alone or as a part of Evans syndrome, with normal number of platelets in remission, and chronic thrombocytopenia, with number of platelets always below normal level [63-65]. In ALPS and WAS, thrombocytopenia is one of the criteria of a particular immunodeficiency type, so this symptom, in chronic form, is constantly present in all patients. However, the chronic form of thrombocytopenia does not exclude the exacerbations with life-threatening low numbers, or even absence of platelets. Therapy with platelets infusions, high dose of immunoglobulins and other immunosuppressive drugs (e.g. steroids, mycophenolate mofetil, sirolimus, classical drugs, rituximab) is effective; however, in majority of patients, this effect is transient. The severe clinical course of ALPS and progressing symptoms of WAS (with time) are indications for HSCT in these patients [40, 44, 45, 47, 48].

In our group of CVID patients with thrombocytopenia, all these forms (acute, chronic, exacerbations of chronic form) were noted, without relation to time of CVID diagnosis and duration. Moreover, in part of patients, thrombocytopenia was diagnosed prior to CVID onset and established diagnosis. Regular substitution of immunoglobulins in replacing dose (0.4 – 0.6 g/kg b.w. intravenously) is not effective in control of platelets number in exacerbation of chronic thrombocytopenia or prevention of acute thrombocytopenia episodes in CVID. The standard therapy of thrombocytopenia with steroids and high-dose immunoglobulins (1.0 - 2.0 g/kg b.w.) is required. Moreover, this immunoglobulins therapy is successful in majority of CVID patients, despite regular substitution of immunoglobulins in replacing dose. After infusion of immunoglobulins in high dose, the regular substitution is continued, supporting the remission of thrombocytopenia. However, there are still problems in management of thrombocytopenia in CVID – short effect of therapy for acute episodes, necessity of maintenance therapy in remission. Long-lasting remission, with normal number of platelets in CVID patients, is similar to patients without CVID, when good results are obtained with high dose of immunoglobulins and/or steroids therapy. However, in part of CVID patients, acute thrombocytopenia showed tendency to chronicity. In chronic form of thrombocytopenia with number of platelets below 100 000/ul, the regular substitution of immunoglobulins in replacing dose seemed to stabilise platelets number, without need for additional therapy, e.g. steroids or azathioprine. Clinical observations of our CVID patients with chronic thrombocytopenia showed increase of platelets number only for few days after infusion of replacing dose immunoglobulins, followed by low decrease during next 3 weeks, although, the platelets number, in nadir, was still higher than in acute episodes of thrombocytopenia. This stable, safety level of platelets, on regular substitution of immunoglobulins (replacing dose) without additional therapy of thrombocytopenia, allows patients to live normally (Table 4) [66].

Patient number	**1 boy**	**2 boy**	**3 boy**	**4 girl**	**5 boy**	**6 boy**	**7 boy**
Diagnosis: CVID thromboc.	6 years 14 years	8 years 4 years	3 years 6 mths, 4 years 10 mths	12 years, 8 years	10 years 11 years	8 years, 7 years	5 years, 13 years
Main symptoms of CVID	Infections of respiratory tract, lymphadeno-pathy, splenomegaly	Thromboc. spleno-megaly	Severe thromboc. lymphadeno-pathy splenomegaly	Thromboc. leukopenia	Thromboc.	Thromboc.	Pneumonias lymphadeno pathy, splenomegaly
Laboratory data at diagnosis of CVID	Low level of IgG IgA, low number of T cells, reverse D4:CD8 ratio, weak response to vaccines	Low level of IgG, IgA, IgM, low number of T, B and NK cells	Low number of T cells, lack of response T cells to stimulation, low level of IgG	Low level of IgG, IgA and IgM, low number of T, B and NK cells	Low level of IgG	Low level of IgG, IgA,	Low level of IgG, IgM, lack of IgA, leukopenia, weak response to vaccines
Other symptoms	Mild leukopenia	leukopenia	Severe haemolytic anaemia	Severe leukopenia	no	No	Agenesis of kidney, LIP, lung fibrosis (progression), bronchiectases

http://dx.doi.org/10.5772/60882

Patient number	1 boy	2 boy	3 boy	4 girl	5 boy	6 boy	7 boy
Dose (g/kg b.w. /month) and response to IgG	0.43-0.38 good, no infections	0.36 good	0.35 – 0.42 good	0.35 – 0.45 weak (increase of platelets 2-3 days)	0.38 – 0.3 good	0.4 – 0.35 good	0.45 – 0.3 weak (low level of IgG)
Complications of therapy	Adverse reaction to IVIG						Severe osteoporosis, overweight, delay of puberty
Other therapies	Steroids before IVIG						Steroids, azathioprine (lung fibrosis) progress
Present status	SCIG	IVIG	No substitution, hematology care	IVIG, hematology care	No substitution, no symptoms	No substitu-tion no symptoms	SCIG, lungs and kidney insufficiency, splenomegaly
Therapy of thrombocyto-penia	steroids (pulses)	IVIG 1.0g/kg b.w. steroids, azathioprine	steroids, azathioprine, IVIG 1.0 g/kg b.w.	steroids	steroids, IVIG 1.0 g/kg b.w.	steroids	steroids
Complications, other symptom	No	No	Severe haemolytic anaemia (Evans syndrome)	Diabetes, severe overweight	No	No	
Lowest number of platelets (/ul)	28 000	0	0	0	27 000	20 000	37 000
Number of platelets at IVIG beginning	253 000	156 000	133 000	15 000	44 000	87 000	126 000
Mean number of platelets during IVIG (/uL)(range)	149 100 (120 000-196 000)	166 000 (141 000-198 000)	131 000 (97 000-154 000)	51 460 (18 000-68 000)	113 500 (56 000-154 000)	172 400 (99 000-264 000)	112 700 (86 000-133 000)
Number and therapy of thromboc. exacerbations	1 IVIG 1.0 g/kg b.w. steroids		3 (1 severe) Steroids, platelets, erythrocytes and plasma	4 IVIG 1.0 g/kg b.w.	1 (severe) Steroids, splenectomy		

Patient number	1 boy	2 boy	3 boy	4 girl	5 boy	6 boy	7 boy
			transfusions, plasmapheresis IVIG (1.0g/kg b.w.)				
Time of observation	12 years	2 years	7 years	4 years	5 years	4 years	11 years

Table 4. Characteristics and course of CVID in patients with thrombocytopenia (thromboc.) [acc.66]

The regular substitution of immunoglobulins in replacing dose not only supplements specific antibodies, but also stimulates maturation of dendritic cells. This activity of immunoglobulins used in substitution was noted in XLA patients with defective dendritic cells phenotype. Similarly, defective phenotype of dendritic cells was found in CVID patients. The dendritic cells play a critical role in predisposition to pathological conditions, e.g. bacterial infections due to impaired antigen presentation and initiating the immune response, induction of autoimmunity process. Stimulation of dendritic cell maturation might be preventing the development of autoimmunity associated with defective function of these cells in immunodeficiency patients. It is believed, that regular substitution of immunoglobulins, even in replacing dose, restores the normal phenotypes of dendritic cells and their proper function [67].

In CVID patients demonstrating refractory thrombocytopenia, recurrent episodes of exacerbations or chronic thrombocytopenia, second-line therapy with immunosuppressive drugs like azathioprine, vincristine, cyclophosphamide and splenectomy is used [63-65]. Moreover, in CVID patients, refractory thrombocytopenia seemed to be more frequent, followed with higher ratio of indications for splenectomy, than in otherwise healthy children. Splenectomy is effective and safe in CVID patients, without higher risk of severe infections due to immunodeficiency. Moreover, the long-lasting results are similar to patients without immunodeficiency [64]. Another therapeutic option for severe thrombocytopenia in CVID patients with normal number of B cells is monoclonal antibody against CD20 (e.g. rituximab) for elimination of B lymphocytes [68, 69]. For these patients with CVID, the risk for severe infections seemed to be higher and substitution of immunoglobulins in replacing dose should be continued every month, without decreasing the dose and/or pause, e.g. for holidays [11, 63, 64, 69]. Thrombocytopenia in CVID patients is considered as unpredictable autoimmune symptom, so a very careful clinical and laboratory monitoring is required.

4.2. Neutropenia/leukopenia, haemolytic anaemia

Neutropenia is very often associated with hyper IgM syndrome (especially in CD40L – X linked and CD40 deficiency type), leading to severe clinical course of infections, e.g. sinusitis, otitis, osteomyelitis [16, 18, 70]. In some patients, recurrent and persistent ulcers of the mucous membrane, e.g. palate, oral cavity, are noted in episodes of deep neutropenia. The symptomatic therapy is based on antibiotics/sulphonamides in prolonged course, granulocyte colony stimulating factor (G-CSF) and immunoglobulin substitution with good effect, but not in all

http://dx.doi.org/10.5772/60882

patients. For hyper IgM patients with severe clinical course, resistance to therapy and episodes of severe bacterial or fungal infections, HSCT is recommended as curative therapy.

In CVID, leukopenia and/or neutropenia, mainly in mild form, is frequently noted. Within our group of CVID children, leukopenia was observed in few patients, but was persistent and refractory to immunoglobulins substitution and without relation to IgG level. However, due to mild clinical form, additional therapy (e.g. G-CSF for neutropenia) is required in singular cases only [71].

It is noted that haemolytic anaemia presents severe clinical symptoms in patients with CVID, hyper IgM, Wiskott-Aldrich syndrome and ALPS. In ALPS, the clinical course of haemolytic anaemia may be life-threatening due to severity and high frequency of episodes. Moreover, these episodes of severe anaemia cause complications, e.g. high level of iron, hepatosplenomegaly (megaspleen), poor general condition of patients. This severe clinical course of ALPS and resistance to steroids, immunoglobulins and immunosuppression therapy are an indication for HSCT as life-saving procedure [47]. Moreover, for patients with milder course of ALPS, symptomatic therapy with good response and careful monitoring of blood parameter are satisfactory.

5. Involvement of the gastrointestinal tract in primary immunodeficiency

5.1. Celiac disease

Celiac disease diagnosed as latent, silent or atypical form, in children older than infants, comprises about 80% of total number of celiac paediatric patients. The clinical symptoms in atypical form of disease are discrete or unspecific, so the diagnosis is often delayed. Moreover, there have been more than 200 symptoms reported in association with gluten sensitivity, which does not facilitate establishing proper, early diagnosis [72]. Low levels of iron, resistant to oral therapy, vitamins (e.g. vit. D), calcium, zinc and other minerals deficiency are symptoms suggesting jejunum dysfunction (malabsorption), typical for celiac disease in children and teenagers [73]. The clinical symptoms of celiac disease may be unspecific (e.g. underweight, inhibition of growth, afts), delicate and overlapping with symptoms characteristic of immunodeficiency (IgAD, CVID without IgA), like abdomen pain, episodes of diarrhoea, chronic diarrhoea, food allergy [72, 73]. The co-existence of IgAD and celiac disease (frequency of celiac disease within IgAD patients is 10–20 times higher than in healthy children) supported the idea of the common genetic background for these two diseases. The study indicated the ancestral haplotype HLA-A1, Cw7, B8, DR3, DQ2 as important for this association of two diseases. However, the frequency of celiac disease within IgAD population is still lower, than expected, based on common genetic background, so this hypothesis remains without confirmation [73]. The other explanation is based on persistent stimulation of immune system associated with mucous membrane, by gluten and gliadin in absence of IgA, which leads to the damage of jejunum and onset of clinical symptoms. Stimulation of immune system, including B lymphocytes, was represented by increased expression of B lymphocyte stimulator (BLyS) and a proliferation-inducing ligand (APRIL) in patients with IgAD and celiac disease, although, the difference between IgAD patient with and without celiac disease was non-significant. Stimulation of B lymphocytes (increased APRIL level) might be important for compensatory local production of IgG and IgM [74]. The number of T lymphocytes TCR γ/δ infiltrating epithelial cells (IEL) was higher in IgAD patients than in healthy people, but lower than number of IEL TCR γ/δ noted in IgAD with co-existent celiac disease [75].

5.2. Leśniowski-Crohn's disease and ulcerative colitis

Chronic diarrhoea as typical clinical symptom of gastrointestinal involvement is seen in a wide range of adult patients (10–50%) with CVID [8, 27, 55, 76]. In children with CVID and IgAD, chronic diarrhoea is much less frequent, but clinical data are based on relatively small number of patients. In IgAD children, the IBD was noted sporadically, with clinical course similar to children without IgAD. In CVID patients, the IBD remains a significant problem for 19–32% of patients [27]. In adults with Leśniowski-Crohn's disease and CVID, besides typical changes of intestine wall and surface, the formation of granulomas is noted. Furthermore, the substitution of immunoglobulins does not inhibit and/or reverse the symptoms of chronic colitis [77, 78]. A variety of explanations are proposed, but the hypothesis that IgG from immunoglobulin preparations are not able to reach the epithelium of intestine, even intact, seems to be interesting. It might explain higher incidence of small bowel inflammation, with severe and progressing course, especially in patients with CVID without IgA, treated with regular immunoglobulins substitution in replacing dose. The other possible mechanisms explaining the differences in Leśniowski-Crohn's course between CVID patients and healthy people are associated with Treg defects, inflammation supported by activated T lymphocytes, and different list of cytokines produced locally within intestine wall [77]. The role of T lymphocytes is postulated based on different histology of infiltrates within wall of small intestine in CVID. The main difference in proportion between T and B lymphocytes within infiltrates is lack of plasmocytes. The remaining phenomena, e.g. the villi flattening, increased number of IEL and lymphocytes in lamina propria, and increased epithelial apoptosis, were observed in CVID patients similar to patients without CVID [27, 77, 78]. The distinct pathway of inflammation in CVID depends also on cytokine profile, when the production of IL-23, IL-17 and TNF is lower in CVID than in Leśniowski-Crohn's patients without CVID [77].

5.3. Autoimmune hepatitis

The exact aetiology of autoimmune hepatitis, similar to other autoimmune diseases, is unknown, but viral infections, especially hepatotropic, and drugs may be the trigger. In etiopathology, the immunological mechanisms involved the function of Treg cells, IgA defence against gastrointestinal pathogens, including viruses [79, 80]. In adult patients with CVID, autoimmune chronic hepatitis is noted in about 10% [78]. The study of autoimmune paediatric liver disease showed association between IgAD and autoimmune hepatitis type 2 with slower progression to cirrhosis than in hepatitis type 1 [81]. This association might facilitate autoimmune hepatitis in patients with IgAD and CVID with low IgA. In patients with hyper IgM syndrome (mainly X-linked), typical liver involvement is associated with *Cryptosporidium parvum* infection. After gastroenteritis, this pathogen infected the epithelium of bile vessels system. In this immune deficiency, T lymphocytes are enable to destroy the infected cells, which results in persistence of pathogen, chronic inflammation, development of sclerosing cholangitis and chronic hepatitis followed by liver failure [7, 11, 78]. One of our patients with X-linked hyper IgM syndrome showed clinical symptoms of sclerosing cholangitis and progressing liver insufficiency. After successful HSCT from MHC-matched healthy sister, the symptoms of cholangitis and cryptosporidiasis resolved. Now, he is free from immunodeficiency and liver symptoms and living normally [personal communication].

5.4. Other autoimmune diseases in patients with immunodeficiency

In adult patients diagnosed with CVID, the autoimmunity presented a different pattern as compared to children. Rheumatoid arthritis, systemic lupus erythematodes are more frequent than gastrointestinal tract disease; however, the haematologic symptoms are equally frequent in children and adult CVID patients [27, 82]. Rheumatoid arthritis is noted in hyper IgM patients and, what seemed unusual, in X-linked agammaglobulinemia [83, 84]. The explanation of this phenomenon is based on detection of small population of immature B cells in peripheral blood. These B cells are often autoreactive, which suggests that the central and peripheral mechanisms of tolerance have failed [11]. One of our boys with XLA developed eosinophilic fasciitis of right crus, with poor response to immunoglobulins in high dose and non-steroidal anti-inflammatory drugs. Now, the improvement was obtained with steroids in high dose (intravenous pulses), followed with steroids in maintenance dose and MTX in prolonged therapy. However, immunosuppression with MTX was complicated with pneumonia (twice) due to XLA, so MTX was changed to mycophenolate mofetil with good response and hope for fewer side effects and better tolerance by immune system. The partial remission (mild symptoms without pain) obtained with MTX continues and, now, the boy is attending school normally, extra effort being the only limitation.

6. Diagnosis and management of primary immunodeficiency with autoimmunity

6.1. Substitution of immunoglobulins

The main goal of regular substitution of immunoglobulin IgG (intravenous or subcutaneous) in X-linked agammaglobulinemia, hyper IgM syndrome and CVID is supply of the specific antibodies. The immunoglobulins, mainly IgG with trace of IgA witout IgM, are separated and purified from serum of healthy blood donors. The antibodies, important for immunodeficient patients, are active against common pathogens and vaccines antigens, so they are able to prevent infections, but with spectrum of common pathogens. The regular substitution of immunoglobulins should be provided according to standard indications for patients with low but basic levels of IgG in serum. The substitution for XLA, hyper IgM patients, in first moment after diagnosis is individualised depending on clinical state and present infections. For patient without infections, but with IgG level below detection, intravenous substitution (IVIG) should be introduced in higher dose (e.g. 0.75 g/kg b.w.) in 2 weeks period, up to the safety level of

IgG in patient's serum (5.0–5.5 g/l). The standard schedule of IVIG is based on half-life of IgG (21–24 days), so the dose 0.4– 0.6 g/kg b.w. is regularly infused every month. The clinical observations of effects of immunoglobulins substitution showed the 6–8 months period as time required for patient's stabilisation ("steady state"). However, in some CVID patients, obtained IgG level within normal value for age is not enough to prevent recurrent infections. For these patients, the "through level" is used as indication for individualised dose of immunoglobulins substitution [27, 39, 77, 85-87]. The modifications of IVIG includes shorter time between the infusion or higher level in singular infusion, due to bacterial infections, wound healing or other causes leading to overconsumption of immunoglobulins. In XLA without infections, the lower dose (0.2–0.3 g/kg b.w.) in longer period (e.g. 6 weeks) may be used. Moreover, adults with complications like chronic lung disease, chronic sinusitis or gastrointestinal disease may require the individual schedule of substitution ("patient-tailored therapy"). These modifications are based not only on clinical patient status, but on careful, precise monitoring of IgG level [27]. The immunoglobulins offered as substitution should prevent the occurrence of infections, at least, to decrease their frequency, soften the clinical course and improve the response to therapy. Moreover, the regular substitution of IgG in replacing dose, seemed to be effective (stabilising) in chronic thrombocytopenia and chronic neutropenia in some patients with this type of autoimmunity [77]. This effect is probably associated with anti-inflammatory activity of IgG, even in replacing dose, although, the precise mechanisms are not described. One interesting observation showed the activation of monocytes subpopulation in patients with CVID after immunoglobulins infusion in replacing dose [88]. It might be that the regular, long-term continued substitution may lead to accumulation of small, repeated effects of IgG, resembling the anti-inflammatory activity of this immunoglobulin in low replacing dose. The mechanisms responsible for anti-inflammatory activity of IgG preparations used in high dose of immunoglobulins (1.0–2.0 g/kg b.w.) for autoimmune diseases therapy (e.g. acute thrombocytopenia, Kawasaki disease, Guillain-Barre syndrome, myasthenia crisis) are well defined and mainly based on regulatory activity [27, 86, 89].

The adverse reactions of IVIG may occur immediately, during the infusion or after, up to 4 days. The symptoms of adverse reactions are mild or severe, including anaphylactic shock as most severe reaction, occurring often very quickly, after few drops of immunglobulins' solution. Fever, chills, pain (headache, abdominal pain) and cough are noted in children as mild symptoms resolved with appropriate symptomatic therapy. The late, severe reactions are the consequence of immunoglobulins distribution into tissues, especially into central nervous system. Severe and progressive headache, vomiting, disturbances of vision, speech and balance are neurological symptoms typical for this reaction. Intensive hydration (decrease of IgG level, filling the vessels) and steroids (anti-oedematic activity) given intravenously are effective as therapy [77, 90, 91]. In case of severe adverse reactions, the subcutaneous way of immunoglobulins substitution (SCIG) is recommended. The amount of immunoglobulins given monthly is divided in four portions (0.1– 0.2 g/kg b.w. per week), administered with special pump in children or with syringe only ("rapid push") in adults. The effectiveness of SCIG is similar to IVIG, but the adverse reactions are very rare and limited to the place of injection. SCIG is a form of home therapy, very comfortable for patients, offering independence from hospital. In XLA, CVID diagnosed in adults, hyper IgM syndrome, the regular substitu-

http://dx.doi.org/10.5772/60882

tion of immunoglobulins is for life, so the SCIG form of immunoglobulins substitution is preferred for these patients avoiding the pain associated with poor vein access after years of IVIG. The exception from indication for "substitution for life" is patients with X-linked hyper IgM syndrome treated with HSCT [92-94]. In children with CVID, the developing immune system gives the opportunity to hang off the substitution after reaching the stable, normal level of IgG, low frequency of infections with good response to therapy, resembling the immune system maturation.

6.2. Symptomatic therapy and prophylaxis of infections

In part of children with CVID, the effect of regular immunoglobulins substitution (IVIG or SCIG) is weak and infections, mainly in respiratory tract, are still present. With time, in some of these patients, the lymphocytic interstitial pneumonia (LIP, or GLILD – granulomatous lymphocytic insterstitial lung disease), chronic sinusitis and bronchiectases develop, progressing lung fibrosis and persistent leukopenia (neutropenia) are noted, so prophylaxis with antibiotics is recommended. The 3–4 months' period of antibiotics or time-to-prime in prophylactic dose is commonly used as effective schedule of supportive therapy, improving clinical status of patients. However, the therapy with antibiotics is still a matter of discussion and different approaches to this therapy are suggested depending on clinical centre and severity of patients' symptoms. The specific and unique recommendation for antibiotics prophylaxis is aimed at prevention of endocarditis following invasive procedures in immunodeficient patients [39]. In our clinical management of more than 200 immunodeficient patients, such complication was not observed, but because of the severity of this symptom, prophylaxis should be considered.

6.3. Monitoring and therapy of co-existent autoimmunity

Therapy of common autoimmune diseases, e.g. thrombocytopenia, neutropenia, haemolytic anaemia, in patients with immunodeficiency is based on standard therapy of such symptoms; the use of immunoglobulins in high dose, steroids, immunosuppression with methrotrexate, vincristine, azatioprine, but special therapy is required for some of immunodeficient patients. In ALPS, the use of sirolimus is suggested, as possibility to induce apoptosis, helping in elimination of double-negative T lymphocytes. Sirolimus is preferentially used in these patients for resolving symptoms (e.g. lymphadenopathy, splenomegaly) and diminish the severity of clinical course. The expected effect of sirolimus is to diminish the spleen volume (megaspleen), one of most danger symptom in children with ALPS [44-47].

The therapeutic approach to immunodeficient patients with Leśniowski-Crohn's disease is generally similar to therapy of patients without immunodeficiency; although, inflammation process in CVID might be resistant to therapy. In these patients, the process of intestine inflammation is active despite immunosuppression (e.g. azathioprine, cyclosporine) used as second line of therapy, after systemic steroids, budesonite and anti- inflammatory non-steroidal drugs without remission. Therapy with the monoclonal antibodies against TNF (infliximab, etanercept) is effective in inductions the remission in patients with immunodeficiency, similar to patients without immunodeficiency. However, CVID patients are more prone to infections during such therapy, so very careful monitoring of this group of patients is recommended, not only for bacterial, but fungal and viral infections, due to defects of T lymphocyte function [8].

The frequency of UC in CVID and IgAD patients is not known, but it seems that in children it is even less frequent than in adult CVID and IgAD patients. In a large group of CVID patients (248 children and adults), UC was noted in 7 patients; however, the unspecific significant malabsorption symptoms were observed in other10 patients [26]. It shows the problem of overlapping symptoms, difficulties in establishing the precise diagnosis and requirement for wide differential diagnostic procedures performed in these patients [26].

7. Progress in therapy of autoimmunity

7.1. Indications for monoclonal antibodies

Monoclonal antibodies are used for elimination of target cell population, cytokine or blocking of determinants on cell surface. Humoral immune deficiency is based on B-cell intrinsic deficiency and disturbances of B-cell ontogeny. Autoimmunity in patients with very low number of B lymphocytes is associated with relatively high number of autoreactive B cells within this small B-cell population. Following this hypothesis of autoimmunity in humoral immunodeficiency, the therapy with monoclonal antibodies against B lymphocytes seems to be logical and reasonable. Use of rituximab (monoclonal antibody against CD20 determinant restricted to mature B lymphocytes) in autoimmune cytopenias in CVID, ALPS and hyper IgM syndrome (as alternative to HSCT) was successful [19, 44, 45, 95].

The therapy of autoimmune diseases characterised by chronic inflammatory process (SLE, rheumatoid arthritis, IBD) with important role of cytokines and T lymphocytes includes monoclonal antibodies against cytokines (TNF), IL-2 receptor on T lymphocytes (CD25 as activation marker) and others. Within CVID patients, celiac disease is often refractory to GFD (RCD), leading to malabsorption syndrome and severe clinical conditions [11, 27, 96, 97], which suggests different mechanism present in these patients. Careful observation and studies showed different forms: type I with T lymphocytes with normal phenotype (expression of CD3 and CD8 determinants, normal polyclonal T-cell receptor (TCR) arrangement) and type II with aberrant T lymphocyte phenotype, intracellular presence of CD3, monoclonal TCR rearrangement [8, 96, 98]. Type II of progressing celiac disease in spite of GFD and some cases of Crohn-like disease are associated with poor prognosis with increased mortality, due to progressing malabsorption syndrome and T-cell lymphoma in reasonable number of such patients [77, 96]. After standard therapy without effect, the second-line therapy with immunosuppression (azathioprine) and/or monoclonal antibodies against TNF (infliximab, etanercept, humira) is required for patients with active, progressive disease [99].

7.2. Suppressive therapy

The first line of immunosuppressive therapy in patients with or without immune deficiency includes steroids, in individual doses, for all autoimmune symptoms and diseases. For cytopenias, especially thrombocytopenia, the schedule with high doses of steroids given intravenously every month ("pulses") is often used to increase the number of platelets. Chronic thrombocytopenia is controlled with maintenance dose of steroids, but the side effects of steroids are the main limitation for this therapy. The second-line therapy includes typical immunosuppressants, e.g. azathioprine, metotrexate, vincristine, cyclophophamide, cyclosporine A. In ALPS, sirolimus and mycophenolate mofetil are suggested, with good clinical response in majority of patients. Moreover, this therapy is well tolerated, without severe side effects, even in infants and babies with ALPS. Regular substitution of immunoglobulins (recommended in intravenous form) is important to diminish the risk of infections associated with prolonged immunosuppression [7, 77, 78, 95].

7.3. Indications for haematopoietic stem cells transplantation (HSCT)

Historically, the first group of patients who underwent HSCT as a life-saving and curative therapy were newborn babies diagnosed with SCID. The following group of patients transplanted with HSCT were children with X-linked immunodeficiency, e.g. hyper IgM syndrome, WAS, chronic granulomatous diseases (CGD) [100-104]. The increasing number of children cured from SCID, improvement of transplantation procedure (low risk factor) and post-transplant care, is encouraging transplantologists and immunologists to offer this therapy for patients with other types of primary immunodeficiency. Now, patients with ALPS, X-linked lymphoproliferative diseases, haemophagocytic lymphohistiocytosis are transplanted in increasing numbers [102]. Successful HSCT in SCID patients, after matched donor transplant, in Europe is 90% survival; non-SCID immunodeficiency patients – about 80%, which means real, great progress in treatment of patients with severe clinical forms of immunodeficiency [101].

The hyper IgM syndrome, ALPS, Wiskott-Aldrich syndrome may represent mild clinical course with satisfactory symptomatic therapy, so HSCT is not a first-line therapy. The indications for HSCT in these patients are based on severe clinical course, progress of symptoms associated with immunodeficiency leading to poor prognosis for life [47, 100-104]. The symptomatic therapy in these syndromes include steroids for severe autoimmunity symptoms, regular substitution of immunoglobulins, antibiotics and antimycotic drugs as prophylaxis, and treatment for existent bacterial, fungal and viral infections. This therapy is necessary up to the time of HSCT, as good clinical state of patient decreases the risk of complications after HSCT. The CVID with typical clinical course is not an indication for HSCT, due to satisfactory effects of symptomatic therapy, much more save, than HSCT. However, in individual cases with progressing, severe complications, like RCD, IBD, leading to malnutrition, this procedure is recommended [97]. Within our CVID children, HSCT was performed with success in girl with severe malnutrition due to malabsorption in celiac disease resistant to GFD. She was treated for few years with restricted GFD, antibiotics, steroids, anti-TNF monoclonal antibodies, immunosuppression (cyclosporin A) without effect, so HSCT was the life-saving procedure. HSCT was performed in our 3 patients (children below age of 3 years) with severe course of ALPS, when therapy with steroids, immunoglobulins, mycophenolate mofetil and sirolimus was without long-lasting remission and progression of the autoimmune symptoms [47].

8. Other problems

8.1. Granulomatous and lymphocytic interstitial lung disease (GLILD) – autoimmunity or not

GLILD (former name – lymphoid interstitial pneumonia) is a rare clinical entity with unknown aetiology and pathophysiology. The diffuse infiltration of lymphoid cells localised mainly in the interstitial tissue is a typical histopathological feature. LIP is typically associated with autoimmunity, e.g. Sjogren syndrome, autoimmune thyroid disease, SLE, but also with immunodeficiency, mainly CVID and AIDS [105, 106]. LIP is noted in about 10% of CVID patients, which could indicate the association between these clinical features. This type of interstitial pneumonia is an independent factor of poor prognosis with negative impact on the survival of patients due to lung fibrosis, followed by recurrent episodes of pneumonia with infiltrations. Clinical symptoms of GLILD overlap with chronic bronchitis or bronchiectases, signalled by prolonged cough. Moreover, the regular substitution of immunoglobulins, in replacing dose, is not effective in prevention and resolving of these lung symptoms. Therapy included prolonged steroids and/or immunosuppression (azathioprine, cyclophosphamide) in individual combination, depending on patient immune system and clinical symptoms. Prolonged therapy with steroid or immunosuppression is difficult in CVID patients, due to increased risk of infections, potentiating of leukopenia/neutropenia and thrombocytopenia. Among our patients with CVID, treated with regular substitution of immunoglobulins, LIP was noted in 3 children. The clinical course of CVID was severe due to RCD in girl (later on transplanted with HSCT), leukopenia (neutropenia) and thrombocytopenia in both boys. Moreover, one of these boys diagnosed with LIP, demonstrated hepatomegaly, splenomegaly and lymphadenopahty localised in lungs hilus and in mesenterium. Therapy of LIP included, in first line, only steroids, followed by azathioprine (because of severe adverse reaction after steroids and lack of effect), with good results in second boy. The resolving of LIP symptoms was slow, taking 2–3 years of immunosuppressive therapy and regular substitution of immunoglobulins in 0.5g/kg b.w. The frequency of infections during this therapy was not higher, but the course of the few infections that occurred was prolonged, requiring antibiotic therapy.

9. Conclusions and general remarks

Autoimmune diseases are a large group of heterogeneous diseases characterised by an unpredictable course with variable response to immunosuppressive therapy, from very good (long-lasting remission), to poor with progression of severe and life-threatening symptoms. Autoimmune diseases in immunodeficiency syndromes can develop prior or after the onset of immunodeficiency, during the regular substitution of immunoglobulins.

The management of patients with autoimmunity associated with immunodeficiency is more difficult than patients without immunodeficiency due to various reasons: the production of autoantibodies, the generally used marker of autoimmunity, is weaker in immunodeficiency;

the clinical symptoms may overlap with basic symptoms of immunodeficiency; the response to therapy is often poorer than in patients without immunodeficiency. The level of autoantibodies, below limit of positive results, due to immunodeficiency, should be considered as significant for diagnosis of autoimmune disease in PID. The interpretation of laboratory results in these patients need very careful and different attitude than usual. The resistance to therapy, severe, and progressing symptoms of autoimmunity, as complication of immunodeficiency (e.g. CVID, ALPS) are the indications for HSCT as life-saving procedure.

Acknowledgements

I would like to thank our immunologists' team (Prof. Danuta Kowalczyk, Prof Maciej Siedlar, Dr Anna Szaflarska, Dr Anita Błaut-Szlósarczyk, Dr Katarzyna Zwonarz) for taking care of our patients with primary immunodeficiencies and transplantologists' team (Prof. Assist, Jolanta Goździk, Prof Assist. Szymon Skoczeń, Dr. Aleksandra Krasowska-Kwiecień, Dr Agnieszka Dłużniewska) for closed cooperation and help in saving our patients' life with HSCT procedure.

Author details

Anna Pituch-Noworolska

Address all correspondence to: mipituch@cyf-kr.edu.pl

Department of Clinical Immunology, Polish-American Institute of Pediatrics, Jagiellonian University, Medical College, Kraków, Poland

References

[1] Al-Herz W, Bousfiha A, Casanova J-L, Chapel H, Conley ME, Cunningham-Rundles Ch, Etzioni A, Fischer A, Franco JL, Geha RS, Hammarstrom L, Nonoyama S, Notaranghelo LD, Ochs HD, Puck JM, Roifman ChM, Seger R, Tang MLK (2011) Primary immunodeficiency diseases: an update on the classification from the International Union of Immunological Societies Expert Committee for primary immunodeficiency. *Front Immunol.* 2; art. 54.

[2] Bousfiha AA, Jeddane L, Ailal F, Al Herz W, Conley ME, Cunnigham-Rundles Ch, Etzioni A, Fischer A, Franco JL, Geha RS, Hammastrom L, Nonoyama S, Ochs HD, Roifman ChM, Seger R, Tang MLK, Puck JM, Chapel H, Notarangelo LD, Casanova J-L (2013) A phenotypic approach for IUIS PID classification and diagnosis: guidelines for clinicians of the bedside. *J Clin Immunol.* 33; 1078-1087.

[3] Chinen J, Notarangelo LD, Shearer WT (2013) Advances in basic and clinical immunology in 2012. *J Allergy Clin Immunol.* 131; 675-682.

[4] Coutinho A, Carneiro-Sampaio M (2008) Primary immunodeficiencies unravel critical aspects of the pathophysiology of autoimmunity and of the genetic in autoimmune disease. *J Clin Immunol.* 28; suppl.1, S4-S10.

[5] Notarangelo LD, Fischer A, Geha RS, Casanova J-L, Chapel H, Conley ME, Cunningham-Rundles Ch, Eztioni A, Hammarstrom L, Nonoyama S, Ochs HD, Puck J, Roifman Ch, Seger R, Wedgwood J (2009) Primary immunodeficiencies: 2009 update.*J Allergy Clin Immunol* 124; 1161-1678.

[6] de Vries E, Driessen G (2011) Primary immunodeficiencies in children: a diagnostic challenge. *Eur J Pediatr* 170; 169-177.

[7] Arkwright PD, Abinun M, Cant AJ (2002) Autoimmunity in human primary immunodeficiency diseases. *Blood.* 99; 2694-2702.

[8] Agarwal S, Cunningham-Rundles C (2009) Autoimmunity in common variable immunodeficiency. *Curr Allergy Asthma Rep.* 9; 347-352.

[9] Oksenhendler E, Gerard L, Fieschi C, Malphettes M, Moulliot G, Jaussaud R, Viallard J-F, Gardembas M, Galicier L, Schleinitz N, Suarez F, Soulas-Sprauel P, Hachulla E, Jaccard A, Gardeur A, Theodorou I, Rabian C, Debre P (2008) Infections in 252 patients with common variable immunodeficiency. *Clin Infect Dis.* 46; 1547-1554.

[10] Arason GJ, Jorgensen GH, Ludviksson BR (2010) Primary immunodeficiency and autoimmunity. *Scand J Immunol.* 71; 317-328.

[11] Cunningham-Rundles Ch (2011) Autoimmunity in primary immune deficiency: taking lessons from our patients. *Clin Exp Immunol.* 164: 6-11.

[12] Schroeder HW, Szymańska-Mroczek E (2013) Primary antibody deficiencies. In: *Fourth Edition Clinical Immunology.* Eds: Rich RR, Fleicher TA, Shearer WT, Schroeder HW, Frew AJ, Weyand CM. Elsevier. pp. 421-436.

[13] Bao Y, Zheng J, Han Ch, Jin J, Han H, Liu Y, Lau Y-L, Tu W, Cao X (2012) Tyrosine kinase btk is required for NK cells activation. *J Biol Chem.* 287; 23769-23778.

[14] Pituch-Noworolska A, Zwonarz K, Błaut-Szlósarczyk A, Szaflarska A, Kowalczyk D, Siedlar M (2013) T lymphocytes and NK cells in X-linked agammaglobulinemia. *Przegl Lek* 70; 1048-1050.

[15] Ochs HD, Smith C (1996) X-linked agammaglobulinemia. *Medicine (Baltimore)* 75; 287-299.

[16] Notarangelo LD, Hayward AR (2000) X-linked immunodeficiency with hyper IgM (XHIM). *Clin Exp Immunol.* 120; 399-405.

[17] Pituch-Noworolska A, Kowalczyk D, Macura-Biegun A, Szaflarska A (2007) The clinical features of hyper-IgM syndrome. *Centr Eur J Immunol.* 32; 105-112.

[18] Davies EG, Thrasher AJ (2010) Update on the hyper immunoglobulin M syndrome. *Brit J Haematol.* 49; 167-180.

[19] Hennig Ch, Happle Ch, Hansen G (2011) "A bad wound may heal, but a bad name can kill" – lessons learned from "hyper IgM syndrome". *J Allergy Clin Immunol.* 128; 1380-1382.

[20] Aghamohammadi A, Cheragi T, Gharagozlou M, Movahedi M, Rezaei N, Yeganeh M, Parvaneh N, Abolhassani H, Pourpak Z, Moin M (2009) IgA deficiency: correlation between clinical and immunological phenotypes. *J Clin Immunol.* 29; 130-136.

[21] Fried AJ, Bonilla FA (2009) Pathogenesis, diagnosis, and management of primary antibody deficiencies and infections. *Clin Microbiol Rev.* 22; 396-414.

[22] Yel L (2010) Selective IgA deficiency. *J Clin Immunol.* 30; 10-16

[23] Notarangelo LD (2009) Primary immunodeficiencies (PIDs) presenting with cytopenias. *Hematology Am Soc Hematol Educ Program.* 139-144.

[24] Vale AM, Schroeder HW (2010) Clinical consequences of defects in B-cell development. *J Allergy Clin Immunol.* 125; 78-787.

[25] Jacob CMA, Pastorino AC, Fahl K, Carneiro-Sampaio M, Monteiro RC (2008) Autoimmunity in IgA deficiency. *J Clin Immunol.* 28; S56-S61.

[26] Cunningham-Rundles Ch, Bodian C (1999) Common variable immunodeficiency. *Clin Immunol.* 92; 34-48.

[27] Cunningham-Rundles Ch (2010) How I treat common variable immune deficiency. *Blood.* 116; 7-15.

[28] Chapel H, Cunningham-Rundles Ch (2009) Update in understanding common variable immunodeficiency disorders (CVIDs) and the management of patients with these conditions. *Brit J Haematol.* 145; 709-727.

[29] Glocker E, Ehl S, Grimbacher B (2007) Common variable immunodeficiency in children. *Curr Opin Pediatr.* 19; 685-692.

[30] Llobet MP, Soler-Palacin P, Detkova D, Hernandez M, Caragol I, Espanol T (2009) Common variable immunodeficiency: 20-years experience at a single centre. *Pediatr Allergy Immunol.* 20; 113-118.

[31] Urschel S, Kaykci L, Wintergerst U, Nothes G, Jansson A, Belochradsky BH (2009) Common variable immunodeficiency disorders in children: delayed diagnosis despite typical clinical presentation. *J Pediatr.* 154; 888-894.

[32] Alachkar H, Taubenheim N, Haenay MR, Dyrandy A, Arkwright PD (2006) Memory switched B cell percentage and not serum immunoglobulin concentration is associat-

ed with clinical complications in children and adults with specific antibody deficiency and common variable immunodeficiency. *Clin Immunol.* 120; 310-318.

[33] Huck K, Feyen O, Ghost S, Beltz K, Bellert S, Niehues T (2009) Memory B-cells in healthy and antibody deficient children. *Clin Immunol.* 131; 50-59.

[34] Notarangelo LD (2010) Primary immunodeficiencies. *J Allergy Clin Immunol.* 125, S182-S194.

[35] Wehr C, Kivioja T, Schmitt Ch, Ferry B, Witte T, Eren E, Vlkova M, Hernandez M, Detkova D, Bos PR, Poerksen G, von Bernuth H, Baumann U, Goldacker S, Gutenberger S, Schlesier M, Bergeron-van der Cruyssen F, Le Garff M, Debre P, Jacobs R, Jones J, Bateman E, Litzman J, van Hagen PM, Plebani A, Schmidt RE, Thon V, Quinti I, Espanol T, Webster AD, Chapel H, Vihinen M, Oksenhendler E, Peter HH, Warnatz K (2008) The EUROclass trial: defining subgroups in common variable immunodeficiency. *Blood.* 111; 77-85.

[36] Warnatz K, Voll RE (2012) Pathogenesis of autoimmunity in common variable immunodeficiency. *Front Immunol.* 3; art. 210.

[37] Chase NM, Verbsky JW, Hintermeyer MK, Waukau AT, Casper JT, Singh S, Shahir KS, Tisol WB, Nugent ML, Rao NR (2013) Use of combinations chemotherapy for treatment of granulomatous and lymphocytic interstitial lung disease (GLILD) in patients with common variable immunodeficiency. *J Clin Immunol.* 33; 30-39.

[38] Gathmann B, Mahlaoui N, Gerard L, Oksenhendler E, Warnatz Kschulze I, Kindle G, Kuijpers TW, van Beem RT, Guzman D, Workman S, Soler-Palacin P, De Gracia J, Witte T, Schmidt RE, Lizman J, Hlavackova E, Thon V, Borte M, Borte S, Kumararatne D, Feighery C, Longhurst H, Helbert M, Szaflarska A, Sediva A, Belohradsky BH, Jones A, Baumann U, Meyts I Kutukculer N, Wagstrom P, Galal NM, Roesler J, Farmaki E, Zinovieva N, Ciznar P, Papadopoulou-Alataki E, Bienemann K, Velbri S, Pnahloo Z, Grimbacher B for the European Society for Immunodeficiencies Registry Working Party (2014): Clinical picture and treatment of 2212 patients with common variable immunodeficiency. *J Allergy Clin Immunol.* 133: 1-11.

[39] Bethune CA, Spickett GP (2000) Common variable immunodeficiency. *BioDrug.* 13; 243-253.

[40] Catucci M, Castiello MC, Pala F, Bosticardo M, Villa A (2012) Autoimmunity in Wiskott-Aldrich syndrome. *Front Immunol.* 3; art. 209.

[41] Park JY, Kob M, Prodeus AP, Rosen FS, Shcherbina A, Remold-O'Donnell E (2004) Early deficit of lymphocytes in Wiskott-Aldrich syndrome: possible role of WASP in human lymphocytes maturation. *Clin Exp Immunol.*136; 104-110.

[42] Ochs HD (1998) The Wiskott-Aldrich syndrome. *Semin Hematol.* 35; 332-345.

[43] Albert MH, Notarangelo LD, Ochs HD (2011) Clinical spectrum, pathophysiology and treatment of the Wiskott-Aldrich syndrome. *Curr Opin Hematol.* 18; 42-48

[44] Rao VK, Oliveira JB (2011) How I treat autoimmune lymphoproliferative syndrome. *Blood*. 118; 5741-5751

[45] Teachey DT, Seif AE, Grupp SA (2009) Advances in management and understanding of autoimmune lymphoproliferative syndrome (ALPS). *Brit J Haematol*. 148; 205-216.

[46] Kwon S-W, Procter J, Dale JK, Strus SE, Stroncek DF (2003) Neutrophil and platelets antibodies in autoimmune lymphoproliferative syndrome. *Vox Sanguinis*. 85; 307-312.

[47] Szaflarska A, Pituch-Noworolska A, Błaut-Szlósarczyk A, Zwonarz K (2013) Autoimmune lymphoproliferative syndrome (ALPS) in infants – indications and effects of sirolimus therapy. First International Primary Immunodeficiency Congress, 7-8.11.2013 Estoril, Portugal.

[48] Rieux-Laucat F, Blanchere S, Danielan S, de Villartay JP, Oleastro M, Solary E, Bader-Maunier B, Arkwright P, Pondare C, Bernaudin F, Chapel H, Nielsen S, Berrah M, Fischer A, le Diest F (1999) Lymphoproliferative syndrome with autoimmunity. *Blood*. 94; 2575-2582.

[49] Elkon K, Casali P (2008) Nature and function of autoantibodies. *Nat Clin Pract Rheumatol*. 4; 491-498.

[50] Lindfors K, Kaukinen K (2012) Contribution of celiac disease autoantibodies to the disease process. *Expert Rev Clin Immunol*. 8; 151-154.

[51] Ardesjo B, Portela-Gomez GM, Rorsman F, Gerdin E, Loof L, Grimelius L, Kampe O, Ekwall O (2008) Immunoreactivity against goblet cells in patients with inflammatory bowel disease. *Inflamm Bowel Dis*. 14; 652-661.

[52] Bogdanos DP, Rigopoulou EI, Smyk DS, Roggenbuck D, Reinhold D, Forbes A, Laass MW, Conrad C (2011) Diagnostic value, clinical utility and pathogenic significance of reactivity to the molecular targets of Crohn's disease specific-pancreatic autoantibodies. *Autoimmun Rev*. 11; 143-148.

[53] Papp M, Norman GL, Altorjay I, Lakatos PL (2007) Utility of serological markers in inflammatory bowel diseases: gadget or magic? *World J Gastroenterol*. 14; 2028-2036.

[54] Malamat G, Verkarre V, Suarez F, Viallard J-F, Lascaux A-S, Cosnes J, Bouhnik Y, Lambotte O, Bechade D, Ziol M, Lavergne A, Hermine O, Cerf-Bensussan N, Cellier C 0(2010) The enteropathy associated with common variable immunodeficiency. *Am J Gastroenterol*. 105; 2262-2275.

[55] Agarval S, Smereka P, Harpaz N, Cunnigham-Rundles Ch, Mayer L (2011) Characterization of immunologic defects in patients with common variable immunodeficiency (CVID) with intestinal disease. *Inflamm Bowel Dis*. 17; 251-259.

[56] Pituch-Noworolska A, Zwonarz K (2012) Celiac and inflammatory bowel diseases in children with primary immunodeficiency. In: *Autoimmune Disease*. Ed. Chan J, InTech, chapter 7, pp. 151-172.

[57] Al-Muhsen SZ (2010) Gastrointestinal and hepatic manifestations of primary immune deficiency diseases. *Saudi J Gastroenterol*. 16; 66-74.

[58] Walker MM, Murray JA (2011) An update in the diagnosis of celiac disease. *Histopathology*. 59; 166-179.

[59] Schirbel A, Fiocchi C (2010) Inflammatory bowel disease: established and evolving considerations on its etiopathogenesis and therapy. *J Digest Dis*. 11; 266-276.

[60] Glocker E, Grimbacher B (2012) Inflammatory bowel disease. *Cell Mol Life Sci*. 69; 41-48.

[61] Genre J, Errante PR, Kokron CM, Toledo-Barros M, Camara NOS, Rizzo LV (2009) Reduced frequency of CD4+CD25highFoxP3+ cells and diminished FoxP3 expression in patients with common variable immunodeficiency: a link to autoimmunity? *Clin Immunol*. 132; 215-221.

[62] Kaser A, Zeissig S, Blumberg RS (2010) Inflammatory bowel disease. *Ann Rev Immunol*. 28; 573-621.

[63] Wang J, Cunningham-Rundles C (2005) Treatment and outcome of autoimmune hematologic disease in common variable immunodeficiency (CVID). *J Autoimmun*. 25: 57-62.

[64] Michel M, Chanet V, Galicier L, Ruivard M, Levy Y, Hermine O, Oksenhendler E, Schaeffer A, Bierling P, Godeau B (2004) Autoimmune thrombocytopenic purpura and common variable immunodeficiency. *Medicine*. 83: 254-263.

[65] Cunningham-Rundles Ch (2002) Hematologic complications of primary immune deficiencies. *Blood Rev*. 16; 61-64.

[66] Pituch-Noworolska A, Siedlar M, Kowalczyk D, Szaflarska A, Błaut-Szlósarczyk A, Zwonarz K (2014) The effect of immunoglobulins substitution in common variable immunodeficiency (CVID) with chronic thrombocytopenia. Congress of Polish Society of Clinical and Experimental Immunology, 24-26 June, Wrocław, Poland.

[67] Kaveri SV, Maddur MS, Hadge P, Lacroix-Desmazes S, Bayry J (2011) Intravenous immunoglobulins in immunodeficiencies: more than mere replacement therapy. *Clin Exp Immunol*. 164: 2-5.

[68] Al-Ahmad M, Al-Rasheed M, Al-Muhadi A (2010) Successful use of rituximab in refractory idiopathic thrombocytopenic purpura in a patient with common variable immunodeficiency. *J Investig Allergol Clin Immunol*. 20: 259-262,

[69] Gobert D, Busel JB, Cunningham-Rundles C, Galicier L, Dechartes A, Berezne A, Bonnotte B, DeRevel T, Auzary C, Jaussaud R, Larroche C, LeQuellec A, Ruivard M, Seve P, Smail A, Viallard J-F, Godeau B, Hermine O, Mechel M (2011) Efficacy and safety of rituximab in common variable immunodeficiency-associated cytopenias: a retrospective multicentre study of 33 patients. *Brit J Haematol*. 155: 498-508.

[70] Pituch-Noworolska A (2014) The effect of immunoglobulins substitution in hyper IgM syndrome. 7th International Immunoglobulins Conference 4-5 Apr, Interlaken, Switzerland.

[71] Sokolic R (2013) Neutropenia in primary immunodeficiency. *Curr Opin Hematol.* 20; 55-65

[72] Nejad AR, Rostami K, Pourhoseingholi MA, Mojarad EN, Habibi M, Dabiri H, Zali Mr (2009) Atypical presentation is dominant and typical for celiac disease. *J Gastrointestin Liver Dis.* 18; 285-291.

[73] Valletta E, Fornaro M, Pecori S, Zanoni G (2011) Selective immunoglobulin A deficiency and celiac disease. *J Invest Allergol Clin Immunol.* 21; 242-244.

[74] Fabris M, De Vita S, Visentini D, Fabro C, Picierno A, Lerussi A, Villalta D, Alessio MG, Tampoia MA, Tonutti E (2009) B-lymphocyte stimulator and a proliferation-inducting ligand serum levels in IgA-deficient patients with and without celiac disease. *Ann NY Acad Sci.* 1173; 268-273.

[75] Borrelli M, Maglio M, Agnese M, Paparo F, Gentile S, Colicchio B, Tosco A, Auricchio R, Troncone R (2009) High density of intraepithelial TCR γ/δ lymphocytes and deposits of immunoglobulin (Ig)M anti tissue transglutaminase antibodies in the jejunum of celiac patients with IgA deficiency. *Clin Exp Immunol.* 160; 199-206.

[76] Daniels JA, Lederman HM, Maitra A, Montgomery EA (2007) Gastrointestinal tract pathology in patients with common variable immunodeficiency (CVID). *Am J Surg Pathol.* 31; 1800-1812.

[77] Agarwal S, Mayer L (2013) Diagnosis and treatment of gastrointestinal disorders in patients with primary immunodeficiency. *Clin Gastroenterol Hepatol.* 3; 1050-1063.

[78] Kobrynski LJ, Mayer L (2011) Diagnosis and treatment of primary immunodeficiency disease in patients with gastrointestinal symptoms. *Clin Immunol.* 139; 238-248.

[79] Blutt SE, Conner ME (2013) The gastrointestinal frontiers: IgA and viruses. *Front Immunol.* 4; art. 402.

[80] Makol A, Watt KD, Chowdhary VR (2011) Autoimmune hepatitis: a review of current diagnosis and treatment. *Hepatitis Res Treat.* Art. 390916; 1-11.

[81] Mieli-Vergani G, Vergani D (2008) Autoimmune paediatric liver disease. *World J Gastroenterol.* 14; 3360-3367.

[82] Bergbreiter A, Salzer U (2009) Common variable immunodeficiency: a multifaceted and puzzling disorder. *Expert Rev Clin Immunol.* 5; 167-180.

[83] Verbruggen G, De Backer S, Deforce P, Demetter P, Cuvelier C, Veys E, Elewaut D (2005) X linked agammaglobulinemia and rheumatoid arthritis. *Ann Rheum Dis.* 64; 1075-1078.

[84] Hernandez-Trujillo VP, Scalchunes C, Cunningham-Rundles Ch, Ochs HD, Bonilla FA, Paris K, Yel L, Sullivan KE (2014) Autoimmunity and inflammation in X-linked agammaglobulinemia. *J Clin Immunol.* 34; 627-632.

[85] Blanco-Quiros A, Solis-Sanchez P, Garrote-Adrados JA, Arranz-Sanz E (2006) Common variable immunodeficiency. Old questions are getting clearer. *Allergol Immunopathol.* 34; 263-275.

[86] Nimmerjahn F, Ravetch JV (2008) Anti-inflammatory actions of intravenous immunoglobulin. *Ann Rev Immunol.* 26; 513-533.

[87] Nimmerjahn F, Ravetch JV (2010) Antibody-mediated modulation of immune responses. *Immunological Rev.* 236; 265-275.

[88] Siedlar M, Strach M, Bukowska-Strakova K, Lenart M, Szaflarska A, Węglarczyk K, Rutkowska M, Baj-Krzyworzeka M, Pituch-Noworolska A, Kowalczyk D, Grodzicki T, Ziegler-Heitbrock L, Zembala M (2011) Preparations of intravenous immunoglobulins diminish the number and proinflammatory response of CD14+CD16+ monocytes in common variable immunodeficiency (CVID) patients. *Clin Immunol.* 139;122-132.

[89] Bayry J, Fournier EM, Maddur MS, Vani J, Wootla B, Siberil S, Dimitrov JD, Lacroix-Desmazes S, Berdah M, Crabol Y, Oksenhendler E, Levy Y, Mouthon L, Sautes-Fridman C, Hermine O, Kaveri SV (2011) Intravenous immunoglobulins induces proliferation and immunoglobulin synthesis from patients with common immunodeficiency. *J Autoimmun* 36: 9-15,

[90] Rezaei N, Abolhassani H, Aghamogammadi A, Ochs HD (2011) Indications and safety of intravenous and subcutaneous immunoglobulin therapy. *Expert Rev Clin Immunol.* 7; 301-316.

[91] Pituch-Noworolska A, Błaut-Szlósarczyk A, Zwonarz K (2010) Stosowanie preparatów immunoglobulin ludzkich – objawy niepożądane. In Polish. (The use of human immunoglobulins – adverse reactions). *Polski Merkuriusz Lekarski.* 29; 202-205.

[92] Kobrynski L (2012) Subcutaneous immunoglobulin therapy. *Biologics: Targ Ther.* 6; 277-287.

[93] Pituch-Noworolska A, Błaut-Szlósarczyk A (2010) Immunoglobulins: characteristics, indications for use and clinical effectiveness. *Int Rev Allergol Clin Immunol.* 16; 94-101.

[94] Haddad E, Barnes D, Kafal A (2012) Home therapy with subcutaneous immunoglobulins for patients with primary immunodeficiency diseases. *Transf Apheresis Sci.* 46; 315-321.

[95] Podjasek JC, Abraham RS (2012) Autoimmune cytopenias in common variable immunodeficiency. *Front Immunol.* 3: art. 189; 1-7.

[96] Nijeboer P, van Wanrooij RLJ, Tack GJ, Mulder CJJ, Bouma G (2013) Update of the diagnosis and management of refractory celiac disease. *Rev Gastroenterol Res Pract*. Art. 518 483.

[97] Al-Toma A, Verbeek WHM, Mulder CJJ (2007) The management of complicated celiac disease. *Dig Dis*. 25; 230-236.

[98] Tennyson Ch, Green PHH (2011) The role of capsule endoscopy in patients with nonresponsive celiac disease. *Gastrointest Endosc* 74; 1323-1324.

[99] Sandhu BK, Fell JME, Beattie RM, Mitton SG, Wilson DC, Jenkins H (2010) Guidelines for the management of inflammatory bowel disease in children in the United Kingdom. *J Ped Gastroenterol Nutri*. 50; S1-S13.

[100] Burroughs L, Woolfrey A (2010) Hematopoietic cell transplantation for treatment of primary immune deficiencies. *Cell Ther Transplant*. doi:10.3205/ctt-2010-en-000077.01.

[101] Cole TS, Johnstone IC, Pearce MS, Fulton B, Fulton B, Cant AJ, Gennery AR, Slatter MA (2012) Outcome of children requiring intensive care following haematopoietic SCT for primary immunodeficiency and other non-malignant disorders. *BMT* 47; 40-45.

[102] Gennery AR, Slatter MA, Grandin L, Taupin P, Cant AJ, Veys P, Amrolia PJ, Gaspar B, Davies EG, Friedrich W, Hoenig M, Notarangelo LD, Mazzolari E, Porta F, Bredius RGM, Lankester AC, Wulffraat NM, Seger R, Gungor T, Fasth A, Sedlacek P, Neven B, Blanche S, Fischer A, Cavazzana-Calvo, Landais P (2010) Transplantation of haematopoietic stem cells and long-term survival for primary immunodeficiencies. *Eur J Allergy Clin Immunol*. 126; 602-610.

[103] Filipovich AH (2008) Hematopoietic cell transplantation for correction of primary immunodeficiencies. *BMT* 42; S49-S52.

[104] De la Morena MT (2013) Recent advances in transplantation for primary immune deficiency diseases. *Clin Rev Allergy Immune*. doi: 10.1007/s12016-013-8379-6.

[105] Cha S-I, Fessler MB, Cool CD, Schwarz MI, Brown KK (2006) Lymphoid interstitial pneumonia: clinical features, associations and prognosis. *Eur Respir J*. 28; 364-369.

[106] Matsubara M, Koizumi T, Wakamatsu T, Fujimoto K, Kubo K, Honda T (2008) Lymphoid interstitial pneumonia associated with common variable immunoglobulin deficiency. Inter Med. 47; 763-767.

Chapter 5

A Concise Review of Autoimmune Liver Diseases

Nwe Ni Than and Ye Htun Oo

Additional information is available at the end of the chapter

http://dx.doi.org/10.5772/60520

1. Introduction

Autoimmune liver disease (AILD) consists of autoimmune hepatitis (AIH), primary biliary cirrhosis (PBC) and primary sclerosing cholangitis (PSC). It is characterised by the immune mediated injury to the hepatocytes and bile ducts. Hepatocyte injury is the predominant features in autoimmune hepatitis and biliary injury is the hallmark of primary biliary cirrhosis (Intrahepatic bile duct injury), primary sclerosing cholangitis or Immunoglobulin (Ig) G4 mediated cholangitis (both intra and extra-hepatic bile duct injury). Overlap or variant syndrome indicates the presence of simultaneous injury to both hepatocytes and cholangiocytes during the course of the disease. Imbalance in effector and regulatory arm of adaptive immune cells had been described as the immunopathogenesis of AILD. Antigenic causative factors are still poorly understood across AILD but genetic, environmental factors and microbiota play a major role in disease pathology.

1.1. Aims

The aim of the chapter is to describe in depth of each disease entity in regard to their immunopathogenesis, diagnosis, investigations and management strategies including standardised care as well as future novel therapies.

1.2. Concerns

Long term global immunosuppressive therapy in AIH with multiple side effects and lack of definitive treatment to tackle the underlying immunopathology in PBC and PSC are major challenging aspects in AILD. Thorough understanding of causative antigens, immunopathogenesis, OMIC profiles (genomic, metabolomics, proteomic and microbiomic) of AILD patients will direct clinicians for stratification and individualized personal care. Novel new immunological based cell and cytokines therapies are urgently warranted in defined unique group of AILD patients.

The diagnosis and management of AILD can be constantly challenging due to the presence of overlap features at diagnosis or gradual evolution in phenotype of diseases from one spectrum (typical AIH) to others (overlap of AIH/PBC and AIH/PSC) during the disease process. Therefore, the continuous assessment of the disease presentations are essential in follow up of patients with AILD.

2. Background

An autoimmune liver disease (AILD) is an umbrella term for diseases caused by immune mediated reaction to either hepatocytes or bile ducts. Regulatory T cells (Treg) play an important and essential role in the maintenance of homeostasis and prevention of autoimmune responses [1]. Autoimmune hepatitis (AIH) is caused by an immune mediated injury of the hepatocytes and characterised by presence of lobular and interface hepatitis on liver histology, presence of hypergammaglobulinaemia and high titre of antinuclear antibodies (ANA) in the serum with transaminitis on liver biochemistry. The main aim of treatment is to suppress the immune system globally and the first line therapies used are prednisolone and azathioprine. Second line therapies such as tacrolimus and mycophenolate mofetil are also used in AIH patients. Two commonly used biologics in difficult-to-treat AIH patients are anti- tumour necrosis factor (anti-TNF) for example Infliximab and anti-CD20 monoclonal antibody therapy as in Rituximab. New novel antigen-specific autologous regulatory T cells therapy development is also in progress for future treatment of autoimmune hepatitis.

Primary biliary cirrhosis (PBC) is an injury to the intra-hepatic biliary ducts and tends of present in 4th to 6th decade of life. The main therapy is ursodeoxycholic acid (UDCA) but new therapies for PBC such as Obeticholic acid have been emerged recently. Patients with PBC tend to suffer with significant itch and management of itch can be challenging at times. There are therapies available for itch from the spectrum to cholestyramine to immunoglobulins infusion treatment.

Primary sclerosing cholangitis (PSC) is an immune mediated injury, mainly to biliary system either intrahepatic or extrahepatic or both. PSC is common in young, male patient and commonly associated with inflammatory bowel disease (IBD), especially ulcerative colitis. There is a significant risk of developing cancer such as cholangiocarcinoma or gall bladder cancer or bowel cancer in these groups of patients and hence surveillance is important. There are no targeted treatments available for PSC and liver transplantation is necessary in end stage PSC.

Detailed summary of three autoimmune liver disease (autoimmune hepatitis, primary biliary cirrhosis and primary sclerosing cholangitis) are documented in table 1.

http://dx.doi.org/10.5772/60520

	AUTOIMMUNE HEPATITIS (AIH)	PRIMARY BILIARY CIRRHOSIS (PBC)	PRIMARY SCLEROSIS CHOLANGITIS (PSC)
AGE	Any age	Any age, common over 40 years	Around 40 years of age
GENDER	Female predominance (4:1)	Female predominance (9:1)	Male predominance (7:3)
ASSOCIATED CONDITIONS	Other autoimmune conditions, commonly thyroid disorders, diabetes mellitus, coeliac disease and inflammatory arthritis	Other autoimmune conditions, commonly thyroid disorders, diabetes mellitus, coeliac disease and inflammatory arthritis	Inflammatory bowel disease, mainly ulcerative colitis
TRANSAMINASE LEVELS (ALT OR AST)	Raised (>5x ULN) ↑↑↑	Raised (stable) ↑	Raised (fluctuating) ↑
ALP OR GGT	Raised ↑	Raised (stable) ↑↑↑	Raised (fluctuating)- (> 3 fold increase) ↑↑↑
IMMUNOLOGICAL PROFILE	Raised ANA, ASMA or LKM Raised Ig G	Raised AMA (anti-gp 210, anti-Sp 100) Raised Ig M	None
BILIARY INVOLVEMENT	No	Yes (small duct)	Yes (small to large duct)
LIVER HISTOLOGY [1]			
INTERFACE HEPATITIS	Yes	May be	May be
PORTAL INFLAMMATION	Lymphoplasmacytic infiltrate	Lymphocytic infiltrate	Lymphocytic infiltrate
GRANULOMAS	No	Yes	Rare (<10% of cases)
RESPONSE TO STEROIDS/ OTHER IMMUNOSUPPRESIONS	Yes	No	No
RESPONSE TO UROSDEOXYCHOLIC ACID (UDCA)	No	Yes	Maybe
PROGNOSIS	If untreated, patient have poor prognosis with 5 and 10 year survival rates of 50 and 10% [2].	Prognosis is excellent in patients who achieved biochemical response with UDCA therapy	Median survival without transplantation is 12 to 15 years [3]

ANA: Anti-nuclear antibodies, ASMA: anti smooth muscle antibodies, LKM: Liver- kidney-microsomal antibodies, g G: Immunoglobulin G, Ig M: Immunoglobulin M, Anti-gp 210: Antibodies against the nuclear pore membrane glycoprotein (anti-gp210), Anti-Sp 100: Antibodies against the nuclear protein Sp100, ULN: Upper limit of normal, UDCA: Ursodeoxycholic acid

Adapted from 1) Trivedi, P.J. and G.M. Hirschfield, Review article: overlap syndromes and autoimmune liver *disease.* Aliment Pharmacol Ther, 2012. 36(6): p. 517-33. 2) Strassburg, C.P. and M.P. Manns, *Therapy of autoimmune hepatitis.* Best Pract Res Clin Gastroenterol, 2011. 25(6): p. 673-87.3) Yimam, K.K. and C.L. Bowlus, Diagnosis and classification of primary sclerosing cholangitis. Autoimmun Rev, 2014. 13(4-5): p. 445-50.

Table 1. Summary of Autoimmune liver disease

3. Autoimmune hepatitis

3.1. Epidemiology

Autoimmune hepatitis (AIH) is an immune mediated, chronic inflammatory disease of unknown aetiology, mainly affecting the hepatocytes. It was first defined in 1950 by Waldenström when he described a chronic hepatitis in young woman which eventually lead to liver cirrhosis [2]. It is characterised by the morphological changes of interface hepatitis on liver biopsy, hypergammaglobulinaemia and the presence of high circulating ANA in the serum [3, 4]. It is more common in women (around 75%) and can affect at any age from young to elderly. It is also associated with other autoimmune conditions such as hypothyroidism, ulcerative colitis, type 1 diabetes mellitus, rheumatoid arthritis, coeliac disease or skin disorders such as vitiligo. Therefore, obtaining a detailed history especially family history of autoimmune conditions are important in the assessment of patients with potential AIH diagnosis.

There is limited evidence regarding the incidence and prevalence of AIH. From the data so far, it has been estimated that the prevalence of AIH is around 5 to 20 cases per 100,000 among the Caucasian population in Western Europe [5]. AIH accounts for up to 20% of chronic hepatitis among the Caucasian population of North America and Western Europe [5]. AIH prevalence and clinical expression appear to vary according to ethnicity. Previous studies showed that black patients tend to have more aggressive disease [6] whereas Hispanic populations had a higher prevalence of cirrhosis [7]. Asian patients develop the disease later in life and have a poorer survival [7] and Alaskan native patients presented more frequently with acute AIH [8].

Clinically, there are three forms of AIH. Type 1 AIH is common in adults and characterised by the presence of ANA and/or anti smooth muscle antibodies (ASMA) with raised Immunoglobulin-G (Ig G). Type 2 is seen mostly in children and characterised by the presence of anti-liver-kidney-microsomal (LKM) antibodies directed against cytochrome P450 (CYP-2D6) [9, 10] and with lower frequency against UDP-glucuronosyltransferases (UGT) [2, 11]. Antibodies against soluble liver or liver-pancreas (SLP) antigens are common in type 3 AIH. Around 19% of patients can present with seronegative disease at the time of diagnosis [12].

3.2. Pathogenesis

The exact aetiopathogenesis of AIH is still unknown. It is a complex process interlinking environmental and genetic factors in a susceptible host. The most common environmental trigger thought to cause AIH is viral infection. Drug induced AIH is a recognised entity and the commonly associated drugs are anti-TNF treatment such as Adalimumab, antibiotics such as minocycline or nitrofurantion or statins such as rosuvastatin [13-15]. Both T cells and B cells play an important role in the adaptive immune response to both self and non-self-antigen. T cells, both CD4 and CD8 T cells, play a major role in the immnuopathogenesis with effector responses mediated by Natural Killer (NK) cells and macrophages [16]. Regulatory T cells (Treg) play an essential role in the homeostasis and prevention of autoimmune conditions [1]. They are classified as CD4+ $CD25^{high}$ $CD127^{Low}$ and represent the 2 % of the CD3 subset [17]. Foxp3 (forkhead box P3) is a transcription factor which controls the phenotype, development and function of Treg [18]. Commitment to Treg lineage primary occurs in the thymus as a result of presenting self- antigens by medullary thymic epithelium. In AIH, the number of Tregs is normal but their function is impaired [19]. Reduction in frequency of Treg has also been reported [17, 20].

Type 1 AIH is associated with human leukocyte antigen (HLA) DR3 (HLA-DRB1*0301) and DR4 (HLA-DRB1*0401) in white North Europe and North American patients [21, 22]. It has been suggested the presence of DR3 is associated with poorer response to treatment and hence requires liver transplantation (LT) [21, 22]. On the other hand, patients with DR4 are usually older and more responsive to treatment with steroid [21]. A recent geno-wide association study of type 1 AIH in Netherlands showed that type 1 AIH is associated with the rs3184504*A allele in the SH2B3 gene [22]. These single nucleotide polymorphisms (SNP) represent the first genetic AIH locus outside the Major Histocompatibility Complex (MHC) region [22]. It encodes a missense variant in exon 3 of the Scr homology 2 adaptor protein 3 (SH2B3) genes located in the 12q24 region [22]. SH2B3 is a negative regulator of T-cell activation, tumour necrosis factor, and Janus kinase 2 and 3 signalling, and plays an essential role in normal haematopoiesis [22]. Capcase recruitment domain family member 10 (CARD 10) gene with allele rs6000782 has been shown to be associated with type 1 AIH [22]. CARD 10 is a scaffold protein and induces pro-inflammatory nuclear factor kB activation and it is widely expressed in a variety of non-haematopoietic tissue including hepatocytes [22].

Proposed pathway of pathogenesis in AIH has been shown in Figure 1.

3.3. Clinical presentations and diagnosis of AIH

Most patients present with nonspecific symptoms such as fatigue, arthralgia and anorexia at the time of presentation. About 25% of patient present asymptomatically [23] and the majority of patients present late with symptoms of portal hypertension and decompensated cirrhosis. Recent systematic review mentioned that around 25 % of elderly patients (age 60 to 65) were more likely to present asymptomatically, they are more likely to be HLA-DR4 positive and cirrhotic at initial presentation [24]. They are less likely to be HLA-DR3-positive and to relapse after treatment withdrawal after complete remission [24]. AIH can also present during pregnancy or postpartum period. Physical examination can either be normal, or show hepatomegaly, splenomegaly or signs of chronic liver disease. In some patients, AIH present as acute severe hepatitis and rarely, they progress to fulminant form and require liver transplantation [2].

Blood tests can show signs of hepatitis with raised alanine transaminase (ALT, U/L) (usually less than 500 U/L), aspartate transaminase (AST, U/L) and occasionally bilirubin (umol/L). Typical immunology profile in AIH patients are raised Ig G with positive ANA, ASMA (in type 1 AIH) and LKM (in type 2 AIH). Patients with acute presentation of AIH should be monitored for synthetic function such as international normalised ratio (INR) and albumin as well as mental status or sign of hepatic encephalopathy since some patients can progress to acute liver failure rapidly and will need liver transplantation. Viral hepatitis, toxins, drugs should be excluded in patient presenting with acute or chronic form of hepatitis. Men with AIH appear to have a higher relapse rate and younger age of disease onset [25, 26]. Cirrhosis at presentation [27, 28] and presence of SLA antibodies are poor predictive outcomes in type 1 AIH patients [29, 30].

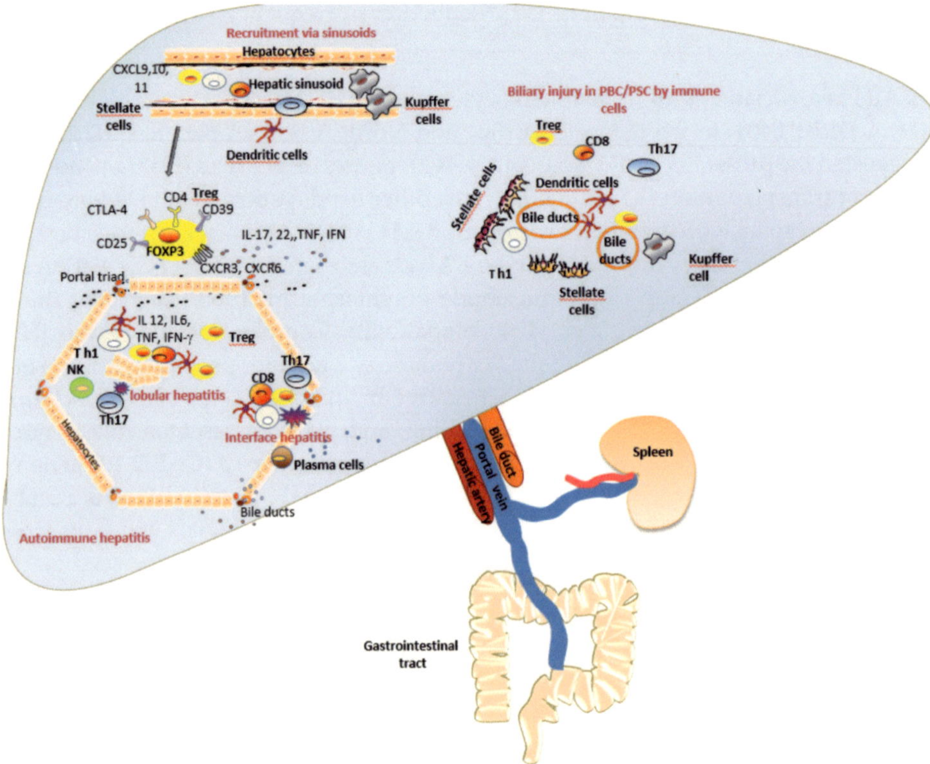

CXCL: chemokine (C-X-C motif) ligand 1, CTLA-4: Cytotoxic T-lymphocyte-associated protein 4, CD: Cluster of Differentiation, CXCR: C-X-C chemokine receptor type, FOXP3: Forkhead box P3, IL: Interleukin, NK: Natural killer, T-reg: T regulatory cells, TNF: Tumour necrosis factor, IFN: Interferon, Th: T helper.

Figure 1. Pathogenesis of Autoimmune hepatitis. Autoimmune hepatitis (AIH) is initiated by the presence of auto antigen peptide onto antigen presenting cells (APC) which activates T helper cells (Th0) due to interleukins (IL) 2 and 4. Upon activation of Th0, it can differentiate into Th1 and Th2 cellular pathway. Th1 produces IL2 and Interferon-gamma (IFN-r) which subsequently activates CD8 lymphocytes.

Liver biopsy is recommended at the time of presentation to establish the diagnosis as well as to guide the treatment, however in patients presenting with acute hepatitis who has suspicious diagnosis of AIH, the treatment should not be delayed [31]. The histological hallmarks of AIH is a lymphoplasmacytic peri-portal infiltrate invading the limiting plate, also called piecemeal necrosis or "interface hepatitis" and eventually lead to lobular hepatitis (Figure 2) [13]. Patients with chronic AIH usually have plasma cell- rich mononuclear infiltrate involving portal and peri-portal regions [16] which subsequently lead to peri-portal fibrosis. Up to 30% of patients with AIH had histological features of cirrhosis at the time of presentation [2]. In 17% of patients with peri-portal hepatitis whereas 82% of patients who had bridging fibrosis, cirrhosis develops within 5 years [2].

The diagnosis of AIH is based on multiple investigations and diagnostic criteria was proposed by the international AIH group in 1993 and subsequently updated in 1999 (Table 2) [13, 32,

http://dx.doi.org/10.5772/60520

33]. In 2008, the groups established the simplified scoring system which is more user friendly in day to day clinical care[13] (Table 3). The scoring is based on combination of the serum immunoglobulins titres (ANA, SMA or LKM), serum liver enzymes and liver histology features with absence of viral hepatitis.

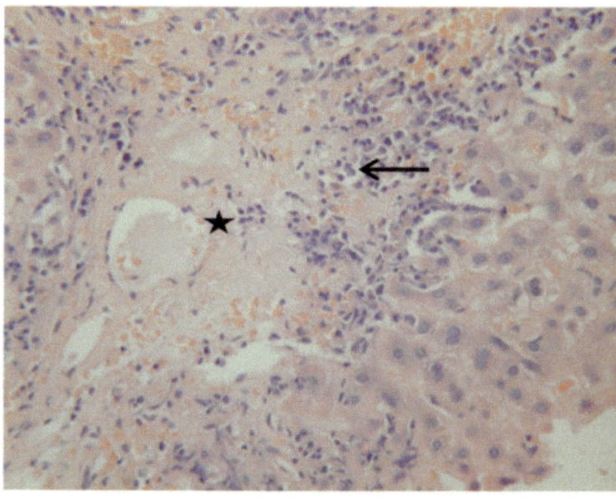

Figure above showed lobular inflammation with mainly plasma rich infiltrates (black arrow) and central peri-venulitis (black star)

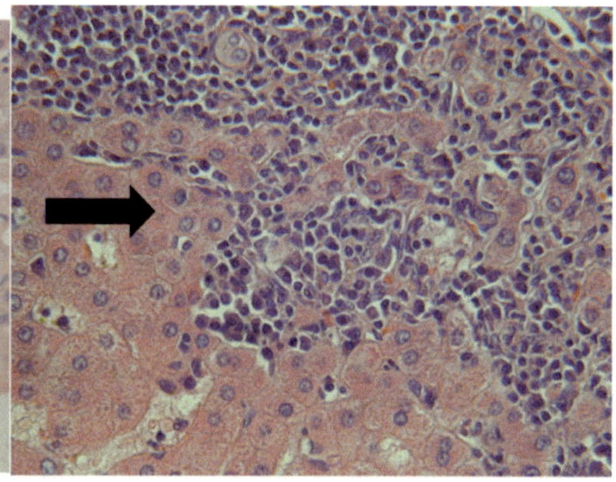

Figure above showed interface hepatitis with rich plasma cell infiltrates (large arrow head).

Figure 2. Histology findings of autoimmune hepatitis

Clinical features	Score
Female	+2
ALP:AST ratio	
• <1.5	+2
• 1.5-3.0	0
• >3.0	-2
Serum globulin or Ig G above normal	
• >2.0	+3
• 1.5-2.0	+2
• 1.0-1.5	+1
• <1.0	0
ANA, SMA or LKM 1	
• >1:80	+3
• 1:80	+2
• 1:40	+1
• <1:40	0
Illicit drug use	
• Positive	-4
• Negative	+1
Average daily alcohol intake	
• <25g/day	+2

Clinical features	Score
• >60g/day	-2
Histological findings	
• Interface hepatitis	+3
• Lymphoplasmacytic infiltrate	+1
• Rosette formation	+1
• None of the above	-5
• Biliary changes	-3
• Other changes	-2
	+2
Other autoimmune disease	
AMA positivity	-4
Viral hepatitis markers	
• Positive	-3
• Negative	+3
Definite AIH	>15
Probable AIH	10-15

ALP: alkaline phosphatase, AST: Aspartate transaminase, Ig: Immunoglobulin, ANA: Antinuclear antibodies, SMA: Smooth muscle antibodies, LKM: Liver kidney microsomal antibodies, AMA: Anti-mitochondrial antibod

Table 2. Revised International Autoimmune Hepatitis Group Scoring System for the Diagnosis of Autoimmune Hepatitis (AIH) (Adapted from Alvarez et al [21] and Chandok et al [22])

Variables	Cut off	Points
ANA or SMA	≥ 1;40	1
	≥ 1:80	2
Or LKM 1	≥ 1:40	2
Or SLA	Positive	1
Ig G	>upper limit of normal	1
	>1.1x upper limit of normal	2
Liver histology	Compatible with AIH	1
	Typical of AIH	2
Absence of viral hepatitis	Yes	2

ANA: anti-nuclear antibodies; SMA: anti-smooth-muscle antibodies; LKM1: liver/ kidney microsomal antibody type 1; SLA: anti-soluble liver antigen.

Definite AIH: A cumulative score ≥7

Probable AIH: A cumulative score =6

Liver histology typical of AIH: interface hepatitis, emperipolesis, hepatic rosette formation

Liver histology compatible with AIH: chronic hepatitis with lymphocytic infiltration, without typical features.

Table 3. Simplified scoring system for autoimmune hepatitis

4. Management/treatment

4.1. Standard therapy

The main aim for treatment of AIH is to suppress the ongoing inflammation and the first line therapies used are steroids (either prednisolone or budesonide) with or without azathioprine (AZA). Steroid side effects such as cosmetic changes, osteopenia, hirsutism, steroid induced diabetes are seen in about 44% of patients within 12 months of treatment and 80% within 24 months of treatment [2]. Budesonide is a preferred choice of treatment for patients who do not tolerate prednisolone due to side effects and in patients with diabetes mellitus. It is a synthetic steroid with high first-pass metabolism in the liver, which is in principle capable of limiting systemic side effects compared to conventional steroids [2]. Due to those side effects mentioned above, the adherence to medication can be an issue and hence, compliance needs to be monitored throughout the treatment period. Patients who need long term steroid therapy (> 3 months) should be started on calcium and vitamin D3 supplements to prevent osteoporosis.

The combination regimen of prednisone and azathioprine is associated with a lower occurrence of corticosteroid-related side effects than the higher dose prednisone regimen (10% versus 44%), and it is the preferred treatment in patients with AIH. AZA side effects include abdominal discomforts, pancreatitis, nausea, cholestatic hepatitis, rashes and leukopenia and they can be seen in 15% of patients who received 50mg of AZA [2]. Azathioprine metabolite and Thiopurine S-Methyl Transferase (TPMT) levels will guide the optimal dose for individual patients. Some patients who cannot tolerate AZA benefit from Mercaptourine. The metabolism of AZA has been demonstrated in Figure 3.

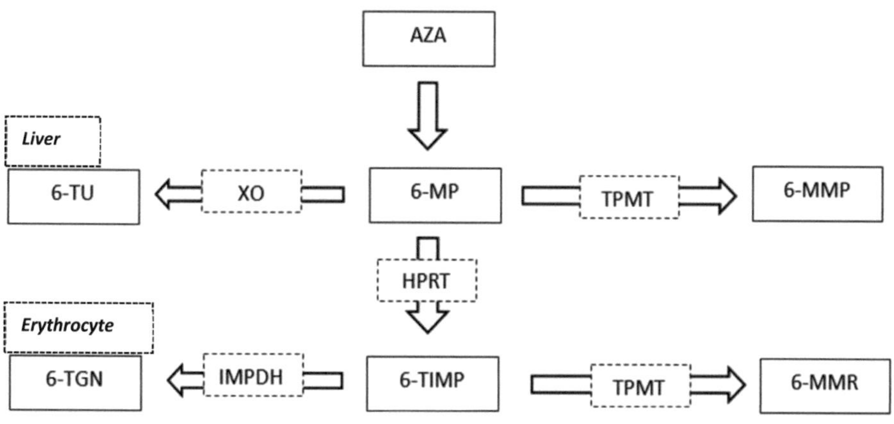

Aza: Azathioprine, MP: Mercaptopurine, TIMP: Thiosine 5 mono phosphate, MMP: Methyl mercaptopurine, MMR: Mehty mercaptopurine ribonucleotides, TU: Thiouric acid, TGN: Thioguanine nucleotide. TPMT: Thiopurine S-methyl transferase, XO: Xanthise oxidase, IMPDH: Inosine monophosphate dehydrogenase, HPRT: Hypoxanthine phosphoribosyltransferase

(Adapted from Dubinsky, M.C., et al., Thioguanine: a potential alternate thiopurine for IBD patients allergic to 6-mercaptopurine or azathioprine. Am J Gastroenterol, 2003. 98(5): p. 1058-63)

Figure 3. Azathioprine metabolism

Around 90% of adult patients respond to therapy within first 2 weeks with improvement in serum immunoglobulins and liver enzymes levels [31]. Treatment should be continued until normalisation of serum immunological and, biological parameters as well as improvement in liver histology. Relapsed AIH is characterized by an increase in the serum aminotransferase levels to at least threefold normal and it occurs in 50% to 86% of patients who previously had complete remission of their disease and usually happens during the first 6 months after the termination of therapy [13, 31]. In patients who has sub-optimal response to initial therapy or relapsed AIH should be considered for more potent treatments such as tacrolimus or mycophenolate mofetil.

4.2. Alternative and future therapies

Alternative therapies include tacrolimus, mycophenolate mofetil (MMF), cyclosporine, methotrexate, cyclophosphamide, ursodeoxycholic acid (UDCA), infliximab and rituximab [14]. Although there are some encouraging results with each of the medications, the treatment has not been implemented into standard management due to lack of randomised control data. Most of the evidence is based on from small, retrospective, single centre case series [34]. Therefore, these treatments should be only commenced in the specialised centre with presence of experienced hepatologists.

Cyclosporine A is a lipophilic cyclic peptide of 11 residues produced by Tolypocladium inflatum that acts on calcium dependent signalling and inhibits T cell function via the interleukin 2 gene [2]. Use of cyclosporine is limited due to its side effects of hirsutism, hypertension, renal insufficiency, hyperlipidaemia, increased risk of infection and malignancy [2]. The evidence of cyclosporine in adult AIH is limited due to a small number of case series arising from single centres. In one study of six patients, cyclosporine normalised ALT in all patients and 3 patients had improvement with liver histology in follow up. Another study of 5 patients with cyclosporine treatment showed biochemical improvement in 4 patients who had not responded to standard therapy [35]. In a study of 8 patients, it showed that cyclosporine is safe and all patients achieved remission [36].

Tacrolimus (Tac) is a macrolide compound and its mechanism is similar to that of cyclosporine A but it binds to a different immunophilin [2]. The main side effect is renal toxicity. Both cyclosporine and tacrolimus are calcineurin inhibitors and can be used as a rescue therapy for difficult to treat AIH patients. Compliance can be monitored by drug level in both drugs. An open label preliminary study in which 21 AIH patients were treated with tacrolimus (Tac) showed reduction of liver enzymes (ALT and AST) in 70-80% of patients who received 3 months of therapy [37]. There are only few studies reported use of Tac in the treatment of AIH although wide experience use of this drug exist in cohort of AIH patients who had liver transplantation (LT) [34]

Mycophenolate Mofetil (MMF) is a non-competitive inhibitor of inosine monophosphate dehydrogenase, which blocks the rate-limiting enzymatic step in de novo purine synthesis. MMF has a selective action on lymphocyte activation, with marked reduction of both T and B lymphocyte proliferation [2]. Many patients experience headache, nausea, diarrhoea, dizziness and neutropenia with MMF therapy [14]. It is contraindicated in pregnancy due to its teratogenic side effects. Recent studies of 59 patients with treatment naïve AIH were treated with MMF and prednisolone as a first line therapies in which the study showed biochemical and immunological parameters improvements in 88% of patients in the first 3 months and 12% had partial response [38]. A study from Canadian group studied 16 patients who failed conventional therapy were given either tacrolimus or MMF [39] and complete response were seen in 50% of patients and 12.5 % had non response to treatment [39]. Another study looking at 36 patients with AIH who were treated with MMF and it showed remission in 39% of patients. The study mentioned in patients who does not respond to AZA, around 75% of those do not respond to MMF either [40].

Infliximab, a recombinant humanized chimeric antibody, has been used in other immunomodulatory conditions such as rheumatoid arthritis and inflammatory bowel disease. However, infliximab has been associated with de novo AIH in some patients with liver transplantation (LT) and therefore, it should be used by the experienced team in specialised centre. A retrospective, single centre review of 11 patients with difficult to treat AIH were treated with infliximab and it showed infliximab led to reduction of inflammation, evidenced by a decrease in transaminases and serum immunoglobulins [41].

Rituximab is an anti-CD20 chimeric monoclonal antibody, a surface marker expressed on B cells, from early pre-B to memory B lymphocytes [42]. Treatment with rituximab leads to B cell depletion through both complement- and antibody-dependent cellular cytotoxicity [42]. AIH is considered to be a T-cell–mediated disease; however, numerous observations would suggest that B cells are also involved in its pathogenesis [43]. Although there were good evidences to suggest that rituximab is effective in autoimmune haemolytic anaemia, cryoglobulinemia and systemic lupus erythematosus, the data on efficacy of rituximab in AIH are limited [44-46]. A study by Burak and colleague showed that Rituximab is well tolerated with no significant side effects and resulted in biochemical response in patients with refractory or intolerant to other treatment [47].

5. Prognosis

Patients with acute, severe AIH who are untreated have poorer short and long term survival compared to treated AIH patients [48-50]. For patients with the severe acute phenotype of AIH, failure to respond to treatment within the first 7–14 days after presentation is associated with a mortality of almost 50% [51]. For patients with established cirrhosis at presentation, treatment can induce remission and improve long-term outcome, with 10-year life expectancies of greater than 90% [52, 53]. Patient with cirrhosis due to AIH usually develop hepatocellular carcinoma at a mean of 9 to 10 years according to previous published case series and hence, routine surveillance with 6 monthly ultrasound scan and alpha feto protein (AFP) is recommended for these cohort of patients [54, 55]. Autoimmune hepatitis is an acceptable reason for liver transplantation, with frequency of survival exceeding 75% at 5 and 10 years after transplant [56, 57]. In summary, the overall prognosis of AIH is good for patient who are treated and responded to immunosuppressive therapy. Therefore, compliance is important which can be achieved by supporting patient and education to the patient. It is also crucial to recognise and treat the patients who are not responsive to standard immunosuppressive therapies with more novel treatments. It is essential to have smooth handover and transition between paediatric and adult hepatology team which will help young patients with AIH to continue with their treatment and follow up.

6. Primary biliary cirrhosis

6.1. Epidemiology

Primary biliary cirrhosis (PBC) is an autoimmune condition and causes a chronic and progressive destruction of intrahepatic bile ducts resulting in chronic cholestasis, portal inflammation, fibrosis and then gradually lead to cirrhosis and liver failure [58]. The disease is predominantly seen in women than men with a ratio of 10:1 [60] and had a prevalence of 1 in 1000 women over the age of 40 [59].

The highest prevalence and incidence rates have been reported in Great Britain, Scandinavia and the northern Midwest region of the USA [5, 61]. It has been suggested that the incidence of PBC is rising and in the United Kingdom (UK), the incidence rate rose from 2.05 cases per 100,000 populations per year in Sheffield from 1980 to 1999 [5, 62] and from 1.1 to 3.2 cases per 100,000 population per year in Newcastle- Upon- Tyne from 1976 to 1994 [63, 64].

6.2. Pathogenesis

Both genetic and environmental factors such as chemical substances, bacterial and viruses play an important role in the pathogenesis of PBC. In general, data indicate that 1 to 6% of PBC cases have at least one other family member presenting with the disease [60]. The concordance rate observed among monozygotic twins for PBC is 63%, among the highest reported in autoimmune diseases [60]. Prior to the advent of genome-wide association studies, only class II HLA loci (HLA-DRB1*08, *11, and *13) had been reproducibly shown to associate with disease [59]. With the application of genome-wide technology, HLA was confirmed as the strongest association and many other risk loci have been identified, with equivalent effect size to HLA, including IL12A, IL12RB2, STAT4, IRF5-TNPO3, 17q12.21, MMEL1, SPIB, and CTLA-4 [59]. These collectively support an important role for innate and adaptive immunity in development of disease [59].

There is an increased auto reactive CD4 pyruvate dehydrogenase complex (PDC)-E2 specific T cells in liver and regional lymph nodes in patients with PBC and CD8 PDC-E2 T cells infiltrates in the liver suggesting that anti-mitochondrial response is either directed to the aetiology or associated with other environmental or genetic trigger [65].

6.3. Clinical presentations and diagnosis

The majority of patients are asymptomatic at the time of diagnosis. With progression of the disease, patients usually develop fatigue and pruritus. Fatigue is the most common symptom and is present in up to 78% of patients with PBC [65]. Fatigue is not associated with disease severity or disease duration or histological findings and it is difficult to manage in most patients. Pruritus is a more specific symptom of PBC than fatigue and formerly occurred in 20%-70% of patients with PBC [65]. It can be local or diffuse, usually worse at night and tend to be in the palms and soles of the feet. Pruritus is often exacerbated by contact with wool, other fabrics, heat, or during pregnancy [65]. Sicca syndrome, hypothyroidism, vitamin D deficiency, osteopenia and hypercholesterolemia are commonly seen in patients with PBC and should be investigated and managed appropriately.

Individuals with abnormal cholestatic liver function tests such as raised alkaline phosphatase (ALP), gamma glutamyl transferase (GGT) and elevated conjugated bilirubin should be investigated for underlying PBC [66]. Immunologically, the majority of patients (around 95%) have positive anti-mitochondrial antibodies (AMA) in their serum and raised levels of immunoglobulins-M (Ig M) [67].

AMA reactivity is classically studied by immunofluorescence and considered positive at a titre of ≥1:40 [66]. The targets of the disease-specific ant mitochondrial response are all members of a family of enzymes, the 2-oxo-acid dehydrogenase complexes and include PDC-E2, branched chain 2-oxo-acid dehydrogenase complex, and 2-oxo-glutaric acid dehydrogenase complex [65]. These enzymes catalyse the oxidative decarboxylation of keto acid substrates and are located in the inner mitochondrial membrane [65].

Patient who had raised ALP and high titre of AMA (tire of ≥ 1:40) or AMA type 2 (M2) can be diagnosed with PBC without liver biopsy as per EASL (European Association for the Study of the Liver) guideline [66]. Positive ANA titres are also found in 30–50% of individuals with PBC (more commonly in the few who are AMA negative), but in this setting ANA reactivity is, in contrast to AIH, often antigen specific (anti gp-210 and anti sp-100) [12, 68].

Stage	Findings
1 (Portal tract Inflammation)	Portal tract inflammation from mainly lymphoplasmacytic infiltrates with or without florid bile duct lesions resulting in septal and interlobular bile ducts.
2 (Peri-portal fibrosis)	Gradual increase of peri-portal lesions extending into the hepatic parenchyma-referred as interface hepatitis.
3 (Bridging fibrosis)	Distortion of the hepatic architecture with numerous fibrous septa. Ductopenia (defined as loss of >50% of interlobular bile ducts) becomes more frequent at this stage.
4 (Cirrhosis)	Cirrhosis with the existence of regenerative nodules.

The stages of PBC are shown in Figure 4.

(Adapted from Lindor KD, Gershwin ME, Poupon R, Kaplan M, Bergasa NV, Heathcote EJ. Primary biliary cirrhosis. Hepatology 2009;50:291-308)

Table 4. Liver histology stages seen in primary biliary cirrhosis

Liver biopsy is rarely needed in the diagnosis of PBC. However, in patients with overlap of AIH/PBC might need liver biopsy to access the degree of the liver injury. In PBC, liver histology is divided into 4 stages (Table 4, Figure 4). Nowadays, the degree of fibrosis can be determined by performing non-invasive procedure such as transient elastography or Fibroscan. Magnetic resonance cholangio-pancreatography (MRCP) and Endoscopic retrograde cholangio-pancreatography (ERCP) are sometimes required to exclude other biliary pathology or PSC.

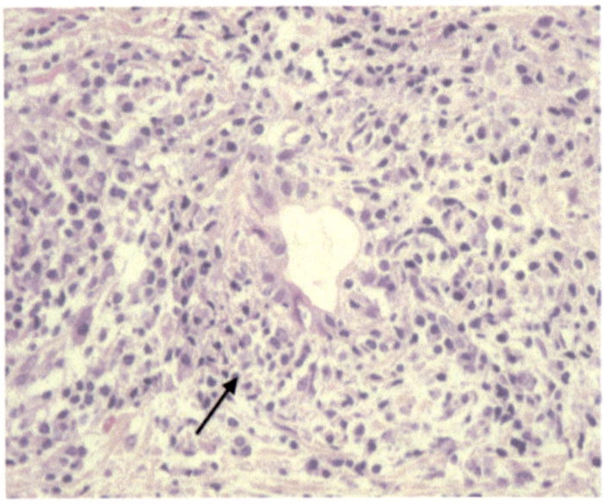

Figure above showed lymphocytic cholangitis seen in PBC (black arrow).

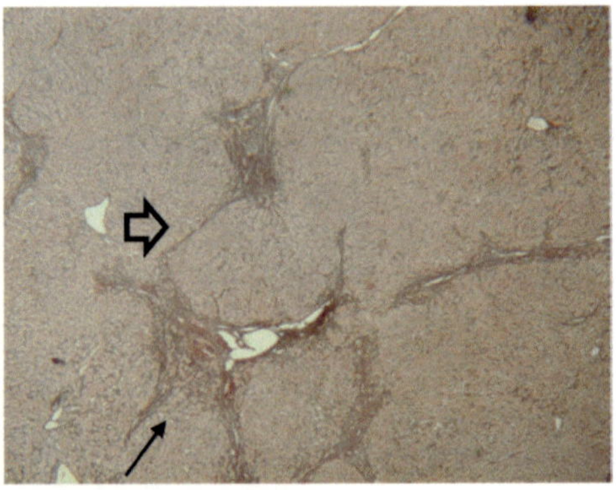

Figure above showed peri-portal (thin arrow) and bridging fibrosis (thick arrow) with reticulin stain

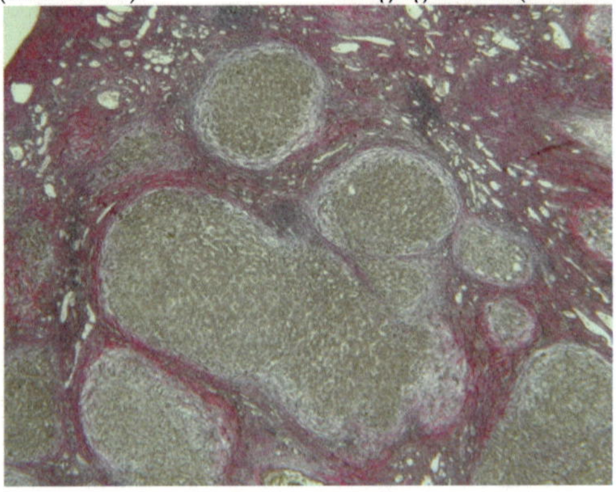

Figure above showed established cirrhosis (Haematoxylin Van Gieson stain)

Figure 4. Histology finding of Primary biliary cirrhosis (PBC)

7. Management/treatment

7.1. Standard therapy

7.1.1. Ursodeoxycholic acid (UDCA)

Ursodeoxycholic acid (UDCA) is the only approved treatment for patients with PBC and shown to be associated with improvement in liver biochemistries, delayed histologic progression of disease, and delayed development of oesophageal varices and prolong transplant free survival [67, 69]. UDCA at a dose of 13-15 mg/kg is proven benefit. Various risk scores have been validated to access the response of UDCA in patients with PBC and these are Barcelona, Paris I and II, Rotterdam and Toronto criteria (table 5) [127-131].

Criteria	Biochemical response
Barcelona	Decrease of serum ALP > 40% or ALP normalisation (after 1 year)
Paris I	ALP ≤ 3 x ULN, AST ≤ 2 x ULN and serum albumin ≤ 1mg/dl (after 1 year)
Paris II	ALP and AST < 1.5 x ULN, serum bilirubin <1mg/dl (after 1 year)
Rotterdam	Normalisation of abnormal serum bilirubin and/or serum albumin (after 1 year)
Toronto	ALP < 1.67 x ULN (after 2 years)

ALP: alkaline phosphatase, AST: Aspartate transaminase, ULN: upper limit of normal

Table 5. Assessment of response to UDCA in patients with PBC

Ursodeoxycholic acid is a hydrophilic bile acid and normally present in about 3% of bile in humans [70]. In patient with cholestasis, there is a decrease in endogenous production of bile acids as well as reduction in the absorption of UDCA [70]. After oral administration of UDCA, it is absorbed in small intestine and colon and transported to liver via portal tract. The absorption of UDCA is increased after meal consumption due to alkaline pH status. Administration of 13-15 mg/kg of UDCA in PBC patients causes enrichment of 40 to 50 % in primary bile acids [70].

Other drugs have been tested, but none have been found as single agents to be of benefit. These include chlorambucil, penicillamine, cyclosporine, corticosteroids, azathioprine, mycophenolate mofetil, thalidomide, methotrexate, malotilate, and colchicine [65].

7.1.2. Treatment for fatigue

Fatigue can be difficult to manage and other underlying conditions such as anaemia, thyroid disorder should be investigated and ruled out. There is no proposed treatment for fatigue and it can sometime persist even after Liver transplantation. A study by Jones et al showed that Modafinil at a dose of 100 to 200 mg/day was associated with a significant improvement in fatigue and improved day time somnolence [71].

7.1.3. Treatment for pruritus

There are few effective treatments available for pruritus in PBC patients. Cholestyramine is a non-absorbable resin and it is the first line therapy in the management of pruritus. The recommended dose of cholestyramine is 4 g per dose to a maximum of 16 g/day given 2-4 hours before or after UDCA [65]. In general, cholestyramine is well tolerated, although some patients report bloating, constipation, and diarrhoea [65].

Rifampicin is a P450 enzyme inducer and used in treatment of pruritus for PBC patients. The recommended dose is 150 mg once daily or twice daily based on the level of bilirubin. Side effects of rifampicin remain a serious concern because cases of hepatitis and hepatic failure, haemolysis and renal impairment and therefore, patient should be closely monitored during the treatment [65]. It should not be used together with serotonin reuptake inhibitor (SSRI) in patient with severe depression since it decrease the effect of SSRI[65].

Opioid antagonist, Naltrexone 50 mg daily, has been shown to be effective in treatment of pruritus in PBC patients. Other agents are SSRI (sertraline), Etarnacept (TNF-alpha inhibitor), Amitriptyline, Anti histamine. Some patient with difficult to treat pruritus can be managed with plasmapheresis.

7.2. Future therapies

Several pilot studies and randomized controlled trials have evaluated various agents in PBC. Trials with mesenchymal stem cells, Rituximab, Ustekinumab, Moexipril which is an angiotensin-converting enzyme (ACE) inhibitor and Abatacept treatments in PBC is currently ongoing (www.clinicaltrials.gov).

There is a suggestion that beta retrovirus might be involved in the pathogenesis of PBC and hence, a randomised controlled trial with lamivudine and zidovudine was studied in PBC patients [72]. There is a good biochemical response seen in patient taking lamivudine and zidovudine but complete biochemical normalisation was not observed [72]. The study did not showed any correlation with virus and biochemical response and as a result, treatment is not recommended in PBC [72].

Recently, fibrates have been thought to be beneficial in PBC since it has anti-inflammatory effect via peroxisome proliferator activated receptor alpha (PPAR-a) [67]. Fenofibrate is a fibric acid and thought to modulate immune response and the cell proliferation and pilot study which treated 20 patients with fenofibrate and UDCA showed significant improvement in liver biochemistry (ALP and ALT) and Ig M although albumin and bilirubin remained unchanged [73]. Larger studies are needed in future. Similar findings were seen in study with bezafibrate.

Obeticholic acid (OCA) is a farnesoid X receptor (FXR) agonist [74]. FXR is expressed in liver, intestine, adrenal glands and kidneys and has an important role in the enterohepatic circulation of bile acids [74, 75]. FXR reduces bile acid synthesis by acting on the enzyme cholesterol 7a hydroxylase and also by down-regulating the expression of the sodium/taurocholate co-transporting peptide, a bile acid uptake protein[75]. Preliminary studies of OCA in patients with PBC have demonstrated marked biochemical improvement when administered in combination with UDCA and alone [74]. Pruritus is the most common side effects and seen at high dose. Currently, there is a phase 3 trial ongoing for OCA treatment in PBC patients.

8. Prognosis

There are many criteria used to assess biochemical response to UDCA (Table 5). The 1-year biochemical response to UDCA provides significant prognostic information even in the early stage of PBC [70]. Early-stage patients who show ALP and AST ◎1.5× upper limit of normal

http://dx.doi.org/10.5772/60520

(ULN), and normal bilirubin level after 1 year of treatment appear to be at very low or no risk of liver failure or progression to cirrhosis. In those patients, they had a 10-year transplant-free survival rate of 90% compared to 51% for those who did not (p <0.001) [76]. About 40% of patients have a suboptimal response to UDCA and subsequently need additional therapy. Liver transplantation is the treatment for patients with decompensated liver cirrhosis and recurrence of PBC is seen in 20% after LT [77].

9. Primary sclerosing cholangitis

9.1. Epidemiology

Primary sclerosing cholangitis (PSC) is a rare autoimmune liver disease and primary affects larger bile ducts. It is caused by chronic inflammation which then leads to fibrotic strictures and dilatation of hepatic biliary system and leading to chronic cholestasis. Chronic cholestasis can subsequently lead to liver cirrhosis with portal hypertension and liver failure [78]. PSC can affect any part of the biliary system including the gallbladder [78].

It is more common in male with median age of around 40 and affects mostly Northern European descendants [79]. The most important underlying risk factor associated with PSC is inflammatory bowel disease and PSC is seen in 75 % of cases of patients with IBD [79]. Around 60 to 80% of patients with PSC have underlying ulcerative colitis, mainly on the right side of the colon and 4% of patients with UC have co-existing PSC [80].

A recent study in UK showed the incidence of PSC to be 0.41 cases per 100,000 populations [81], although the true incidence may be underestimated since it is a relatively rare diseases and needs expertise and invasive procedures to make the diagnosis [79].

9.2. Pathogenesis

The exact mechanism of pathogenesis in PSC is unknown but thought to be multifactorial. It has thought that PSC occurs in individuals with genetic predisposition triggers various environmental stimuli [80]. Patient who has first degree relative with PSC have 9 to 39 fold increased risk of developing PSC and the most associated HLA are HLA DRB1 and DRQ1 [80]. Gut and liver axis theory had been proposed in the pathogenesis of PSC [82]. Manipulation of the intestinal micro flora changes the immune and metabolic pathway [83]. There has been hypothesized that translocation of microbial flora across the inflamed, permeable gut via the portal system to liver and biliary system activate the immune system and cause inflammation of the biliary tree [84-86]. Homing of mucosal lymphocytes which possess (C-C motif chemokine receptor-9) CCR9 and alpha4beta7 in the liver leads to biliary damage in PSC [87, 88]. Recently mucosa associated innate T cells and innate lymphoid cells has been proposed in the pathogenesis of PSC [89]. Although the putative gut-derived trigger(s) of hepatobiliary pathobiology in PSC has not been determined, microbial metabolites or products (i.e., pathogen-associated molecular patterns, PAMPs) such as lipopolysaccharide (i.e., endotoxin,

LPS) and peptidoglycan (i.e., a bacterial cell wall polymer, PG) have been proposed as likely candidates [90].

9.3. Clinical presentations and diagnosis

About 15-40% of patients are asymptomatic during the early stage of the clinical course and at later stage, the most common symptoms are jaundice, pruritus, fatigue and abdominal pain [79]. Any patient who has underlying IBD and abnormal liver blood tests especially raised ALP should be investigated for PSC. In 95 % of cases, ALP rose 3-10 times the upper limit of normal and other liver enzymes ALT and AST were 2-3 times above the normal limit [79]. Bilirubin tends to be within normal range in about 60% of patients. In 69-95% of patients with PSC, 50 to 80% of patients with UC and 10-20% of patients with Crohn's colitis have positive perinuclear antineutrophil autoantibodies (pANCA) [79].

Mayo risk score is used in PSC and the score is calculated using age, bilirubin, albumin, liver transaminase, AST and varcieal bleed and it is used to estimate survival of patient with PSC for up to 4 years [132]. The Mayo Risk Score= (0.0295 * (age in years)) + (0.5373 * (total bilirubin in mg/dL)) - (0.8389 * (serum albumin in g/dL)) + (0.5380 * (AST in IU/L) + (1.2426 * (points for variceal bleeding; 0= No, 1=Yes)). The score of less than or equal to zero is regarded as low risk, between 0 and 2 as intermediate and above 2 as high risk groups.

The diagnosis is best confirmed by MRCP, which is a non-invasive and first line investigation for the diagnosis of PSC. ERCP is used mainly for therapeutic purposes such as stenting, balloon dilatation and biliary brushing in patient with PSC. Contrast cholangiography, which reveals characteristic features of diffuse, multifocal strictures and focal dilation of the bile ducts, leading to a beaded appearance [79]. Liver biopsy is rarely necessary due to good diagnostic yield with MRCP or ERCP investigations except in suspicion of small duct PSC or overlap with AIH. Periductal concentric ("onion-skin") fibrosis is a classic histopathologic finding of PSC, but this observation is infrequent in PSC [91] (Figure 5).

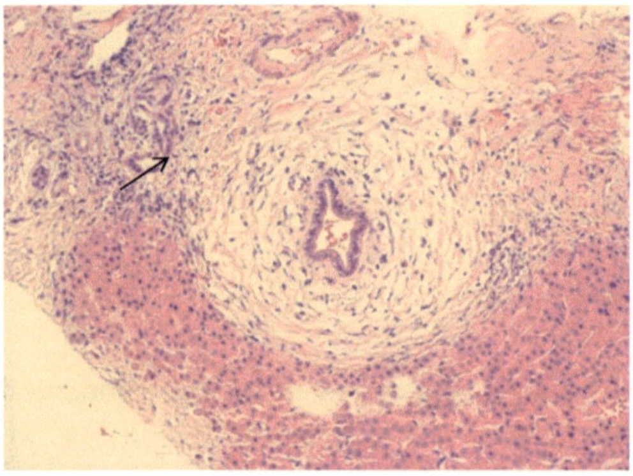

Figure above showed early sign of PSC: peri-ductal fibrosis (black arrow).

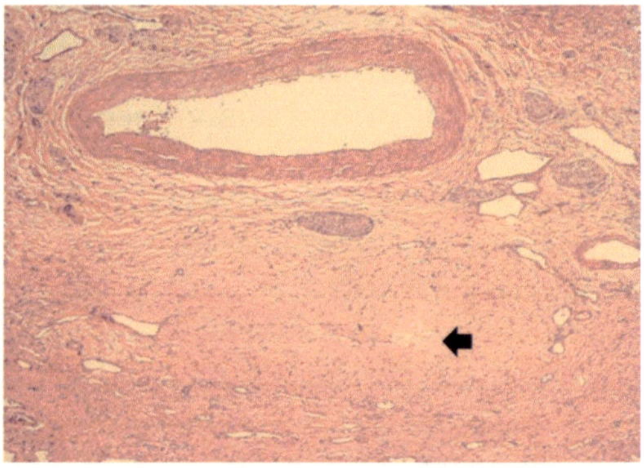

Figure above showed late stage of PSC with fibro-obliterative duct lesion, in which the bile duct is completely filled with fibrosis (large arrow)

Figure 5. Histology findings in Primary Sclerosing Cholangitis (PSC)

http://dx.doi.org/10.5772/60520

In addition to biliary cirrhosis, complications of PSC include dominant strictures of the bile ducts, cholangitis, cholangiocarcinoma, colon dysplasia and cancer in patients with IBD, gallbladder polyps, gallbladder cancer, and hepatic osteodystrophy [79]. Cholangitis occurs in 10 to 15 % of patients with PSC [80]. The cumulative lifetime risk for cholangiocarcinoma in PSC is estimated at 7 to 15% [67]. About half of those cholangiocarcinomas are diagnosed within one year of PSC diagnosis and the rate of cancer development is 0.5 to 1.5% per year subsequently after the first year[67]. Suspected dominant stricture should be investigated by Endoscopic ultrasound scan (EUS) and biopsy along with Positron Emission Tomography (PET) scan.

Immunoglobulin G4 (Ig-G4) associated cholangitis is similar to PSC and is characterized by the presence of biliary strictures, lymphoplasmacytic infiltration and elevated Ig G4 serum levels [92]. Ig G4 elevation is seen in 12% of PSC patients [92]. The biliary features are similar on the cholangiogram in these two conditions and hence, it is important to check Ig G4 level and review the anatomy of pancreas on imaging. Tissue from liver biopsy can be stained using monoclonal anti-human IgG4 antibody. It is important to differentiate between the two because Ig G4 associated cholangitis or pancreatitis responsive to steroids unlike PSC.

10. Management/treatment

10.1. Standard therapy

To date, there are no effective therapies for patients with PSC and the only treatment for end stage PSC is liver transplantation. Timing for liver transplantation is challenging in PSC as these patients sometimes do not fulfil MELD criteria MELD criteria but they can deteriorate rapidly thus early referral to experience centres is essential. UDCA has been used in cholestatic patients with PSC although the data suggested that the medication has not improved overall survival. Studies utilizing doses between 10–15 mg/kg/day were associated with biochemical and histologic improvement [93, 94]. Two previous studies looking at high dose UDCA at a dose of 17-23 mg/kg/day [95] and 28-30 mg/kg/day [96, 97] showed that there were no difference in mortality or LT but increased in adverse events. A recent meta-analysis found no difference in fatigue, mortality, histologic progression or development of cholangiocarcinoma for standard or high dose UDCA [92, 98] and therefore, high dose UDCA is not used in routine clinical practice.

Antibiotics are used in patients with biliary sepsis in the background of PSC and some clinicians used rotating antibiotics in patients with resistant bacteremia. Published data looking into vancomycin or metronidazole treatment suggests that both are efficient in treatment of infection but vancomycin achieved improvement in ALT more than metronidazole with less side effects [99]. A recent randomised pilot study of vancomycin or metronidazole treatment in PSC patients showed that both antibiotics are effective although only vancomycin group reached the primary end point of reduction in ALP at 12 weeks [99].

10.2. Future therapies

There are many ongoing clinical trials in PSC such as obeticholic acid, mitomycin, thalidomide, LUM001: an Apical Sodium-dependent Bile Acid Transporter Inhibitor (ASBTi), GS-6624: a Monoclonal Antibody against Lysyl Oxidase like 2 (LOXL2), Xifaxan, Cladribine and the combination of UDCA and all trans-retinoid acid (ATRA) (www.clnicaltrial.gov). There are ongoing phase 1 and 2 trials on anti-fibrotic therapies in PSC.

11. Overlap syndrome

The term 'overlap syndrome' described co-existence of AIH with features of PBC or PSC [12]. The diagnosis can be challenging and there is no single test available to diagnose. Therefore, it is important to revisit clinical history or repeat investigation if there is in doubt with the diagnosis. The diagnosis can be made with combination of tests such as blood biochemistry, immunology with addition of radiology and tissue biopsy. It is assumed that overlap syndrome can be found in 5-20% of cases [12].

11.1. AIH/PBC overlap

AIH/PBC should be considered in patients with mixed pattern of cholestastic and hepatitis features or anyone with suboptimal response to immunosuppressions. It has been reported that AIH/PC occurs in 8% of patients with either AIH or PBC. Some PBC patients express negative AMA with positive ANA serology or SMA serology and hence, diagnosis based on immunology alone can be tricky. In general, IgG elevation is common in AIH and IgM is manly observed in PBC. Treatment should be targeted both AIH and PBC in these patients.

11.2. AIH/PSC overlap

In adults with both AIH and IBD, cholangiographic changes suggestive of PSC are present in up to 44% patients and may affect therapy and prognosis [13]. Those who develop AIH during childhood or Autoimmune sclerosing cholangitis are most common to develop into AIH/PSC overlap. MRCP and repeat liver biopsy is recommended. Treatment should be directed towards PSC and immunosuppression should be slowly weaned off unless they are indicated for inflammatory bowel disease.

12. Liver Transplantation (LT)

Liver transplantation (LT) is the treatment for patients with end stage AIH, PBC or PSC disease. The common indications are decompensated liver cirrhosis as indicated by the presence of refractory or resistant ascites, hepatic encephalopathy or uncontrolled variceal bleeding. Hepatocellular carcinoma, hepatopulmonary syndrome and portopulmonary hypertension are the other indications for LT. Model for End Stage Liver Disease (MELD) score is calculated by using renal function (Creatinine), International Normalised ratio (INR) and Bilirubin. MELD score= [0.957x Log_e (creatinine in mg/dL) + 0.378x Log_e (bilirubin in mg/dL) + 1.120x Log_e (INR) + 0.643) [133]. Patients with MELD score of above 16 with other indication is considered for liver transplant assessment. MELD score was initially developed to predict survival in patients undergoing Trans jugular Porto systemic shunt [100, 101]. In 2002, UNOS (the United Network of Organ Sharing) adapted a new approach to allocate organ giving priority to the sickest patient and the assessment is based on MELD score [102]. Implementation of MELD in 2002 led to an immediate reduction in LT waiting list registrations for the first time in history of LT (12% decrease in 2002) [103] as well as reduction in mortality on the waiting list [104].

Since 1996, listing for transplantation in the United Kingdom was based on the following principles: selecting patients if the expected survival without transplantation was 1 year or less or liver disease that was associated with an unacceptable quality of life and expecting that patients would have an at least 50% survival at 5 years with acceptable quality of life [105]. Serum sodium was associated with a higher risk of mortality independent of the MELD score in patients listed for orthotropic liver transplantation [106]. In United Kingdom, UKLED score (United Kingdom End Stage Liver Disease has been used since 2008 and it is calculated from patient's INR, serum creatinine, serum bilirubin and serum sodium) has been used in assessment of liver transplantation. UKELD score of 49 is the baseline entry criteria for LT assessment. Patients with UKELD score of 49 have 9% one year mortality and score above 60 has mortality of 50% [105].

LT is required in about 10% of patients with AIH and in Europe; 4-6 % of LT are for the indication of AIH [2, 7]. Long-term survival is excellent in AIH patients with 5 year survival being up to 92 % [2]. Recurrence of AIH can occur post LT and the rate of recurrence is between 8-12 % at year 1 and higher after 5 years follow up with the rate of around 36-65% [107]. The treatment should be either increase with the ongoing immunosuppressive therapies or change to alternative therapies such as addition of MMF, replacement of tacrolimus with cyclosporine or the replacement of calcineurin inhibitor (CNI) with sirolimus [108].

In patients with PBC, LT is indicated for decompensated liver cirrhosis, hepatocellular carcinoma and intractable pruritus with unacceptable quality of life. Patient should be referred for LT assessment when the bilirubin reaches around 100 umol/L with MELD >12 and Mayo risk score of 7-8 [134]. PBC can recur in post LT and the median time is 3 to 5.5 years although it can happen within the first year of transplantation [108]. PBC recurs in 15 to 30% of patients after LT and most of the patients do not lose their graft [67]. The treatment of recurrence PBC is UDCA, which causes improvement with ALP and ALT but not the patient or graft survival [109].

In addition to above mentioned indication for LT, some patients with PSC will need LT due to intractable pruritus, recurrent cholangitis in the presence of dominant bile duct strictures that cannot be managed endoscopically and the presence of limited stage cholangiocarcinoma [108]. 5 year survival post LT is around 80%[92]. Recurrence of PSC have been documented among LT recipients and its prevalence ranges from 15 to 30% and the median time for recurrence is between 3 and 5 years post LT [108] and can be associated with poor survival and graft loss [67].

13. De novo autoimmune hepatitis post LT

De novo autoimmune hepatitis (d-AIH) in LT patients whom were transplanted for other reasons than AIH was documented in late 1990 [110]. De novo autoimmune hepatitis occurs in 1-7 % of patients 0.1-9 years after transplantation, especially in children [135]. Risk factors for de novo-AIH had been associated with older age donor, female donor, acute cellular rejection and the use of tacrolimus [111, 112]. The disease is usually characterized by features of acute hepatitis in otherwise stable transplant recipients. The characteristic feature is a marked hypergammaglobulinaemia with positive ANA. Antibodies against glutathione S-transferase T1 (GSTT1) has been reported in patients with de novo immune hepatitis following liver transplantation, thus suggesting that immune system recognizes the Glutathione S-transferase theta-1 (GSTT1) protein as a non-self-antigen, and mount an allo-reactive immune response and molecular mimicries that override self-tolerance[113]. Antibodies against cytokeratin 8/18 in patient with de novo autoimmune hepatitis after living-donor liver transplantation had also been reported thus the changes in cytokeratin 8/18 in hepatocytes might be one of the sources of pathogenesis of de novo autoimmune hepatitis after liver transplantation[114]. A histologic pattern of centri-lobular injury including increased necroinflammatory activity and increased plasma cell infiltration correlates with measurements of autoimmunity in de novo AIH recipients [115]. Treatment with increased dose of steroids or Azathioprine results in an improved outcome. However, maintenance therapy is usually required [116]. Standard liver tests do not reflect the extent of these changes, so protocol liver biopsies may be required to detect these changes [117].

14. Pregnancy and AILD

Pregnancy constitutes a major challenge to the maternal immune system. AIH tends to improve after the second trimester of pregnancy, allowing a decrease in immunosuppressive therapy. It is due to a variety of immunological alterations that are induced by pregnancy in order to protect the semi-allogeneic fetus from rejection. Immuno-regulation induced by pregnancy polarizes the immune system to T-Helper (TH)-2 predominant phenotype. The increase of circulating inhibitors of pro-inflammatory cytokines occurring in pregnancy could act as a potent anti-inflammatory agent in AIH. T regulatory (Treg) cells are a recently discovered subset of T-lymphocytes with potent suppressive activity and pivotal roles in curtailing destructive immune responses and preventing autoimmune disease[118]. Systemic expansion of the maternal T suppressor or CD4+CD25+ regulatory T cell pool during pregnancy suppress an aggressive allogeneic response directed against the fetus[119].

Premature birth is the greatest risk and fetal mortality is reported to be around 21%, perinatal mortality is 4% and maternal mortality is 3% [14]. Poor disease control in the year prior to pregnancy and the absence of drug therapy are associated with poor outcomes [120]. Adverse pregnancy outcomes were highly associated with the presence of antibodies against soluble liver antigen/liver-pancreas (SLA/LP) and Ro/SSA [121] Preconception advice and discussion is important and should be emphasised. More than half of the women reduced or stopped the immune suppression during pregnancy or breastfeeding. AZA is a Food and Drug Administration (FDA) category D drug and safety in pregnancy has not been well established in human studies [14] however, current pharmacological treatment including azathioprine appears to be safe during pregnancy and lactation. There are no reported increased in congenital malformations with AZA and it is safe to use in mother who plan to breast-feed the baby. AIH commonly exacerbates following delivery [122, 123] and therefore, vigilance is required during the postpartum period. Patients with AIH need to be monitored carefully during pregnancy and for several months post partum [124]. Women with advance cirrhosis and portal hypertension have an increased risk of variceal bleed during the pregnancy and therefore, eradication of varices either with banding or pharmaco-therapy are recommended prior to conception. Pregnant women with cirrhosis and portal hypertension should undergo upper GI endoscopy during the second trimester and careful discussion with obstetric team and fetal medicine team is required for the safety of mother and the baby.

There are limited data for pregnancy and PBC. It has been noted that early diagnosis of PBC and early used of UDCA have a favourable outcomes on the pregnancy [125]. PSC rarely occur in female but the condition does not seem to reduce fertility in both men and women according to case series [126].

15. Conclusion

AILD is a spectrum of autoimmune condition mainly affecting liver (in the case of AIH) and biliary system (in PBC and PSC). The diagnosis is guided by clinical, biochemical and immunological parameters, although liver biopsy is still useful especially in patients with AIH to diagnose as well as for the assessment and monitoring of the disease status. In AIH, the aim of the treatment is to suppress the immune system with long term immunosuppressive medications such as azathioprine. There are new therapies emerging on the horizon. In PBC, women are more affected and the current treatment used is UDCA although there are many trials running ongoing in the treatment of PBC and it is an exciting era. For PSC, the definitive treatment is liver transplantation and more research is needed to understand that pathogenesis and treatment in this field of subject.

Acknowledgements

The histology slides were kindly provided by Professor Stefan Hubscher, Liver Histology Department, University Hospital Birmingham NHS Trust, Birmingham, UK. N.N.T is funded by National Institute for Health Research (NIHR) and Y.H. O is funded by Medical research council (MRC).

Author details

Nwe Ni Than[1,2] and Ye Htun Oo[1,2*]

*Address all correspondence to: y.h.oo@bham.ac.uk

1 Centre for Liver Research and NIHR BRU, University of Birmingham, UK

2 University Hospital Birmingham NHS Trust, UK

References

[1] Wang, P. and S.G. Zheng, *Regulatory T cells and B cells: implication on autoimmune diseases.* Int J Clin Exp Pathol, 2013. 6(12): p. 2668-74.

[2] Strassburg, C.P. and M.P. Manns, *Therapy of autoimmune hepatitis.* Best Pract Res Clin Gastroenterol, 2011. 25(6): p. 673-87.

[3] T Zolfino, M.A.H., S Norris, P M Harrison, B C Portmann, I G McFarlane, *Characteristics of autoimmune hepatitis in patients who are not of European Caucasoid ethnic origin.* Gut, 2002. 50: p. 713-717.

[4] Zachou, K., et al., *Review article: autoimmune hepatitis -- current management and challenges.* Alimentary pharmacology & therapeutics, 2013. 38(8): p. 887-913.

[5] Blachier, M., et al., *The burden of liver disease in Europe: a review of available epidemiological data.* J Hepatol, 2013. 58(3): p. 593-608.

[6] Lim, K.N., et al., *Autoimmune hepatitis in African Americans: presenting features and response to therapy.* Am J Gastroenterol, 2001. 96(12): p. 3390-3394.

[7] Wong, R.J., et al., *The impact of race/ethnicity on the clinical epidemiology of autoimmune hepatitis.* J Clin Gastroenterol, 2012. 46(2): p. 155-61.

[8] Hurlburt, K.J., et al., *Prevalence of autoimmune liver disease in Alaska Natives.* Am J Gastroenterol, 2002. 97(9): p. 2402-7.

[9] Manns, M.P., et al., *Major antigen of liver kidney microsomal autoantibodies in idiopathic autoimmune hepatitis is cytochrome P450db1.* J Clin Invest, 1989. 83(3): p. 1066-72.

[10] Manns, M.P., et al., *LKM-1 autoantibodies recognize a short linear sequence in P450IID6, a cytochrome P-450 monooxygenase.* J Clin Invest, 1991. 88(4): p. 1370-8.

[11] Strassburg, C.P., et al., *Autoantibodies against glucuronosyltransferases differ between viral hepatitis and autoimmune hepatitis.* Gastroenterology, 1996. 111(6): p. 1576-86.

[12] Trivedi, P.J. and G.M. Hirschfield, *Review article: overlap syndromes and autoimmune liver disease.* Aliment Pharmacol Ther, 2012. 36(6): p. 517-33.

[13] Makol, A., K.D. Watt, and V.R. Chowdhary, *Autoimmune hepatitis: a review of current diagnosis and treatment.* Hepatitis research and treatment, 2011. 2011: p. 390916.

[14] Liberal, R., et al., *Autoimmune hepatitis: A comprehensive review.* Journal of Autoimmunity, 2013. 41(0): p. 126-139.

[15] Czaja, A.J., *Drug-induced autoimmune-like hepatitis.* Dig Dis Sci, 2011. 56(4): p. 958-76.

[16] Oo, Y., S. Hubscher, and D. Adams, *Autoimmune hepatitis: new paradigms in the pathogenesis, diagnosis, and management.* Hepatology International, 2010. 4(2): p. 475-493.

[17] Muratori, L. and M.S. Longhi, *The interplay between regulatory and effector T cells in autoimmune hepatitis: Implications for innovative treatment strategies.* J Autoimmun, 2013. 46: p. 74-80.

[18] Sakaguchi, S., et al., *Immunologic self-tolerance maintained by activated T cells expressing IL-2 receptor alpha-chains (CD25). Breakdown of a single mechanism of self-tolerance causes various autoimmune diseases.* J.Immunol., 1995. 155(3): p. 1151-1164.

[19] Oo, Y.H., et al., *Distinct roles for CCR4 and CXCR3 in the recruitment and positioning of regulatory T cells in the inflamed human liver.* Journal of immunology, 2010. 184(6): p. 2886-98.

[20] Longhi, M.S., et al., *Impairment of CD4(+)CD25(+) regulatory T-cells in autoimmune liver disease.* Journal of Hepatology, 2004. 41(1): p. 31-37.

[21] Verma, S., M. Torbenson, and P.J. Thuluvath, *The impact of ethnicity on the natural history of autoimmune hepatitis.* Hepatology, 2007. 46(6): p. 1828-35.

[22] de Boer, Y.S., et al., *Genome-wide association study identifies variants associated with autoimmune hepatitis type 1.* Gastroenterology, 2014. 147(2): p. 443-52.e5.

[23] Liberal, R., et al., *Diagnostic criteria of autoimmune hepatitis.* Autoimmun Rev, 2014. 13(4-5): p. 435-40.

[24] Chen, J., G.D. Eslick, and M. Weltman, *Systematic review with meta-analysis: clinical manifestations and management of autoimmune hepatitis in the elderly.* Aliment Pharmacol Ther, 2014. 39(2): p. 117-24.

[25] Al-Chalabi, T., et al., *Impact of gender on the long-term outcome and survival of patients with autoimmune hepatitis.* Journal of Hepatology, 2008. 48(1): p. 140-147.

[26] Al-Chalabi, T., et al., *Impact of gender on the long-term outcome and survival of patients with autoimmune hepatitis.* J Hepatol, 2008. 48(1): p. 140-7.

[27] Feld, J.J., et al., *Autoimmune hepatitis: effect of symptoms and cirrhosis on natural history and outcome.* Hepatology, 2005. 42(1): p. 53-62.

[28] Panayi, V., et al., *The natural history of autoimmune hepatitis presenting with jaundice.* Eur J Gastroenterol Hepatol, 2014. 26(6): p. 640-5.

[29] Montano-Loza, A.J., et al., *Prognostic implications of antibodies to Ro/SSA and soluble liver antigen in type 1 autoimmune hepatitis.* Liver Int, 2012. 32(1): p. 85-92.

[30] Czaja, A.J., P.T. Donaldson, and A.W. Lohse, *Antibodies to soluble liver antigen/liver pancreas and HLA risk factors for type 1 autoimmune hepatitis.* Am J Gastroenterol, 2002. 97(2): p. 413-9.

[31] Manns, M.P., et al., *Diagnosis and management of autoimmune hepatitis.* Hepatology, 2010. 51(6): p. 2193-2213.

[32] Alvarez, F., et al., *International Autoimmune Hepatitis Group Report: review of criteria for diagnosis of autoimmune hepatitis.* J Hepatol, 1999. 31(5): p. 929-38.

[33] Chandok, N., M.G. Silveira, and K.D. Lindor, *Comparing the simplified and international autoimmune hepatitis group criteria in primary sclerosing cholangitis.* Gastroenterol Hepatol (N Y), 2010. 6(2): p. 108-12.

[34] Yeoman, A.D., M.S. Longhi, and M.A. Heneghan, *Review article: the modern management of autoimmune hepatitis.* Aliment Pharmacol Ther, 2010. 31(8): p. 771-87.

[35] Fernandes, N.F., et al., *Cyclosporine therapy in patients with steroid resistant autoimmune hepatitis.* Am J Gastroenterol, 1999. 94(1): p. 241-8.

[36] Sciveres, M., et al., *Effectiveness and safety of ciclosporin as therapy for autoimmune diseases of the liver in children and adolescents.* Aliment Pharmacol Ther, 2004. 19(2): p. 209-17.

[37] Van Thiel, D.H., et al., *Tacrolimus: a potential new treatment for autoimmune chronic active hepatitis: results of an open-label preliminary trial.* Am J Gastroenterol, 1995. 90(5): p. 771-6.

[38] Zachou, K., et al., *Mycophenolate for the treatment of autoimmune hepatitis: prospective assessment of its efficacy and safety for induction and maintenance of remission in a large cohort of treatment-naive patients.* J Hepatol, 2011. 55(3): p. 636-46.

[39] Chatur, N., et al., *Transplant immunosuppressive agents in non-transplant chronic autoimmune hepatitis: the Canadian association for the study of liver (CASL) experience with mycophenolate mofetil and tacrolimus.* Liver Int, 2005. 25(4): p. 723-7.

[40] Hennes, E.M., et al., *Mycophenolate mofetil as second line therapy in autoimmune hepatitis?* Am J Gastroenterol, 2008. 103(12): p. 3063-70.

[41] Weiler-Normann, C., et al., *Infliximab as a rescue treatment in difficult-to-treat autoimmune hepatitis.* J Hepatol, 2013. 58(3): p. 529-34.

[42] Casal Moura, M., et al., *Management of autoimmune hepatitis: Focus on pharmacologic treatments beyond corticosteroids.* World J Hepatol, 2014. 6(6): p. 410-8.

[43] D'Agostino, D., A. Costaguta, and F. Alvarez, *Successful treatment of refractory autoimmune hepatitis with rituximab.* Pediatrics, 2013. 132(2): p. e526-30.

[44] Fernandez-Nebro, A., et al., *Multicenter longitudinal study of B-lymphocyte depletion in refractory systemic lupus erythematosus: the LESIMAB study.* Lupus, 2012. 21(10): p. 1063-76.

[45] Ferri, C., et al., *Treatment with rituximab in patients with mixed cryoglobulinemia syndrome: results of multicenter cohort study and review of the literature.* Autoimmun Rev, 2011. 11(1): p. 48-55.

[46] Penalver, F.J., et al., *Rituximab is an effective and safe therapeutic alternative in adults with refractory and severe autoimmune hemolytic anemia.* Ann Hematol, 2010. 89(11): p. 1073-80.

[47] Burak, K.W., et al., *Rituximab for the treatment of patients with autoimmune hepatitis who are refractory or intolerant to standard therapy.* Can J Gastroenterol, 2013. 27(5): p. 273-80.

[48] Cook, G.C., R. Mulligan, and S. Sherlock, *Controlled prospective trial of corticosteroid therapy in active chronic hepatitis.* Q J Med, 1971. 40(158): p. 159-85.

[49] Kirk, A.P., et al., *Late results of the Royal Free Hospital prospective controlled trial of prednisolone therapy in hepatitis B surface antigen negative chronic active hepatitis.* Gut, 1980. 21(1): p. 78-83.

[50] Heneghan, M.A., et al., *Autoimmune hepatitis.* The Lancet. 382(9902): p. 1433-1444.

[51] Miyake, Y., et al., *Clinical characteristics of fulminant-type autoimmune hepatitis: an analysis of eleven cases.* Aliment Pharmacol Ther, 2006. 23(9): p. 1347-53.

[52] Schvarcz, R., H. Glaumann, and O. Weiland, *Survival and histological resolution of fibrosis in patients with autoimmune chronic active hepatitis.* J Hepatol, 1993. 18(1): p. 15-23.

[53] Kanzler, S., et al., *Duration of immunosuppressive therapy in autoimmune hepatitis.* J Hepatol, 2001. 34(2): p. 354-5.

[54] Montano-Loza, A.J., H.A. Carpenter, and A.J. Czaja, *Predictive factors for hepatocellular carcinoma in type 1 autoimmune hepatitis.* Am J Gastroenterol, 2008. 103(8): p. 1944-51.

[55] Yeoman, A.D., et al., *Evaluation of risk factors in the development of hepatocellular carcinoma in autoimmune hepatitis: Implications for follow-up and screening.* Hepatology, 2008. 48(3): p. 863-70.

[56] Duclos-Vallee, J.C., et al., *A 10 year follow up study of patients transplanted for autoimmune hepatitis: histological recurrence precedes clinical and biochemical recurrence.* Gut, 2003. 52(6): p. 893-7.

[57] Roberts, M.S., et al., *Survival after liver transplantation in the United States: a disease-specific analysis of the UNOS database.* Liver Transpl, 2004. 10(7): p. 886-97.

[58] Bowlus, C.L. and M.E. Gershwin, *The diagnosis of primary biliary cirrhosis.* Autoimmun Rev, 2014. 13(4-5): p. 441-4.

[59] Hirschfield, G.M. and P. Invernizzi, *Progress in the genetics of primary biliary cirrhosis.* Semin Liver Dis, 2011. 31(2): p. 147-56.

[60] Selmi, C., et al., *Genomic variants associated with primary biliary cirrhosis.* Genome Med, 2010. 2(1): p. 5.

[61] Czaja, A.J., et al., *Clinical distinctions and pathogenic implications of type 1 autoimmune hepatitis in Brazil and the United States.* J Hepatol, 2002. 37(3): p. 302-8.

[62] Ray-Chaudhuri, D., et al. *Epidemiology of primary biliary cirhosis (PBC) in Sheffield updated: Demographics and relationship to water supply.* in *HEPATOLOGY.* 2001. WB SAUNDERS CO INDEPENDENCE SQUARE WEST CURTIS CENTER, STE 300, PHILADELPHIA, PA 19106-3399 USA.

[63] James, O.F., et al., *Primary biliary cirrhosis once rare, now common in the United Kingdom?* Hepatology, 1999. 30(2): p. 390-4.

[64] Myszor, M. and O.F. James, *The epidemiology of primary biliary cirrhosis in north-east England: an increasingly common disease?* Q J Med, 1990. 75(276): p. 377-85.

[65] Lindor, K.D., et al., *Primary biliary cirrhosis.* Hepatology, 2009. 50(1): p. 291-308.

[66] *EASL Clinical Practice Guidelines: management of cholestatic liver diseases.* J Hepatol, 2009. 51(2): p. 237-67.

[67] Zein, C.O. and K.D. Lindor, *Latest and emerging therapies for primary biliary cirrhosis and primary sclerosing cholangitis.* Curr Gastroenterol Rep, 2010. 12(1): p. 13-22.

[68] Bogdanos, D.P. and L. Komorowski, *Disease-specific autoantibodies in primary biliary cirrhosis.* Clin Chim Acta, 2011. 412(7-8): p. 502-12.

[69] Corpechot, C., et al., *Biochemical response to ursodeoxycholic acid and long-term prognosis in primary biliary cirrhosis.* Hepatology, 2008. 48(3): p. 871-7.

[70] Paumgartner, G. and U. Beuers, *Ursodeoxycholic acid in cholestatic liver disease: mechanisms of action and therapeutic use revisited.* Hepatology, 2002. 36(3): p. 525-31.

[71] Jones, D.E. and J.L. Newton, *An open study of modafinil for the treatment of daytime somnolence and fatigue in primary biliary cirrhosis.* Aliment Pharmacol Ther, 2007. 25(4): p. 471-6.

[72] Mason, A.L., et al., *Clinical Trial: Randomized controlled trial of zidovudine and lamivudine for patients with primary biliary cirrhosis stabilized on ursodiol.* Aliment Pharmacol Ther, 2008.

[73] Levy, C., et al., *Pilot study: fenofibrate for patients with primary biliary cirrhosis and an incomplete response to ursodeoxycholic acid.* Aliment Pharmacol Ther, 2011. 33(2): p. 235-42.

[74] Silveira, M.G. and K.D. Lindor, *Obeticholic acid and budesonide for the treatment of primary biliary cirrhosis.* Expert Opin Pharmacother, 2014. 15(3): p. 365-72.

[75] Parés, A., *Treatment of primary biliary cirrhosis: Is there more to offer than ursodeoxycholic acid?* Clinical Liver Disease, 2014. 3(2): p. 29-33.

[76] Kuiper, E.M., et al., *Improved prognosis of patients with primary biliary cirrhosis that have a biochemical response to ursodeoxycholic acid.* Gastroenterology, 2009. 136(4): p. 1281-1287.

[77] Poupon, R., *Primary biliary cirrhosis: A 2010 update.* Journal of Hepatology, 2010. 52(5): p. 745-758.

[78] Karlsen, T.H., E. Schrumpf, and K.M. Boberg, *Update on primary sclerosing cholangitis.* Digestive and Liver Disease, 2010. 42(6): p. 390-400.

[79] Yimam, K.K. and C.L. Bowlus, *Diagnosis and classification of primary sclerosing cholangitis.* Autoimmun Rev, 2014. 13(4-5): p. 445-50.

[80] Eaton, J.E., et al., *Pathogenesis of primary sclerosing cholangitis and advances in diagnosis and management.* Gastroenterology, 2013. 145(3): p. 521-36.

[81] Card, T.R., M. Solaymani-Dodaran, and J. West, *Incidence and mortality of primary sclerosing cholangitis in the UK: a population-based cohort study.* J Hepatol, 2008. 48(6): p. 939-44.

[82] Tabibian, J.H., S.P. O'Hara, and N.F. Larusso, *Primary sclerosing cholangitis: the gut-liver axis.* Clinical gastroenterology and hepatology : the official clinical practice journal of the American Gastroenterological Association, 2012. 10(7): p. 819; author reply 819-20.

[83] Hirschfield, G.M., et al., *Primary sclerosing cholangitis.* Lancet, 2013. 382(9904): p. 1587-99.

[84] Henriksen, E.K., E. Melum, and T.H. Karlsen, *Update on primary sclerosing cholangitis genetics.* Current opinion in gastroenterology, 2014. 30(3): p. 310-9.

[85] Karlsen, T.H. and K.M. Boberg, *Update on primary sclerosing cholangitis.* Journal of hepatology, 2013. 59(3): p. 571-82.

[86] Tabibian, J.H., S.P. O'Hara, and K.D. Lindor, *Primary sclerosing cholangitis and the microbiota: current knowledge and perspectives on etiopathogenesis and emerging therapies.* Scandinavian journal of gastroenterology, 2014. 49(8): p. 901-8.

[87] Eksteen, B., et al., *Hepatic endothelial CCL25 mediates the recruitment of CCR9+ gut-homing lymphocytes to the liver in primary sclerosing cholangitis.* J Exp Med, 2004. 200(11): p. 1511-7.

[88] Eksteen, B., et al., *Hepatic endothelial CCL25 mediates the recruitment of CCR9+ gut-homing lymphocytes to the liver in primary sclerosing cholangitis.* The Journal of experimental medicine, 2004. 200(11): p. 1511-7.

[89] Berglin, L., et al., *In Situ Characterization of Intrahepatic Non-Parenchymal Cells in PSC Reveals Phenotypic Patterns Associated with Disease Severity.* PloS one, 2014. 9(8): p. e105375.

[90] Tabibian, J.H., J.A. Talwalkar, and K.D. Lindor, *Role of the microbiota and antibiotics in primary sclerosing cholangitis.* Biomed Res Int, 2013. 2013: p. 389537.

[91] Chapman, R., et al., *Diagnosis and management of primary sclerosing cholangitis.* Hepatology, 2010. 51(2): p. 660-78.

[92] Eaton, J.E. and J.A. Talwalkar, *Primary Sclerosing Cholangitis: Current and Future Management Strategies.* Curr Hepat Rep, 2013. 12(1): p. 28-36.

[93] Beuers, U., et al., *Ursodeoxycholic acid for treatment of primary sclerosing cholangitis: a placebo-controlled trial.* Hepatology, 1992. 16(3): p. 707-14.

[94] Lindor, K.D., *Ursodiol for primary sclerosing cholangitis. Mayo Primary Sclerosing Cholangitis-Ursodeoxycholic Acid Study Group.* N Engl J Med, 1997. 336(10): p. 691-5.

[95] Olsson, R., et al., *High-dose ursodeoxycholic acid in primary sclerosing cholangitis: a 5-year multicenter, randomized, controlled study.* Gastroenterology, 2005. 129(5): p. 1464-72.

[96] Lindor, K.D., et al., *High-dose ursodeoxycholic acid for the treatment of primary sclerosing cholangitis.* Hepatology, 2009. 50(3): p. 808-14.

[97] Imam, M.H., et al., *High-dose ursodeoxycholic acid increases risk of adverse outcomes in patients with early stage primary sclerosing cholangitis.* Aliment Pharmacol Ther, 2011. 34(10): p. 1185-92.

[98] Triantos, C.K., et al., *Meta-analysis: ursodeoxycholic acid for primary sclerosing cholangitis.* Aliment Pharmacol Ther, 2011. 34(8): p. 901-10.

[99] Tabibian, J.H., et al., *Randomised clinical trial: vancomycin or metronidazole in patients with primary sclerosing cholangitis - a pilot study.* Aliment Pharmacol Ther, 2013. 37(6): p. 604-12.

[100] Malinchoc, M., et al., *A model to predict poor survival in patients undergoing transjugular intrahepatic portosystemic shunts.* Hepatology, 2000. 31(4): p. 864-71.

[101] Kamath, P.S., et al., *A model to predict survival in patients with end-stage liver disease.* Hepatology, 2001. 33(2): p. 464-70.

[102] Neuberger, J., *Allocation of donor livers — is MELD enough?* Liver Transplantation, 2004. 10(7): p. 908-910.

[103] Wiesner, R., et al., *Model for end-stage liver disease (MELD) and allocation of donor livers.* Gastroenterology, 2003. 124(1): p. 91-6.

[104] Biggins, S.W. and K. Bambha, *MELD-based liver allocation: who is underserved?* Semin Liver Dis, 2006. 26(3): p. 211-20.

[105] Neuberger, J., et al., *Selection of patients for liver transplantation and allocation of donated livers in the UK.* Gut, 2008. 57(2): p. 252-7.

[106] Kim, W.R., et al., *Hyponatremia and mortality among patients on the liver-transplant waiting list.* N Engl J Med, 2008. 359(10): p. 1018-26.

[107] Czaja, A.J., *Diagnosis, pathogenesis, and treatment of autoimmune hepatitis after liver transplantation.* Digestive diseases and sciences, 2012. 57(9): p. 2248-66.

[108] Liberal, R., et al., *Liver transplantation and autoimmune liver diseases.* Liver Transpl, 2013. 19(10): p. 1065-77.

[109] Charatcharoenwitthaya, P., et al., *Long-term survival and impact of ursodeoxycholic acid treatment for recurrent primary biliary cirrhosis after liver transplantation.* Liver Transpl, 2007. 13(9): p. 1236-45.

[110] Kerkar, N., et al., *De-novo autoimmune hepatitis after liver transplantation.* Lancet., 1998. 351(9100): p. 409-413.

[111] Miyagawa-Hayashino, A., et al., *Outcome and risk factors of de novo autoimmune hepatitis in living-donor liver transplantation.* Transplantation, 2004. 78(1): p. 128-35.

[112] Montano-Loza, A.J., et al., *Incidence and risk factors associated with de novo autoimmune hepatitis after liver transplantation.* Liver Int, 2012. 32(9): p. 1426-33.

[113] Aguilera, I., et al., *Antibodies against glutathione S-transferase T1 (GSTT1) in patients with de novo immune hepatitis following liver transplantation.* Clin.Exp.Immunol., 2001. 126(3): p. 535-539.

[114] Inui, A., et al., *Antibodies against cytokeratin 8/18 in a patient with de novo autoimmune hepatitis after living-donor liver transplantation.* Liver transplantation : official publication of the American Association for the Study of Liver Diseases and the International Liver Transplantation Society, 2005. 11(5): p. 504-7.

[115] Sebagh, M., et al., *Histologic findings predictive of a diagnosis of de novo autoimmune hepatitis after liver transplantation in adults.* Transplantation, 2013. 96(7): p. 670-8.

[116] Salcedo, M., et al., *Response to steroids in de novo autoimmune hepatitis after liver transplantation.* Hepatology., 2002. 35(2): p. 349-356.

[117] Syn, W.K., et al., *Natural history of unexplained chronic hepatitis after liver transplantation.* Liver Transpl., 2007. 13(7): p. 984-989.

[118] Oo, Y.H. and D.H. Adams, *Regulatory T cells and autoimmune hepatitis: what happens in the liver stays in the liver.* Journal of hepatology, 2014.

[119] Aluvihare, V.R., M. Kallikourdis, and A.G. Betz, *Regulatory T cells mediate maternal tolerance to the fetus.* Nat Immunol, 2004. 5(3): p. 266-271.

[120] Westbrook, R.H., et al., *Outcomes of pregnancy in women with autoimmune hepatitis.* Journal of autoimmunity, 2012. 38(2-3): p. J239-44.

[121] Schramm, C., et al., *Pregnancy in autoimmune hepatitis: outcome and risk factors.* American Journal of Gastroenterology, 2006. 101(3): p. 556-560.

[122] Samuel, D., et al., *Severe autoimmune hepatitis first presenting in the early post partum period.* Clinical gastroenterology and hepatology : the official clinical practice journal of the American Gastroenterological Association, 2004. 2(7): p. 622-4.

[123] Buchel, E., et al., *Improvement of autoimmune hepatitis during pregnancy followed by flare-up after delivery.* The American journal of gastroenterology, 2002. 97(12): p. 3160-5.

[124] Terrabuio, D.R., et al., *Follow-up of pregnant women with autoimmune hepatitis: the disease behavior along with maternal and fetal outcomes.* Journal of clinical gastroenterology, 2009. 43(4): p. 350-6.

[125] Hammoud, G.M., et al., Liver diseases in pregnancy: liver transplantation in pregnancy. World J Gastroenterol, 2013. 19(43): p. 7647-51.

[126] Wellge, B.E., et al., Pregnancy in primary sclerosing cholangitis. Gut, 2011. 60(8): p. 1117-21.

[127] Parés A, Caballería L, Rodés J. Excellent Long-Term Survival in Patients With Primary Biliary Cirrhosis and Biochemical Response to Ursodeoxycholic Acid. Gastroenterology. 2006;130(3):715-20.

[128] Corpechot C, Abenavoli L, Rabahi N, Chrétien Y, Andréani T, Johanet C, et al. Biochemical response to ursodeoxycholic acid and long-term prognosis in primary biliary cirrhosis. Hepatology. 2008;48(3):871-7.

[129] Corpechot C, Chazouillères O, Poupon R. Early primary biliary cirrhosis: biochemical response to treatment and prediction of long-term outcome. Journal of hepatology. 2011;55(6):1361-7.

[130] Kuiper EMM, Hansen BE, de Vries RA, den Ouden–Muller JW, van Ditzhuijsen TJM, Haagsma EB, et al. Improved Prognosis of Patients With Primary Biliary Cirrhosis That Have a Biochemical Response to Ursodeoxycholic Acid. Gastroenterology. 2009;136(4):1281-7.

[131] Kumagi T, Guindi M, Fischer SE, Arenovich T, Abdalian R, Coltescu C, et al. Baseline Ductopenia and Treatment Response Predict Long-Term Histological Progression in Primary Biliary Cirrhosis. Am J Gastroenterol. 2010;105(10):2186-94

[132] Wiesner RH, Grambsch PM, Dickson ER, Ludwig J, Maccarty RL, Hunter EB, et al. Primary sclerosing cholangitis: Natural history, prognostic factors and survival analysis. Hepatology. 1989;10(4):430-6.

[133] Malinchoc M, Kamath PS, Gordon FD, Peine CJ, Rank J, ter Borg PCJ. A model to predict poor survival in patients undergoing transjugular intrahepatic portosystemic shunts. Hepatology. 2000;31(4):864-71.

[134] European Association for the Study of the L. EASL Clinical Practice Guidelines: Management of cholestatic liver diseases. Journal of Hepatology. 2009;51(2):237-67.

[135] Czaja A. Diagnosis, Pathogenesis, and Treatment of Autoimmune Hepatitis After Liver Transplantation. Dig Dis Sci. 2012;57(9):2248-66.

Chapter 6

Celiac Disease and Other Autoimmune Disorders

M.I. Torres, T. Palomeque and P. Lorite

Additional information is available at the end of the chapter

http://dx.doi.org/10.5772/60695

1. Introduction

Celiac disease (CD) is an autoimmune condition affecting the small intestine, triggered by the ingestion of gluten, the protein fraction of wheat, barley, and rye. There is a strong linkage between CD and HLA-DQ2 and HLA-DQ8 haplotypes. As in other autoimmune diseases, CD results from of an immune response to self-antigens, leading to tissue destruction plus the production of autoantibodies and has a complex pattern of inheritance with influence from both environmental as well as additive and non-additive genetic factors [1, 2]

A significantly increased prevalence of other autoimmune diseases has been reported in individuals with CD and their first-degree relatives as compared to controls. This chapter provides an overview of the pathogenesis of CD and reviews the literature regarding associations between CD and other autoimmune diseases, including the potential effects of gluten-free diet therapy on the prevention or amelioration of associated diseases. It has been speculated that these associations might share a pathogenic basis that involves the same environmental triggers, genetic predisposition, compromise of the intestinal barrier secondary to the failure of tight junctions, leading to greater permeability of the intestine, and perhaps mechanisms yet to be identified [1, 2].

2. Autoimmune disorders

The decline in physiological tolerance against "self" antigens gives rise to autoimmune disorders. While various mechanisms might participate in this process, faulty regulation of B-cell and T-cell activation as well as of inflammation pathways are plausible [3]. Predisposition to autoimmune diseases has been related to genetic, epigenetic, and environmental factors. With modern genetic-analysis techniques, our grasp of autoimmunity is steadily improving.

To date, over 30 genome-wide association studies (GWAS) have examined an array of autoimmune diseases (AID) while studies have identified hundreds of common variants that represent protection or risk [4].

The genetic bases of autoimmunity are just starting to be uncovered, while several susceptibility genes have been identified in the most common autoimmune diseases. In addition, structural variants (insertion/ deletion polymorphisms, copy number variations, etc.) are also likely to play a significant role in determining susceptibility to autoimmune disorders [3-4].

Although on the genetic level, immune-related diseases still differ, e.g. in the number of disease-susceptibility loci, the effect sizes associated with each locus, and the environmental factors involved in the various diseases [5], there is clearly a remarkable overlap of susceptibility factors between various immune-related diseases [6-8]. The complex inheritance pattern implies the involvement of several genes. Despite that the same genes are unlikely to account for susceptibility to all autoimmune disorders, one gene complex (major histocompatibility complex, MHC, in the human leukocyte antigen, HLA) has invariably been involved as a key genetic risk factor and might explain why the autoimmune diseases co-exist [9].

This overlap clearly implies the involvement of shared pathways in multiple autoimmune diseases and, most importantly, suggests that general treatment modalities might be feasible for some immune-related diseases [9].

3. Celiac disease as an autoimmune disorder

Celiac disease (CD) is one of the best-understood immune-related diseases. CD is frequent with a prevalence of about 1:100, and it occurs selectively in individuals expressing HLA-DQ2 or HLA-DQ8. The prevalence of CD in the western world is probably underestimated, since not all cases of CD are symptomatic and thus go undiagnosed [1]. As in patients with organ-specific autoimmune disorders, patients with CD have autoantibodies and suffer from the destruction of a specific tissue-cell type by CD8+ T cells [2, 10]. The presence of highly disease-specific transglutaminase 2 (TG2)-specific autoantibodies allows the diagnosis of the disease. These autoimmune features require the presence of gluten, and HLA-DQ2- or HLA-DQ8-restricted gluten-specific CD4+ T-cell responses have a central role in disease pathogenesis [10, 11]. On the basis of CD, it bears considering that exogenous antigens may drive autoimmune disorders.

The pathogenesis of CD reveals a complex interplay between environmental factors, genetics, the adaptive and innate immune systems, and the presence of autoantigens, in a process which has still not been fully elucidated.

It is a multifactorial disease caused by many different genetic factors acting in concert with non-genetic causes. Similar to other autoimmune diseases, CD is a polygenic disorder for which the MHC locus is the single most important genetic factor. The MHC locus accounts for 40 to 50% of the genetic variance in the disease. A genetic association between CD and the HLA class II genes in the major histocompatibility complex (MHC) has been documented [12,

13]. Although the HLA component of CD susceptibility is well characterized, little is known about the possible role of other genes than HLA [14–16]. Recently, various non-MHC genes have been found to be susceptibility factors. To date, researchers have described 39 loci having 57 independent association signals [17]. Of these genes, many are associated with immunity, especially with T-cell and B-cell function. All these loci together account for an estimated 14% of all genetic variance of CD [17].

These non-HLA genes may be important determinants of disease susceptibility, as indirectly shown by the high disease concordance rate in monozygotic twins (70%) compared with only 30% in HLA identical twins [18]. Mounting evidence suggests a genetic relationship between the *CTLA4* locus and various autoimmune disorders. CTLA4-Ig blockage of T-cell activation may determine some (though not all) immunological aspects of human CD [19]. A French case-control study [20] reported evidence of association between CD and *CTLA4* exon 1 polymorphism. Also, significant evidence for linkage to CD was found in a recent study on family-based linkage of the *CTLA4* region, as well as 39UTR polymorphisms and exon 1 [21].

More than 60% of CD-associated susceptibility loci are shared with at least another autoimmune condition such as type-1 diabetes and rheumatoid arthritis [22], suggesting common pathogenic mechanisms. In particular, the recognition of peptides by HLA molecules, posttranslational modifications required for optimal peptide binding, and immune mechanisms leading to tissue damage have been found [23].

One of the most important factors triggering CD is dietary gluten, a storage protein present in wheat and related grains (hordein in barley, secalin in rye, and avedin in oats). CD is an excellent model for studying the contribution of genetic factors to immune-related disorders because: (1) the environmental triggering factor is known (gluten); (2) as in other autoimmune diseases, in which specific HLA types (HLADQA1 and HLA-DQB1 are critically involved; (3) there is involvement of non-HLA disease-susceptibility loci, many of which are shared with other autoimmune diseases; (4) there is an elevated incidence of other immune-related diseases both in family members and individuals; and (5) both the innate and the adaptive immune responses play a role in CD [24, 25].

The tendency for multiple autoimmune disorders to occur over the lifetime of a CD patient has been well described. The co-existence of autoimmune diseases with CD is striking, and there is an association of the disease with type-1 diabetes, Sjögren's syndrome, autoimmune thyroid disorders, connective-tissue diseases and IgA deficiency. The role of protein complexes formed between exogenous and endogenous proteins in the formation of autoantibodies, and a CD8+ T cell response directed against altered-self and mediated by NK receptors in CD is an autoimmune reaction [8].

3.1. Pathogenesis

The main factors in CD pathogenesis include defective antigen processing by epithelial cells, along with the intrinsic properties of gliadins in addition to the individual's HLA-DQ haplotype [26]. This disorder is closely related to HLA class-II genes which map to the DQ locus. CD has been associated with the expression of both HLA-DQ2 and HLA-DQ8 expression

[27, 28]. A number of studies [29] have shown that most CD patients carry DQ2 (DQA1*05/DQB1*02), while the rest display an association with DQ8 (DQA1*0301/DQB1*0302). These HLA genes collectively represent as much as 50% of the genetic risk of developing CD. Studies on independent genome-wide linkage have found scant overlap among linkage regions, except for the HLA region on chromosome 6p21. According to linkage studies, besides the HLA region, the two likeliest regions are 19p13 and 5q32 [30-32].

The polymorphisms associated with autoimmune diseases appear to be primarily in genes that have immune functions. These polymorphisms have presumably evolved for their advantages in combating pathogens. These polymorphisms, in the presence of foreign antigen gluten, may also help shape the immune response [33].

Gliadin peptide presentation and T-cell activation are critical events in the pathogenesis of CD. The toxic effects of these prolamins include the reduction of F-actin, inhibition of cell growth, premature cell death, the rearrangement of the cytoskeleton, and increased small-intestine permeability [34].

Gastric, intestinal, and pancreatic enzymes do not fully digest gluten peptides in individuals with CD. In these patients, a 33-mer peptide which has been isolated and has been identified as being the prime trigger of inflammation in reaction to gluten [35]. This peptide reacts with tissue transglutaminase (tTG), which is the main CD autoantigen, by which specific glutamine residues of gluten are deamidated to glutamic acid. [12, 36]. Antigen-presenting cells that express molecules of HLA-DQ2 and HLA-DQ8 show greater affinity for deamidated peptides. Afterwards, as the immunogenic peptides generated bind to HLA molecules, peptide complexes form and are capable of activating host-gluten-specific CD4+ T cells found in the lamina propria. When these T cells are activated, a number of cytokines are produced, in turn promoting inflammation and damage to the small-intestine villi from metalloproteinases released by inflammatory cells and fibroblasts [35, 29]. Activated gluten-specific CD4+ T cells are also capable of stimulating B cells to produce anti-gluten and anti-TG2 antibodies. It is believed that the IFN-gamma production from these gluten-specific T cells may be the main cause of mucosal intestinal lesion [35, 12]. Furthermore, shifts in intestinal permeability, secondary to changes in tight junctions or in food-antigen processing, have recently been associated also with a loss of gluten tolerance [29].

3.2. Clinical presentation

The clinical profile of CD is extremely varied. In children, the disorder is often reflected in anemia, abdominal distension, chronic diarrhea, steatorrhea, delayed puberty, and short stature. Common adult symptoms include abdominal distention and pain, chronic diarrhea, malabsorption, and general weakness [9]. Nevertheless, many individuals have few or no gastrointestinal symptoms, but present features such as neurological problems, anemia, osteoporosis, dermatitis herpetiformis, and fertility problems among others [29, 12]. Therefore, instead of primarily a gastrointestinal malady, CD should be considered more as a multisystem disorder. Whereas some non-intestinal symptoms of CD, e.g. osteoporosis or anemia, are due chiefly to nutritional deficiencies resulting from mucosal injury, others imply a far more complex relation to CD involving immunological as well as genetic factors.

http://dx.doi.org/10.5772/60695

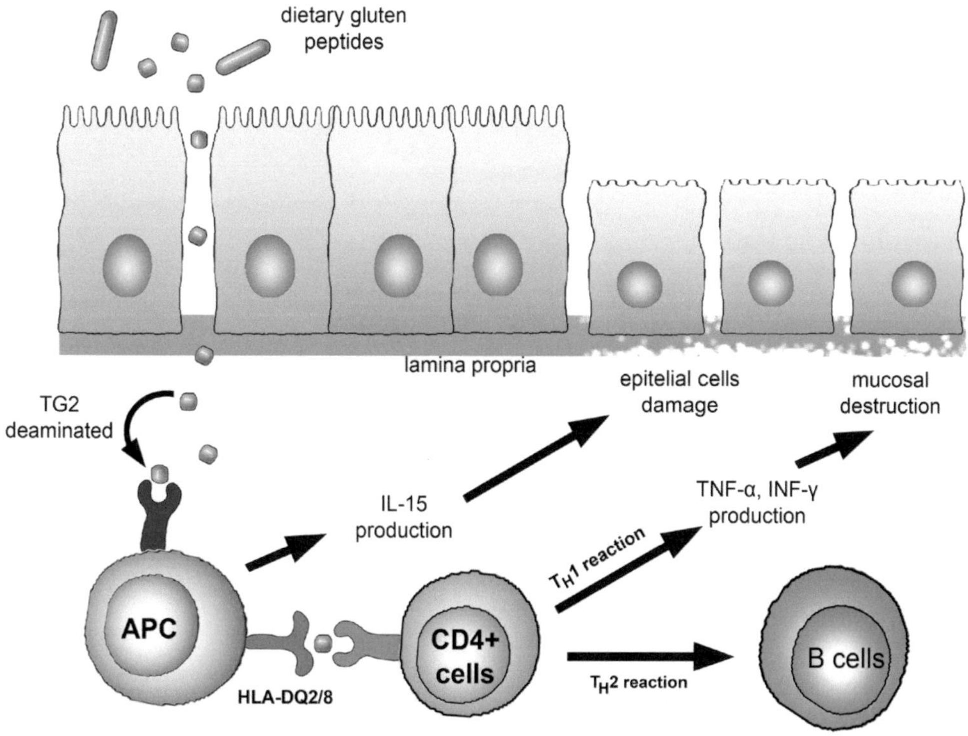

Figure 1. Schematic representation of CD pathogenesis.(*Re-drawn of Sollid LM et al.* Nature Reviews Immunology *13, 294-302. 2013)*

3.3. Diagnosis

CD can be diagnosed according to the current guidelines, given that an intestinal biopsy is the only diagnostic procedure with broad consensus. CD diagnosis should follow the criteria laid out by the North American Society for Pediatric Gastroenterology, Hepatology and Nutrition (NASPGHAN) or the European Society for Paediatric Gastroenterology and Nutrition (ESPGAN) [37].[38]. Figure 2 summarizes CD diagnosis.

3.4. Immune (oral) tolerance

The intestinal tract is the major immunological organ of the human body and plays an essential role in the induction of oral tolerance. Given that immunologically mediated reactions to foods can affect almost all organ systems, some extrinsic factors, such as gluten, can perturb the immune regulation in autoimmune disorders. The immune system of the intestine is exposed to innumerable antigens from foods, and endogenous as well as exogenous microbes [39]. Oral tolerance involves a lack of immune responsiveness towards food and bacterial antigens of the gut flora. Many mechanisms at the cellular and molecular levels participate in regulating this basic aspect of the intestinal immune system [40].

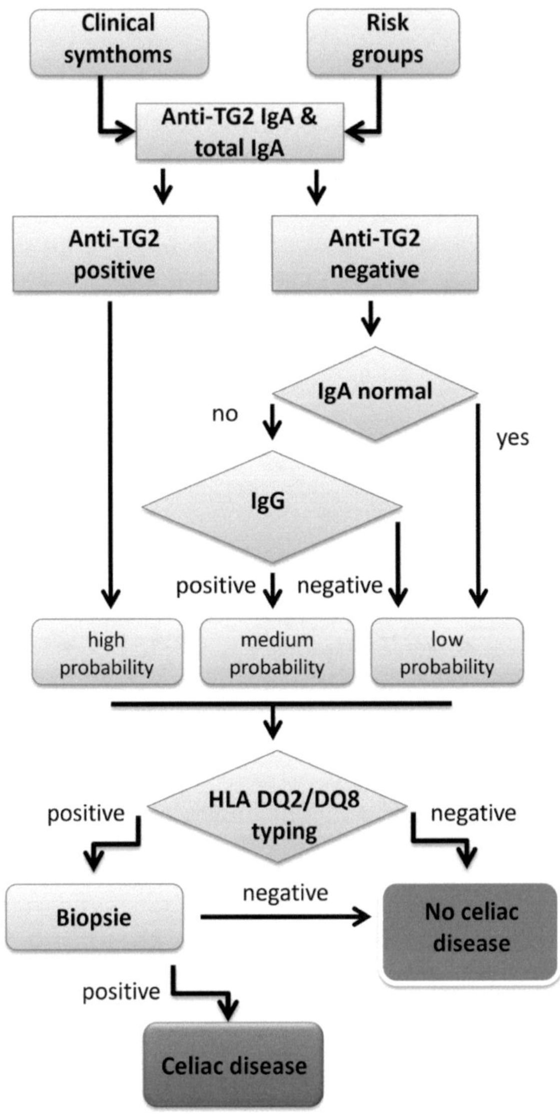

Figure 2. Algorithm for the diagnosis of celiac disease (*Re-drawn of Mayo Foundation for Medical Education and Research (MFMER)*

The most widespread food-sensitivity pathology in humans, CD results from defective immune tolerance (oral tolerance) to gluten (wheat) and the prolamin (rye and barley). Researchers have identified numerous gluten peptides that gut T cells recognize [41]. A major event in the CD pathogenesis involves the activation of gluten-reactive T cells. A high percentage of intraepithelial T cells that bear a gamma-delta chain of antigenic T-cell receptors ($\gamma\delta$ IEL) characterizes the mucosa in CD patients [42].

When ingested, the agent that triggers the disorder, gliadin, may penetrate the epithelial barrier to trigger a harmful immune response mediated by T cells. Immature dendritic cells, having characteristically low MHC class-II expression as well as co-stimulatory molecules, can modulate tolerance apparently by inducing Treg cells (T regulatory cells) [43]. Furthermore, Treg-cell-released IL-10 can mediate the activity of immature dendritic cells, inhibiting their differentiation, and thus locally favoring the presence of "tolerizing dendritic cells" [44]. Anergy of effector T cells is induced by IL-10-modulated dendritic cells through an as yet unknown process that requires contact between cells.

The immune-response shift towards tolerance or immunity is determined by the maturation stage and functional aspects of the dendritic cells. The unresponsiveness stage of immature dendritic cells can be overcome with the participation of gliadin peptides by inducing the functional and phenotypic maturation of dendritic cells, promoting more effective gliadin peptide processing and presentation to specific T lymphocytes [45]

A mouse model that overexpressed IL-15 in the lamina propria, at amounts comparable to those found in CD subjects, in cooperation with retinoic acid, was demonstrated to break oral tolerance to dietary antigens, triggering the differentiation of inflammatory dendritic cells that produce proinflammatory cytokines IL-12p70 and IL-23 and prompting the differentiation of IFN-γ-producing T cells (TH1 immunity)[46]. Also, Type-I IFNs are upregulated in the intestinal mucosa of subjects having active CD [47]. By activating dendritic cells, Type-I IFNs promote TH1-type immunity, causing oral tolerance to be lost, and might be an alternative pathway, triggering the loss of gluten tolerance.

Of special interest in CD is the expression of soluble HLA-G, as this molecule is key in immune-tolerance induction. We suggest that in CD a greater expression of soluble HLA-G could help to restore gluten tolerance. That is, HLA-G appears to interact with an inhibitory receptor (ILT), leading to the development of tolerogenic dendritic cells, inducing immunosuppressive and anergic T cells, and inhibiting dendritic-cell maturation/activation. Inflammatory stimuli and cytokines tightly control the expression of ILT receptors in dendritic cells [48]. Torres MI et al. found a correlation between higher levels of soluble HLA-G expression and CD associated with other autoimmune diseases, this depending on a genetic link of these diseases through HLA genes[48].

3.5. Autoimmune features of celiac disease

3.5.1. Autoantibodies

Untreated CD patients (on a wheat-containing diet) usually have higher levels of antibodies against wheat gluten, several other food antigens, and autoantigens present in the mucosa. In some autoimmune disorders, autoantibodies can specifically interfere with the biologic activities of a specific antigen, while in others they can cause tissue injury by forming immune complexes that activate the complement system. High titers of autoantibodies against tissue transglutaminase 2 (TG2) in patient sera TG2-specific immunoglobulin A (IgA) is the most characteristic aspect of CD and can be used to diagnose the disorder, reaching specificity and sensitivity of almost 100%. Even subjects with negative serum TG2-specific antibodies still seem to produce these antibodies locally, as reflected by small-intestine deposits [49]. In the small-intestine mucosa of untreated cases, it has in fact been demonstrated that, with CD, roughly 10% of all plasma cells prove to be TG2-specific [50]. The anti-TG2 antibodies in CD have been shown to be capable of interfering with TG2 activity and hamper the differentiation of epithelial cells [51, 52]. In addition, anti-TG2 antibodies also reportedly increased the permeability of epithelial cells in an intestinal cell line and activated monocytes on binding to Toll-like receptor 4, perhaps contributing to gut injury [53].

In CD subjects, although autoantibodies are directed mainly against the activated Ca2+ (extracellular) form of TG2, calreticulin and actin antibodies also appear [54, 55]. Antibodies to TG2 include IgA as well as IgG isotypes, whereas IgA antibodies are more specific than IgG antibodies, and it is also though that this Ab is produced primarily in the mucosa of the intestine [56]. A weak inhibitory effect of the antibodies on certain TG2-catalyzed reactions has been reported [57, 58]. TG2 is involved in the formation of active TGF-β by the crosslinking of the TGF-β binding protein. Indirect inhibition of TGF-β activation can have broad effects, including dysregulation of enterocytes and immune cells [59]. TG2 participates in the motility as well as attachment of fibroblasts and monocytes through interactions with fibronectin and integrins. The cause of CD villous atrophy could be the activity of TG2 autoantibodies upsetting fibroblast and epithelial cell migration to the tips of the villi from the crypts [60].

Also, anti-TG2 antibodies may play a part in certain non-intestinal symptoms of CD, by interacting with TG2, in addition to cross-reaction with other transglutaminases. Deposits of anti-transglutaminase antibody have in fact been detected in the brainstem and cerebellum of a patient showing cerebellar ataxia, and, in fact, gluten sensitivity. In certain idiopathic, neurological, and psychiatric disorders, these antibodies proliferate, moving some researchers to examine the potential of their cross-reactivity to neural antigens. In addition, anti-gliadin antibodies reportedly bind to neural cells and also cross-react specifically with synapsin I [61].

3.5.2. Autoreactive intraepithelial lymphocytes

Leukocyte accumulation is common in autoimmune lesions. Similarly, leukocyte infiltration occurs in CD lesions, in the lamina propria as well as in the epithelium [62]. CD8+ T cells, called intraepithelial cytotoxic lymphocytes (IE-CTLs), predominantly infiltrate the epithelium. The lamina propria shows greater density of different cell types, including antigen-presenting cells (dendritic cells and monocytes), plasma cells, and CD4+ T cells.

Inhibitory and activating NKG2 natural killer (NK) receptors tightly regulate normal intraepithelial lymphocytes (IELs). These receptors recognize non-classical HLA molecules, which are induced by IFN-β (HLA-E) and stress (MIC) exerted on epithelial cells of the intestine [63, 64]. CD, when untreated, characteristically has increasing density of proliferating TCRgd+ CD8_ CD4_ and TCRab+ CD8+ CD4_ cells in the villous epithelium, and this upregulates the selectively activating NKG2 receptors [63, 65]. The upregulation of these NKG2 receptors seems to be driven by IL-15, which is expressed by CD enterocytes [63, 66]. IL-15 seems to play a critical role in the expansion of IELs [66], and in the induction of MIC molecules on intestinal epithelial cells [67].

As suggested by Sollid *et al.*, in order for IE-CTLs to kill, need two independent but related changes in the mucosa of the intestine: 1) a epithelium that is under stress and expresses high IL-15 levels and non-classical MHC class-I molecules; and 2) activated gluten-specific CD4+ T cells [68]. The way in which B-cell immunity, an adaptive anti-gluten T-cell immunity, epithelial stress, and TG2 activation interact to determine the acquisition of a killer phenotype by IE-CTLs remains to be elucidated.

3.5.3. Gluten-free diet and autoimmune disorders

Numerous papers have investigated the effect of CD treatment on the incidence and prognosis of various autoimmune disorders [69]. A prospective study by Ventura et al. examining 90 adults with biopsy-proven CD determined the autoimmune antibody levels associated with type-1 diabetes (glutamic acid decarboxylase, islet cell, anti-insulin) as well as autoimmune thyroiditis (anti-thyroperoxidase); the examination was at CD diagnosis, and later, while on a gluten-free diet (GFD), at intervals of as much as 2 years [70]. As all antibodies normalized after 2 years without gluten intake, the authors concluded that a GFD was therapeutic against related autoimmunity [70]. In a study by Cosnes et al., autoimmune-disease incidence proved lower in the gluten-free-diet group compared to the gluten-intake group [71]. In the same study, subjects with their first CD diagnosis at more than 36 years of age displayed a lower cumulative risk of autoimmune disorders vs. subjects diagnosed at 16 to 36 or under 16 years of age. The authors suggest that because CD manifests autoimmune dysregulation, celiac patients who are older may be less prone to autoimmunity or CD [71]. Also, a later onset of CD is related to greater intestinal-barrier integrity, thus diminishing antigen triggers in the case of several autoimmune diseases. Other large-scale prospective studies would be helpful to elucidate the way in which CD is related to other autoimmune conditions and to clarify the possible influence that GFD exerts in this context. Further clarification of these relationships would provide a fuller comprehension of specific disorders and of general autoimmunity.

4. Other autoimmune disorders associated

4.1. Associated autoimmune endocrine diseases

4.1.1. Type 1 Diabetes (T1D)

The association between CD and autoimmune insulin-dependent diabetes mellitus is one of the most intensely studied relationships. The prevalence of CD among patients with type-1 diabetes has been estimated in approximately 4% and this risk is highest with diabetes onset in childhood but also with a longer diabetes duration. It is known that T1D and CD both have autoimmune origins [72]. Also, both disorders have been associated with the major histocompatibility complex class-II antigen DQ2 encoded by the alleles, DQA1∗501 and DQB1∗201, this offering a genetic basis in common for the expression of these disorders. A recent study has also demonstrated that 7 shared non-HLAloci are associated with T1D as well as CD, including a 32-bp insertion-deletion variant on chromosome 3p21, *CTLA4* on chromosome

2q33, *SH2B3* on chromosome 12q24, *PTPN2* on chromosome 18p11, *TAGAP* on chromosome 6q25, *IL18RAP* on chromosome 2q12, and *RGS1* on chromosome 1q3 [73].

The ADA (American Diabetes Association) recommends screening T1D patients for CD and placing all children with a confirmed diagnosis of CD on a gluten-free diet (GFD) [74]. The screening of T1D patients for CD and a GFD is recommended by the NASPGHAN (the North American Society for Pediatric Gastroenterology and Hepatology) for children without symptoms but with an associated condition such as T1D. However, the ADA recognizes that meager evidence exists for suggesting that a GFD provides short-term improvement of diabetes. Furthermore, it remains to be clarified whether asymptomatic patients derive long- or short-term health benefits, or both, from a GFD [75]. No clinical studies available have monitored the natural progress of CD in asymptomatic patients, so that no beneficial effects for asymptomatic CD and T1D patients strictly following a GFD are known. A GFD may affect the lipid profile, HbA1c, glycemic values, insulin needs, and perhaps even diabetes complications over the long term. Furthermore, GFD could alter, for example, growth rate, body-mass index (BMI), height, and/or weight, although no consensus is available on the ultimate results of such a diet. Hence, it is important to evaluate the impact of a GFD on metabolic control, growth and nutritional status in children with TID and CD [76]

4.1.2. Thyroid diseases

In subjects having autoimmune thyroid disease (i.e. Hashimoto's thyroiditis and Grave's disease), the CD rate reportedly accelerates, and its prevalence ranges between 2% and 7%. Similar findings have been reported in CD patients, whose serological signs of autoimmune thyroid disease (AITD) reached 26%, and in whom the detection of thyroid dysfunction reached 10% of the cases, and thyroid disease risk was some 3-fold higher than in control. Increased CD prevalence is known to occur in children and young adults who have AITD was caused by enrichment with patients with other co-morbidities associated with CD. In the absence of these co-morbidities or gastrointestinal symptoms, the prevalence of CD in AITD may not be sufficient to justify serological screening for CD in patients with AITD. A prevalence of positive tTG-IgA titers in patients with AITD was found to be higher than in a healthy population and a greater prevalence (2.3%) of biopsy-confirmed CD was noted in patients having AITD. [77]

The coexistence of CD and AITD has been explained by several mechanisms such as common genetic predisposition and the association of both diseases with the gene-encoding *CTLA4*, a gene causing susceptibility to thyroid autoimmunity. Several studies have suggested that *CTLA4* gene polymorphisms may be linked to autoimmune diseases, including TID, CD, Addison's disease, and autoimmune thyroid disorders [78, 79]. CTLA4 CT60 A/G polymorphism was reported to be strongly associated with autoimmune thyroid disease (AITD and an increased risk to develop a subsequent autoimmune disease in CD children [80].This study in an Italian population showed that the risk of AITD in children with CD was substantially modified by the CTLA4 CT60 A/G polymorphism, with the G allele in the homozygous state being the high-risk genotype. In this sense, CTLA4 CT60 A/G polymorphism evaluation may

http://dx.doi.org/10.5772/60695

be useful for stratifying the frequency of testing celiac children for antibodies indicative of AITD [80].

4.2. Associated autoimmune liver disease

Autoimmune hepatitis (AIH), primary biliary cirrhosis (PBC) and primary sclerosing cholangitis (PSC) are all considered to be autoimmune liver diseases, in which the end result is immune-mediated hepatocellular or hepatobiliary injury [81]. Clinical observations have demonstrated a link between CD and all three major autoimmune liver diseases, the association with primary biliary cirrhosis (PBC) being greatest. Disturbances in mucosal immunity may also be responsible for the hepatic manifestations of graft vs. host disease (GVHD) and IgG4-associated autoimmune pancreatitis [81].

The breakdown of gut-liver axis equilibrium plays a central role in the development of immune disorders involving the small bowel and liver in the context of genetic predisposition, and/or gut inflammation. Comsmensals or pathogenic bacteria may stimulate immune responses that fail to be suppressed by regulatory networks resulting in liver disease as a consequence of a breakdown in self-tolerance driven by molecular-mimicry or activation of innate immune pathways [82]. In celiac disease, immunologically active molecules generated from the cross-linking between tTG and food/bacterial antigens reach the liver through the portal circulation owing to the increased intestinal permeability and may contribute to triggering immune hepatic damage. This enterohepatic pathway is facilitated by the aberrant expression of adhesion molecules and chemokines that under normal conditions are restricted to either the gut or liver.

Celiac disease and primary biliary cirrhosis have several features in common, such as greater incidence in the female population, specific autoantibodies, and autoimmune comorbidities. For both diseases, reciprocal screening is advised, because early diagnosis followed by adequate treatment can enhance the outlook for such patients [82].

4.3. Associated autoimmune dermatological diseases

4.3.1. Dermatitis herpetiformis

Dermatitis herpetiformis (DH) is an inflammatory cutaneous disease with typical histopathological and immunopathological findings, clinically characterized by intensely pruritic polymorphic lesions with chronic relapse. DH patients reportedly undergo changes in the small intestine; later, these abnormalities prove similar to those found in subjects with CD. Currently this is considered more common than specific cutaneous manifestations of CD [83].

Although all DH patients present gluten sensitivity, a great majority are asymptomatic in terms of digestive symptoms [84]. The intestinal biopsy performed in DH patients could reveal signs of gluten sensitivity in 60% to 75%, ranging from normal-appearing epithelium to a flat mucosa (Marsh I to III). DQ8 and HLA DQ2 prevalence is the same level as in CD, giving strength to the idea that DH can be considered a cutaneous manifestation of CD. In fact HLA DQ2 is expressed in some 90% of DH patients (approx. 20% of controls), the other 10% being DQ8. It is extremely rare to find patients who do not have the two predisposing HLA types [85]. These two types typify this disease, and consequently a lifelong strictly gluten-free diet is the most effective cure.

An additional worthwhile observation refers to CD patients who have DH. That is, these patients not only have anti-TG2 antibodies but also have antibodies which target TG3, this being a transglutaminase expressed only in the dermal papillae of patients with dermatitis herpetiformis [86]

4.3.2. Psoriasis

Psoriasis is a chronic inflammatory disease characterized by well-demarcated, erythematous, scaly plaques. Epidemiological and clinical studies suggest that psoriasis is associated with celiac disease and celiac disease markers. Bhatia et al. [87] performed a meta-analysis to show that psoriatic populations have an approximately 2.4-fold increased risk of elevated levels of AGA compared with control subjects. These authors showed that IgA AGA antibodies were positive in about 14% of patients with psoriasis vs. 5% of healthy control subjects. CD antibody positivity has been positively correlated with psoriasis severity or psoriatic arthritis. Notably, these psoriasis patients with high counts of CD antibodies did not necessarily show a correspondence to biopsy-confirmed diagnosis of celiac disease [87].

The pathogenesis of psoriasis and celiac disease involves the interplay among multiple gene-susceptibility loci, the immune system, and various environmental factors and may involve shared biological mechanisms. Genome-wide association studies of psoriasis and CD have revealed that these two diseases share genetic-susceptibility loci at 8 genes, including at *TNFAIP3*, *RUNX3*, *ELMO1*, *ZMIZ1*, *ETS1*, *SH2B3*, *SOCS1*, and *UBE2L3*. [88-90]. Adaptive and innate immune responses are regulated by these genes. Despite that autoantibody formation that typifies the Th2 axis is associated with CD, immunological studies of CD show that gamma-delta T cells, Th17 cells, Th1 cells, and natural killer-like cells have key importance in disease pathogenesis [91-94]. Similarly, psoriasis has been related to gamma-delta T cells, Th17 cells, and T helper (Th1) cells. Further hypotheses that link CD to psoriasis involve greater intestinal permeability under both conditions, and the proposal that, in patients with CD, vitamin-D deficiency can provoke psoriasis [95-97].

Regarding the benefit of a GFD in patients with psoriasis, some case reports showed a decrease in serologic markers of celiac disease after GFD and a significant reduction in the Psoriasis Area Severity Index score. These case reports documented resolution of psoriasis after GFD [98].

4.4. Associated rheumatological disorders and connective-tissue diseases

4.4.1. Systemic lupus erythematosus

Systemic lupus erythematosus (SLE) is a multisystem disorder with manifestations including rash, arthritis, cytopenia, and renal disease. Some case reports have suggested the association between CD and SLE. Patients with CD were at a 3-fold increased risk of SLE compared to the

http://dx.doi.org/10.5772/60695

general population. Although this excess risk remained more than 5 years after CD diagnosis, absolute risks were low. SLE is a complex autoimmune disease characterized by dysregulated interactions between autoreactive T and B lymphocytes and the development of antinuclear antibodies [99].

This is striking because both disorders share the human leukocyte *HLA-B8* and *HLA-DR3* histocompatibility antigens, and a variety of antibodies including the detection of tTG IgA as well as antinuclear and anti-stranded DNA antibodies [100]. Picceli et al. found a significantly higher frequency of anti-endomysium antibodies (IgA-EmA) in SLE patients than in controls, although the titers of antibodies were predominantly low [101].

4.4.2. Rheumatoid arthritis

Celiac disease (CD) and rheumatoid arthritis (RA) are two autoimmune diseases characterized by distinct clinical features but increased co-occurrence in families and individuals. In fact, rheumatoid arthritis shares many major features that have been identified in CD, such as HLA association, T-cell infiltration in target organs, disease-specific autoantibodies, and the specific targeting of modified antigens *in vivo* [102]. Therefore, case studies of CD should help in identifying disease-relevant T-cell epitopes in rheumatoid arthritis.

More specifically, key enzymes catalyzing the post-translational modification of different amino-acid residues in antigenic structures play a major role both in CD as well as RA— that is, distinct peptidyl arginine deiminase (PAD) isoforms in RA [104] and TG2 in CD [103]. These enzymes plus other features shared by CD and RA, include immune targeting of modified proteins, target organ T-cell infiltration, autoimmune phenomena, HLA association, and the importance of post-translational modification regarding peptide binding to disease-associated HLA molecules.

Also, in CD as well as in RA, genome-wide association studies (GWAS) have identified the HLA region and 26 non-HLA genetic-risk loci. Research has demonstrated that, of the 26 CD and 26 RA risk loci, six are common to the two disorders, including *TAGAP, TNFAIP3, IL2-IL21, ICOS-CTLA4, REL,* and *MMEL/TNFRSF14* eliminate, and [105-107]

5. Conclusions

Celiac disease is categorized as an autoimmune disorder. In this context, it is noteworthy that celiac disease has been associated with various autoimmune disorders, but there are no reliable data to establish a cause and effect relationship between celiac disease, gluten, and these autoimmune conditions. In any case, there are more similarities between celiac disease and typical autoimmune diseases, such as type-1 diabetes and rheumatoid arthritis, than previously suspected. It has been proposed that such relationships might be accounted for by the common pathogenesis that involves similar environmental triggers, genetic predisposition, and the loss of intestinal barrier secondary to dysfunction of tight junctions leading to greater gut permeability, and perhaps other mechanisms yet to be discovered.

Acknowledgements

Supported by Junta de Andalucía throughout the program "Ayudas a grupos de investigación", group BIO-220.

Author details

M.I. Torres*, T. Palomeque and P. Lorite

*Address all correspondence to: mitorres@ujaen.es

Department of Experimental Biology. University of Jaén, Spain

References

[1] Sollid LM, Jabri B. Is celiac disease an autoimmune disorder? Cur Op Immunol 17:595–600. 2005

[2] Green PH, Cellier C. Celiac disease. N Engl J Med. 357:1731–1743. 2007

[3] Baranzini SE. The genetics of autoimmune diseases: a networked perspective. CurrOpilmmunol 21 (6): 596–60. 2009

[4] Hindorff LA, Sethupathy P, Junkins HA, et al. Potential etiologic and functional implications of genome-wide association loci for human diseases and traits. ProcNatlAcadSci USA 106:9362-9367. 2009

[5] Visscher PM, Brown MA, McCarthy MI et al. Five years of GWAS discovery. Am J Hum Genet 90(1):7–24. 2012

[6] Zhernakova A, Alizadeh BZ, BevovaM, et al. Novel association in chromosome 4q27 region with rheumatoid arthritis and confirmation of type 1 diabetes point to a general risk locus for autoimmune diseases. Am J Hum Genet 81 (6):1284–1288.2007

[7] Trynka G, WijmengaC, Van Heel DA.A genetic perspective on coeliac disease. Trends Mol Med 16(11):537–550. 2010

[8] Gutierrez-Achury J, Coutinho de Almeida R, et al. Shared genetics in coeliac disease and other immune-mediated diseases. J Intern Med 269(6):591–603. 2011

[9] Fernando MMA, Stevens CR, Walsh EC.Defining the Role of the MHC in Autoimmunity: A Review and Pooled Analysis.PLoS Genet 4(4): e1000024. 2008

[10] Dieterich W, Ehnis T, Bauer M, et al. Identification of tissue transglutaminase as the autoantigen of celiac disease. Nat Med 3:797-801. 1997

[11] Herzog J, Maekawa Y, Cirrito TP et al. Activated antigen-presenting cells select and present chemically modified peptides recognized by unique CD4 T cells. ProcNatlAcadSci USA 102:7928-7933. 2005

[12] Alaedini A, Green PH. Narrative review: celiac disease: understanding a complex autoimmune disorder. Ann Intern Med 142:289–98. 2005

[13] Louka AS, Sollid LM. HLA in coeliac disease: unravelling the complex genetics of a complex disorder. Tissue Antigens 61:105–17. 2003

[14] Mazzilli MC, Ferrante P, Mariani P et al. A study of Italian pediatric celiac disease patients confirms that the primary HLA association is to the DQ (a1*0501, b1*0201) heterodimer. Hum Immunol33: 133–139. 1992

[15] Sollid LM, Markussen G, Ek J et al. Evidence for a primary association of celiac disease to a particular HLA-DQ a/b heterodimer. J Exp Med 169: 345–350. 1989

[16] Tighe MR, Hall MA, Barbado M et al. HLA class II alleles associated with celiac disease susceptibility in a southern European population. Tissue Antigens40: 90–97. 1992

[17] Trynka G, Hunt KA, Bockett NA, et al. Dense genotyping identifies and localizes multiple common and rare variant association signals in celiac disease. Nature Genet. 43:1193–1201. 2011

[18] Mearin ML, Pena AS. Clinical indications of HLA typing and measurement of gliadin antibodies in coeliac disease.Neth J Med31: 279–285. 1987

[19] Maiuri L, Auricchio S, Coletta S et al. Blockage of T-cell costimulation inhibits T-cell action in celiac disease. Gastroenterology115: 564–572. 1998

[20] Djilali-Saiah I, Schmitz J, Harfouch-Hammoud E *et al*. CTLA-4 gene polymorphism is associated with predisposition to coeliac disease. Gut 43: 187–189. 1998

[21] Holopainen P, Arvas M, Sistonen P et al. CD28/CTLA4 gene region on chromosome 2q33 confers genetic susceptibility to celiac disease. A linkage and family-based association study. Tissue Antigens53: 470–475. 1999

[22] Zhernakova A, Stahl EA, Trynka Get al. Meta-analysis of genome-wide association studies in celiac disease and rheumatoid arthritis identifies fourteen non-HLA shared loci. PLoS Genet. 7:e1002004. 2011

[23] Kumar V, Wijmenga C, Withoff S. From genome-wide association studies to disease mechanisms: celiac disease as a model for autoimmune diseases. SeminImmunopathol 34:567–580. 2012

[24] Zhernakova A, Van Diemen CC, Wijmenga C.Detecting shared pathogenesis from the shared genetics of immune-related diseases. Nat Rev Genet 10(1):43–55. 2009

[25] Van Heel DA, Hunt K, Greco L. Genetics in coeliac disease. Best Pract Res ClinGastroenterol 19(3):323–339. 2005

[26] Robins G, Howdle PD. Advances in celiac disease. CurrOpinGastroenterol21: 152-161. 2005

[27] Kim CY, Quarsten H, Bergseng E, et al. Structural basis for HLA-DQ2-mediated presentation of gluten epitopes in celiac disease. ProcNatlAcadSci USA101: 4175-4179. 2004

[28] Louka AS, Sollid LM. HLA in coeliac disease: unravelling the complex genetics of a complex disorder. Tissue Antigens61: 105-117. 2003

[29] Torres MI, López Casado MA, et al. New aspects in celiac disease.World J Gastroenterol13(8): 1156-1161. 2007

[30] Greco L, Corazza G, Babron MC, et al. Genome search in celiac disease.Am J Hum Genet 62:669-675. 1998

[31] Babron MC, Nilsson S, Adamovic S, et al. Meta and pooled analysis of European coeliac disease data. Eur J HumGenet 11:828-834. 2003

[32] Van Belzen MJ, Meijer JW, Sandkuijl LA, et al. A major non-HLA locus in celiac disease maps to chromosome 19. Gastroenterology125:1032-1041. 2003

[33] Rioux JD, Abbas AK. Paths to understanding the genetic basis of autoimmune disease. Nature 435:584-589. 2005

[34] Clemente MG, De Virgiliis S, Kang JS, et al. Early effects of gliadin on enterocyte intracellular signalling involved in intestinal barrier function. Gut.52:218–223. 2003

[35] Sollid LM. Coeliac disease: dissecting a complex inflammatory disorder. Nat Rev Immunol2: 647-655. 2002

[36] Kim CY, Quarsten H, Bergseng E, et al. Structural basis for HLA-DQ2-mediated presentation of gluten epitopes in celiac disease. ProcNatlAcadSci USA101: 4175-4179. 2004

[37] Husby S, Koletzko S, Korponay-Szabó IR et al. European society for pediatric gastroenterology, hepatology and nutrition guidelines for the diagnosis of coeliac disease. JPGN 54(1):136-160.2012

[38] Guideline for the diagnosis and treatment of celiac disease in children: recommendations of the North American society for pediatric gastroenterology, hepatology and nutrition. JPGN 40:1-19. 2005

[39] Briani C, Samaroo D, Alaedini A. Celiac disease: From gluten to autoimmunity. Autoimmunity Reviews 7: 644–650. 2008

[40] Dubois B, Goubier A, Joubert G, et al. Oral tolerance and regulation of mucosal immunity. Cell Mol Life Sci. 62:1322–1332. 2005

[41] Arentz-Hansen H, McAdam SN, Molberg Ø, et al.Celiac lesion T cells recognize epitopes that cluster in regions of gliadins rich in proline residues. Gastroenterology. 123:803–809. 2002

[42] Ebert EC. Intra-epithelial lymphocytes: interferon-gamma production and suppressor/cytotoxic activities. ClinExpImmunol82:81–85. 1990

[43] Alpan O, Rudomen G, Matzinger P. The role of dendritic cells, B cells, and M cells in gut-oriented immune responses.J Immunol.166:4843–4852. 2001

[44] Steinman RM, Turley S, Mellman I, et al. The induction of tolerance by dendritic cells that have captured apoptotic cells.J ExpMed191:411–416. 2000

[45] Palová-Jelínková L, Rozková D, Pecharová B, et al. Gliadin fragments induce phenotypic and functional maturation of human dendritic cells. J Immunol.175:7038–7045. 2005

[46] DePaolo RW, Abadie V, Tang Fet al. Co-adjuvant effects of retinoic acid and IL-15 induce inflammatory immunity to dietary antigens. Nature 471:220–224. 2011

[47] Monteleone G, Pender SL, Alstead E, et al. Role of interferon αin promoting T helper cell type 1 responses in the small intestine in coeliac disease. Gut. 48:425–429. 2001

[48] Torres MI, López-Casado MA, Luque J, et al. New advances in coeliac disease: serum and intestinal expression of HLA-G. IntImmunol18:713–718. 2006

[49] Maglio M, Tosco A, Auricchio R, et al. Intestinal deposits of anti-tissue transglutaminase IgA in childhood celiac disease. Dig Liver Dis 43:604–608. 2011

[50] Di Niro R, Mesin L, Zheng NY, et al. High abundance of plasma cells secreting transglutaminase 2-specific IgA autoantibodies with limited somatic hypermutation in celiac disease intestinal lesions. Nat Med 18:441–5. 2012

[51] Esposito C, Paparo F, Caputo I, et al. Antitissuetransglutaminase antibodies from coeliac patients inhibit transglutaminase activity both in vitro and in situ. Gut 51:177–81. 2002

[52] Halttunen T, Maki M. Serum immunoglobulin A from patientswithceliac disease inhibits human T84 intestinal crypt epithelial cell differentiation.Gastroenterology 116:566–572. 1999

[53] Zanoni G, Navone R, Lunardi C, et al. In celiac disease, a subset of autoantibodies against transglutaminase binds toll-like receptor 4 and induces activation of monocytes. PLoSMed 3:e358. 2006

[54] Sanchez D, Tuckova L, Sebo P et al. Occurrence of IgA and IgG autoantibodies to calreticulin in coeliac disease and various autoimmune diseases. J Autoimmun 15:441-449. 2000

[55] Clemente MG, Musu MP, Frau F, et al. Immune reaction against the cytoskeleton in coeliac disease. Gut 47:520-526. 2000

[56] Marzari R, Sblattero D, Florian F, et al. Molecular dissection of the tissue transglutaminase autoantibody response in celiac disease. J Immunol 166:4170-4176. 2001

[57] Esposito C, Paparo F, Caputo I, et al. Anti-tissue transglutaminase antibodies from coeliac patients inhibit transglutaminase activity both in vitro and in situ. Gut 51:177-181. 2002

[58] Dieterich W, Trapp D, Esslinger B, et al. Autoantibodies of patients with coeliac disease are insufficient to block tissue transglutaminase activity. Gut 52:1562-1566. 2003

[59] Nunes I, Gleizes PE, Metz CN, et al. Latent transforming growth factor-β binding protein domains involved in activation and transglutaminase-dependent cross-linking of latent transforming growth factor-β. J Cell Biol 136:1151-1163. 1997

[60] Akimov SS, Belkin AM. Cell surface tissue transglutaminase is involved in adhesion and migration of monocytic cells on fibronectin. Blood 98:1567-1576. 2001

[61] Alaedini A, Okamoto H, Briani C, et al. Immune cross-reactivity in celiac disease: anti-gliadin antibodies bind to neuronal synapsin I. J Immunol 178:6590–6595. 2007

[62] Sollid LM. Molecular basis of celiac disease.Annu Rev Immunol.18:53–81.2000

[63] Roberts AI, Lee L, Schwarz E, et al. NKG2D receptors induced by IL-15 costimulate CD28-negative effector CTL in the tissue microenvironment. J Immunol167:5527-5530. 2001

[64] Jabri B, De Serre NP, Cellier C, et al.Selective expansion of intraepithelial lymphocytes expressing the HLA-E-specific natural killer receptor CD94 in celiac disease. Gastroenterology 118:867-879. 2000

[65] Meresse B, Chen Z, Ciszewski C, et al. Coordinated induction by IL15 of a TCR-independent NKG2D signaling pathway converts CTL into lymphokine-activated killer cells in celiac disease. Immunity 21:357-366. 2004

[66] Mention JJ, Ben Ahmed M, Begue B, et al. Interleukin 15: a key to disrupted intraepithelial lymphocyte homeostasis and lymphomagenesis in celiac disease. Gastroenterology 125:730-745. 2003

[67] Hü ES, Mention JJ, Monteiro RC, et al. A direct role for NKG2D/MICA interaction in villous atrophy during celiac disease. Immunity 21:367-377. 2004

[68] Sollid LM, Jabri B. Triggers and drivers of autoimmunity: lessons from coeliac Disease. Nat Rev Immunol. 13(4):.294-302. 2013

[69] Denham JM, Hill ID. Celiac Disease and Autoimmunity: Review and Controversies. CurrAllergyAsthmaRep 13:347–353. 2013

[70] Ventura A Neri E, Ughi C, et al. Gluten-dependent diabetes-related and thyroidrelated autoantibodies in patients with celiac disease.J Pediatr. 137(2):263–5. 2000

[71] Cosnes J, Cellier C, Viola S et al. Incidence of autoimmune diseases in celiac disease: protective effect of the gluten-free diet. ClinGastroenterolHepatol. 6(7):753–8. 2008

[72] Smyth DJ, Plagnol V, Walker NM, *et al*. Shared and distinct genetic variants in type 1 diabetes and coeliac disease. N Eng J Med 359: 2767-77. 2008

[73] Knip M, Veijola R, Virtanen SM, et al. Environmental triggers and determinants of type 1 diabetes.Diabetes.54(2):S125–36. 2005

[74] Hill ID, Dirks MH, Liptak GS, et al. "Guideline for the diagnosis and treatment of celiac disease in children: recommendations of the North American Society for Pediatric Gastroenterology, Hepatology and Nutrition, " JPGN 40(1):1–19. 2005.

[75] Sanchez-Albisua I, Wolf J, Neu A, et al. "Coeliac disease in children with type 1 diabetes mellitus: the effect of the gluten-free diet, " Diabetic Medicine 22(8): 1079–1082. 2005.

[76] Scaramuzza AE, Mantegazza C, Bosetti A, et al. Type 1 diabetes and celiac disease: The effects of gluten free diet on metabolic control. World J Diabetes15; 4(4): 130-134. 2013

[77] Sattar N, Lazare F, Kacer M, et al.Celiac Disease in Children, Adolescents, and Young Adults with Autoimmune Thyroid Disease J Pediatr 158:272-275. 2011

[78] Kristiansen OP, Larsen ZM, Pociot F. CTLA-4 in autoimmune diseases—a general susceptibility gene to autoimmunity? Genes Immun 1:170–84. 2000

[79] Turpeinen H, Laine AP, Hermann R, et al. A linkage analysis of the CTLA4 gene region in Finnish patients with type 1 diabetes.Eur J Immunogenet 30:289–93. 2003

[80] Tolone C, Cirillo G, Papparella A, et al. A. common CTLA4 polymorphism confers susceptibility to autoimmune thyroid disease in celiac children. Dig Liver Dis41:385-389. 2009

[81] Trivedi PJ, Adams DH. Mucosal immunity in liver autoimmunity: A comprehensive review. Journal of Autoimmunity 46: 97-111.2013

[82] Volta U, Caio G, Tovoli F, *et al.* Gut-liver axis: an immune link between celiac disease and primary biliary cirrhosis. Expert Rev GastroenterolHepatol. 7(3): 253-61. 2013

[83] Alonso-Llamazares J, Gibson LE, Rogers RS. Clinical, pathologic, and immunopathologic features of dermatitis herpetiformis: review of the Mayo Clinic experience. Int J Dermatol. 46:910-9. 2007

[84] Herrero-González JE. Clinical guidelines for the diagnosis and treatment of dermatitis herpetiformis].ActasDermosifiliogr. 101:820-6. 2010

[85] Collin P, Reunala T. Recognition and manegment of cutaneous manifestations of celiac disese: a guide for dermatologists. Am J ClinDermatol. 4:13-20. 2003

[86] Sardy M, Karpati S, Merkl B, et al. Epidermal transglutaminase (TGase 3) is the autoantigen of dermatitis herpetiformis. J Exp Med 195:747-757. 2002

[87] Bhatia BK, Millsop JW, Debbaneh M, et al. Diet and psoriasis, part II: Celiac disease and role of a gluten-free diet. J Am AcadDermatol 71:350-8. 2014

[88] Tsoi LC, Spain SL, Knight J, et al. Identification of 15 new psoriasis susceptibility loci highlights the role of innate immunity Nat Genet, 44: 1341–1348. 2012

[89] Trynka G, Hunt KA, Bockett NA, *et al.* Dense genotyping identifies and localizes multiple common and rare variant association signals in celiac disease. Nat Genet, 43: 1193–1201. 2011

[90] Lu Y, Chen H, Nikamo P, et al. Association of cardiovascular and metabolic disease genes with psoriasis. J Invest Dermatol, 133: 836–839. 2013

[91] Salvati VM, MacDonald TT, Bajaj-Elliott M, et al. Interleukin 18 and associated markers of T helper cell type 1 activity in celiac disease Gut, 50: 186–190. 2002

[92] Cianci R, Cammarota G, Frisullo G, et al.Tissue-infiltrating lymphocytes analysis reveals large modifications of the duodenal "immunological niche" in celiac disease after gluten-free diet. ClinTranslGastroenterol, 13;3:e28. doi: 10.1038/ctg.2012.22.. 2012

[93] Kupfer SS, Jabri B. Pathophysiology of celiac disease. GastrointestEndoscClin N Am 22: 639–660. 2012

[94] Humbert P, Bidet A, Treffel P et al. Intestinal permeability in patients with psoriasis.J DermatolSci, 2: 324–326. 1991

[95] Montalto M, Cuoco L, Ricci R et al. Immunohistochemical analysis of ZO-1 in the duodenal mucosa of patients with untreated and treated celiac disease Digestion 65 : 227–233. 2002

[96] Holick MF. Vitamin D: a millenium perspective. J Cell Biochem 88:296-307. 2003

[97] Bhatia BK, Millsop JW, Debbaneh M, et al.Diet and psoriasis, part II: Celiac disease and role of a gluten-free diet. J Am AcadDermatol 71:350-8. 2014

[98] Ludvigsson JF, Rubio-Tapia A, Chowdhary V, et al. Increased Risk of Systemic Lupus Erythematosus in 29, 000 Patients with Biopsy-verified Celiac Disease.JRheumatol 39(10):1964-1970. 2012

[99] Marau I, Shoenfeld Y, Bizarro N, et al. IgA and IgG tissue transglutaminase antibodies in systemic lupus erythematosus.. Lupus 13: 241–244. 2004

[100] Picceli VF, Skare TL, Nisihara R, et al. Spectrum of autoantibodies for gastrointestinal autoinmune diseases in systemic lupus erythematosus patients. Lupus 22: 1150–1155. 2013

[101] Molberg Ø and Sollid LM.A gut feeling for joint inflammation –using coeliac disease to understand rheumatoid arthritis. Trends Immunol.27(4): 188-194. 2006

[102] Esposito, C. and Caputo, I.Mammalian transglutaminases.Identification of substrates as a key to physiological function and physiopathological relevance. FEBS J. 272: 615–631. 2005

[103] Vossenaar, E.R. et al. PAD, a growing family of citrullinating enzymes: genes, features and involvement in disease. Bioessays 25: 1106–1118. 2003

[104] Zhernakova A, Stah EA, Trynka G, et al. Meta-Analysis of Genome-Wide Association Studies in Celiac Disease and Rheumatoid Arthritis Identifies Fourteen Non-HLA Shared Loci. Plos Genetics February 7(2)| e1002004. 2011

[105] Stahl EA, Raychaudhuri S, Remmers EF, et al. Genome-wideassociation study meta-analysis identifies seven new rheumatoid arthritis riskloci. Nat Genet 42: 508–514.

[106] Hunt KA, Zhernakova A, Turner G, et al. Newly identified genetic risk variants for celiac disease related to the immune response. Nat Genet 40: 395–402. 2008

Chapter 7

Vitiligo – A Complex Autoimmune Skin Depigmenting Disease

Mitesh Dwivedi, Naresh C. Laddha,
Anthony P. Weetman, Rasheedunnisa Begum and
Helen Kemp

Additional information is available at the end of the chapter

http://dx.doi.org/10.5772/59762

1. Introduction

Vitiligo is an acquired, non-contagious disease in which progressive, patchy loss of pigmentation from the skin, overlying hair and oral mucosa results from the loss of melanocytes from the involved areas [1]. Clinically, two large subsets of vitiligo are distinguished namely focal or segmental vitiligo and non-segmental or generalised vitiligo [2]. Focal vitiligo presents with a limited number of small lesions while segmental vitiligo is typified by an asymmetric distribution involving segments of the skin surface, sometimes in a dermatomal fashion, by depigmented macules. Non-segmental vitiligo corresponds to all generalised, usually symmetrical, forms including acrofacial vitiligo. The course of the disease is unpredictable but is often episodically progressive with phases of stabilised depigmentation. Extending vitiligo with enlarging macules or the development of new lesions is classified as the active form of the disease [3].

Although vitiligo might be viewed as minor disorder, skin depigmentation can cause psychological stress in patients with respect to self-esteem and social interactions. This is particularly true for individuals with deeply pigmented skin [4], and for women who in some cultures face social and marital stigma [5]. The prevalence of vitiligo has been reported to be 0.5 to 1% of the world population [6,7]. In India, the prevalence varies from 0.5 to 2.5 % [8], although the states of Gujarat and Rajasthan have a prevalence of 8.8% [9]. Vitiligo affects all with no predilection for gender or race. The disease usually starts in childhood or young adulthood: the clinical manifestation begins before 20 years of age in 50% of cases, while in 25% of cases the onset is before the age of 14 years [10].

Many factors have been implicated in the aetiology and pathogenesis of the vitiligo including infections [11], stress [12], neural abnormalities [13], defective melanocyte adhesion [14], and genetic susceptibility (Figure 1) [15]. The biochemical hypothesis argues that melanocyte destruction is due to the accumulation of toxic metabolites from melanogenesis, the breakdown of free-radical defence and an excess of hydrogen peroxide [16-18]. In addition, many studies have indicated a role for both cellular [19] and humoral [20] immunity in the pathogenesis of vitiligo. This chapter will focus on the available evidence which supports the involvement of autoimmunity in the aetiology and pathogenesis of vitiligo.

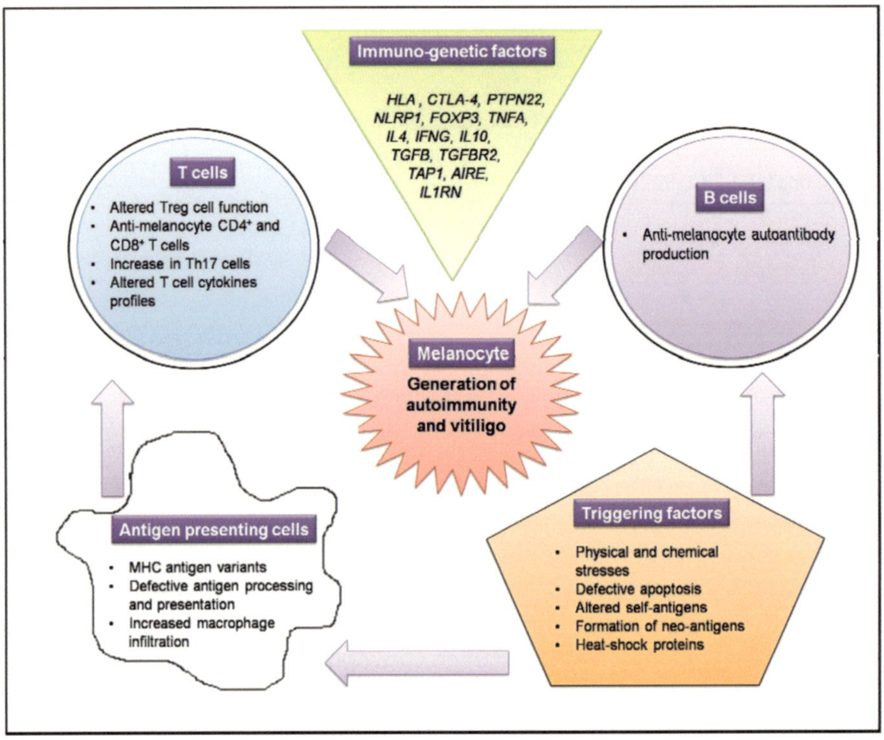

Figure 1. The generation of autoimmune responses against melanocytes in vitiligo. Depigmentation in vitiligo results from a hyperactive response of the immune system against melanocytes. A complex interaction of immune cells and immuno-genetic factors is the most likely aetiology. In particular, defects of T cell subsets as well as altered melanocyte antigens may give rise to increased autoreactive $CD8^{+}$and $CD4^{+}$T cells and the generation of anti-melanocyte autoantibodies. The triggering factors involved in generation of autoimmunity in vitiligo patients are still not clearly defined, although physical trauma and melanocyte oxidative stress have been implicated.

2. Association with autoimmune diseases

Vitiligo is frequently associated with other autoimmune disorders, particularly autoimmune thyroid disease [21]. Patients with vitiligo are also more likely to suffer from autoimmune conditions than those in the general population [22]. For example, a survey of more than 2,600 unselected Caucasian vitiligo patients indicated elevated frequencies of autoimmune thyroid disease, Addison's disease, systemic lupus erythematosus and pernicious anaemia, and, indeed, approximately 30% of patients were affected by at least one other autoimmune disease [23]. Furthermore, the same autoimmune diseases were found at an increased prevalence in the first-degree relatives of vitiligo patients [23] and in multiplex vitiligo families [24]. Such findings indicate that vitiligo can be part of a specific group of autoimmune diseases to which individuals can be genetically predisposed, and are also evidence for its autoimmune pathogenesis.

3. Immuno-regulatory genes

The involvement of immune-regulatory genes with vitiligo development has been extensively documented [15]. For example, the association of certain major histocompatibility complex (MHC) alleles with vitiligo has suggested an important link between the aetiology of the disease and aberrant presentation of self-antigens to the immune system. Most recently, alleles of human leukocyte antigen (HLA) genes *HLA-A*33:01*, *HLA-B*44:03*, and *HLA-DRB1*07:01* have been reported to be significantly more prevalent in Indian vitiligo patients as compared with healthy controls [25]. In the European-derived white population, vitiligo shows primary association with *HLA-A* in the class I region [26], specifically *HLA-A*02:01* [27], and in the class II region upstream of *HLA-DRA* and located between *HLA-DRB1* and *HLA-DQA1*. Furthermore, studies of Chinese have shown MHC associations in the class I region, between *HLA-B* and *HLA-C* [28] and in the class III region [29].

Other immune-regulatory genes that contain single nucleotide polymorphisms associated with vitiligo susceptibility include *PTPN22* (lymphoid-specific protein tyrosine phosphatase, non-receptor type 22), *IL2RA* (interleukin-2 receptor alpha chain), *UBASH3A* (ubiquitin-associated and SH3 domain–containing A protein), and *C1QTNF6* (C1q and tumour necrosis factor–related protein) [26].

4. Immunological features of melanocytes

Several studies have shown abnormal expression of MHC class II antigen HLA-DR and increased expression of intercellular adhesion molecule-1 (ICAM-1) by perilesional melanocytes in vitiligo compared with melanocytes from normal skin [30-32]. These molecules have important roles in antigen presentation and in the activation of T helper cells, so their expression by melanocytes could contribute to the anti-melanocyte cellular immune responses that are observed in vitiligo [19,33].

Both vitiligo and normal melanocytes are also capable of expressing MHC class I molecules [31], which could allow interaction with destructive cytotoxic T cells. Indeed, melanocytes have an antigen processing and presenting capability which can make them target cells for T cell-mediated cytotoxicity [34]. Finally, in perilesional vitiligo biopsies, melanocytes express macrophage markers CD68 and CD36 [32] and reduced levels of membrane regulators of complement activation, including decay acceleration factor and membrane cofactor protein [35], which suggests a vulnerability of these cells to attack by macrophages and the complement system, respectively.

5. Autoantibodies

Melanocyte autoantibodies have been detected in the sera of vitiligo patients at a significantly higher frequency than in healthy individuals [20,36]. They are associated with the extent of vitiligo, being present in 93% of patients with 5-10% of skin area involvement, and in 50% of patients with less than 2% of skin depigmentation [37]. In addition, patients with active vitiligo have increased levels of melanocyte autoantibodies compared to those with stable disease [38,39]. Characterisation of melanocyte autoantibodies has demonstrated that they belong to the subclasses IgG1, IgG2 and IgG3 [40], although studies have also found that IgA levels of melanocyte autoantibodies are associated with disease activity [41]. Several melanocyte-specific autoantibody targets have been identified including tyrosinase [42-44], tyrosinase-related protein (TRP)-1 [45], dopachrome tautomerase (or TRP-2) [46,47], PMEL [48] and GTP-binding protein Rab38 [49].

Autoantibodies against targets not specifically expressed by melanocytes have also been detected in patients with vitiligo including the melanin-concentrating hormone receptor 1, gamma-enolase, alpha-enolase, heat-shock protein 90, osteopontin, ubiquitin-conjugating enzyme, translation-initiation factor 2, tyrosine hydroxylase and laminA [49-51]. In addition, organ-specific autoantibodies, particularly against the thyroid, adrenal glands, gastric parietal cells, and pancreatic islet cells are commonly found in vitiligo patients [52], along with anti-nuclear autoantibodies and IgM-rheumatoid factor [53]. Keratinocyte autoantibodies which correlate with vitiligo extent and activity have been reported [54].

With respect to pathogenicity, vitiligo patient autoantibodies can mediate complement damage and antibody-dependent cellular cytotoxicity against melanocytes and melanoma cells *in vitro* and *in vivo* [55-57]. Passive immunisation of nude mice grafted with human skin has also indicated that IgG from vitiligo patients can induce the destruction of melanocytes [58]. Furthermore, melanocyte autoantibodies from vitiligo patients can induce HLA-DR and ICAM-1 expression on and release of interleukin (IL)-8 from melanocytes [59]. Such changes enhance the antigen-presenting activity of melanocytes allowing antigen-specific immune effector cell attack. More recent work has found that 69% of vitiligo patient sera tested induced melanocyte detachment in a reconstructed epidermis model, although this was unrelated to either the extent or the activity of the disease [60]. Finally, melanocyte autoantibodies isolated from vitiligo patients, but not from healthy controls, are able to penetrate cultured melanocytes and trigger them to engage in apoptosis [61].

6. CD4⁺helper and CD8⁺cytotoxic T cells

The first evidence for a possible role for T cells in the pathogenesis of vitiligo came from studies on inflammatory vitiligo [62]. Since then, circulating autoreactive $CD8^+$cytotoxic T that recognise melanocyte antigens (MART1, PMEL and tyrosinase) have been detected in vitiligo patients [33,63-66]. Peripheral $CD8^+$T cells are more prevalent in active cases of vitiligo as compared to stable cases, and their frequency correlates with the extent of depigmentation [53,67]. They also express high levels of the skin-homing receptor cutaneous lymphocyte-associated antigen and display cytotoxic reactivity towards melanocytes [33].

Histological studies of skin biopsies from vitiligo patients have demonstrated that infiltrating cytotoxic and helper T cells are most prominent at the periphery of vitiligo lesions [32,68]. Moreover, a significant increase in the number of $CD4^+$and $CD8^+$T cells are detected in the marginal skin in both stable and active vitiligo cases [69]. These perilesional T cells exhibit a predominantly type-1-like cytokine secretion profile of tumour necrosis factor (TNF)-alpha and interferon (IFN)-gamma, the latter enhancing T cell trafficking to the skin by increasing ICAM-1 expression on target cells [70,71]. The majority of infiltrating T cells are activated, as indicated by the expression of the MHC class II antigen HLA-DR [32,68] and the presence of granzyme $B^+$and $perforin^+$cytotoxic T lymphocytes [32]. There is also evidence for down-regulation of the T helper 2 cell-dependent CDw60 molecules in the vitiliginous epidermis. This observation correlates with infiltrating T cells exhibiting a T helper 1 cell-type cytokine production pattern consistent with cell-mediated organ-specific autoimmunity [72].

Using a skin explant model to investigate the effector functions of perilesional $CD8^+$T cells, the latter, which are enriched for cytotoxic T lymphocytes that recognise melanocyte antigens (MART1, PMEL and tyrosinase), infiltrate normally pigmented skin and eradicate melanocytes [19]. The capacity of cytotoxic T cells for damaging melanocytes has also been observed in an experimental murine model of vitiligo: melanocytes were destroyed by $CD8^+$T cells recognising a single H2-Kb-binding peptide derived from dopachrome tautomerase [73].

7. T helper 17 cells

Increased numbers of T helper $17A^+$cells are found in the leading edge of vitiligo lesions as shown by immunohistochemistry and immunofluorescence [74,75]. Elevated levels of IL-17A mRNA are also present in the same locality [75], evidence that signifies active T helper 17 cells in vitiligo lesions. *In vitro*, T helper 17 cell-related cytokines directly affect melanocyte activity and function, including the down-regulation of melanin production and the shrinkage of melanocytes [74]. In terms of the local cytokine network in the skin, IL-17A dramatically induces production of IL-1beta, IL-6, and TNF-alpha by skin-resident cells such as keratinocytes and fibroblasts [74].

8. Regulatory T cells

Natural Treg cells play a key role in maintaining peripheral tolerance through the active suppression of self-reactive T cell activation and expansion [76], thereby preventing the development of the autoimmune responses. To date, several studies have indicated perturbations in Treg cell numbers and/or function in vitiligo patients [67,77-79]. Such alterations might lead to the reported higher levels and activation of cytotoxic T cells in individuals with the disease [67,77].

Assessment of circulating Tregs by flow cytometric analysis has revealed a decrease in their numbers in vitiligo patients compared to controls [67,77,78]. Reduced peripheral Treg cell numbers have also been reported in early age-of-onset patients (1-20 years) compared to those with late onset vitiligo, and decreased circulating Treg cell counts have been demonstrated in patients with active vitiligo as compared to those with stable disease [67]. Moreover, a striking reduction in the number of Tregs in the marginal and lesional skin of vitiligo patients has been observed [69,80]. Interestingly, some studies have demonstrated that peripheral or lesional skin $CD4^{+}CD25^{+}FoxP3^{+}$Treg cell numbers remain unaltered in vitiligo [81-83], and even that either may be increased [67,84]. Interestingly, discrepancy between the relative abundance of Treg cells present in the circulation of vitiligo patients as compared to their skin was reported to be due to reduced expression of the chemo-attractant CCL22 within vitiligo patient skin so impairing migration of Tregs into the tissue [83].

As well as defects in Treg cell numbers, their function can also be impaired in vitiligo patients. Indeed, the suppressive effects of Tregs in vitiligo cases are significantly reduced as indicated by their impaired ability to inhibit proliferation and cytokine production from autologous $CD8^{+}$T cells [77,78]. In line with this, the expression of FoxP3 (the dedicated mediator of the genetic program governing Treg cell development and function) in $CD4^{+}CD25^{hi}$ Tregs is significantly decreased in vitiligo patients compared to controls [67]. Moreover, the mean percentage area of positive immunostaining in skin biopsies and peripheral blood levels of FoxP3 are significantly lower in vitiligo patients compared to controls [85]. Vitiligo area scoring index, vitiligo disease activity and stress score also correlate negatively with FoxP3 levels [85]. The expression of CTLA-4 (a T cell surface molecule involved in regulation of T cell activation) is also decreased in vitiligo patients, an impairment that could perturb the normal suppressive capacity of Treg cells [86]. Furthermore, decreased serum and tissue levels of transforming growth factor (TGF)-beta (important for imposing a Treg cell phenotype) are observed in individuals with vitiligo [87]. Reduced levels of TGF-beta also correlate with increased disease activity [88] and the percentage of involved body area [89]. Moreover, lowered IL-10 (contributes to Treg cell-mediated immunosuppression) levels are present in active cases of vitiligo [88,90]. Finally, and importantly, in a mouse model of vitiligo, the adoptive transfer of melanocyte-specific Tregs was found to induce a lasting remission of the disease [91], thus proposing Treg cells as a potential therapeutic target.

9. Macrophages

Macrophage infiltration has been demonstrated in vitiligo lesions, with increased numbers present in perilesional compared with normal skin [32,92]. There is evidence that macrophages are involved in the clearing of apoptosed melanocytes from the skin in vitiligo patients [93]. In addition, macrophages expressing activating Fc-gamma receptors have been shown to mediate depigmentation in a mouse model of autoimmune vitiligo [94]. Moreover, macrophage migration inhibitory factor, which is a potent activator of macrophages and is considered to play an important role in cell-mediated immunity, has been found at significantly higher levels in vitiligo patients compared to controls [95].

10. Dendritic cells

Enhanced populations of CD11c^{+}myeloid dermal dendritic cells and CD207^{+}Langerhans cells have been observed in the leading edges of vitiligo lesions [75,96,97]. Dendritic cell-LAMP^{+}and CD1c^{+}sub-populations were also found to be significantly expanded in the lesional edges of vitiligo skin [75]. More recently, dendritic cell-mediated destruction of melanocytes has been demonstrated *in vivo* and *in vitro* [96,98]. This process was related to the release by stressed melanocytes of heat-shock protein 70, a molecule which in turn induced the expression of membrane tumour necrosis factor-related apoptosis-inducing ligand (TRAIL) on dendritic cells as well as the activation of dendritic cell effector functions directed against stressed melanocytes exhibiting elevated TRAIL death receptor expression [96,98].

11. Natural killer cells

Alterations in natural killer (NK) cells have been demonstrated in vitiligo patients indicating a role for them in the pathogenesis of the disease [99]. The percentages of NK cells with activatory receptors, as denoted by the expression of CD16^{+}CD56^{+}and CD3^{+}CD16^{+}CD56^{+}, are significantly increased in vitiligo patients compared with the controls, while the percentage of NK cells expressing the inhibitory receptor CD158a^{+}is significantly reduced.

12. Cytokines

Various studies have implicated cytokine involvement in the pathogenesis of vitiligo [100]. For example, increased serum levels of soluble IL-2 receptor are associated with vitiligo activity, indicating T cell activation [101], and elevated production of IL-6, which can induce ICAM-1 expression on melanocytes thereby facilitating leukocyte interactions, and IL-8, which can attract neutrophils to amplify destructive inflammatory responses, are found in vitiligo patients [102]. In addition, other pro-inflammatory cytokines including IL-1, IL-4, IFN-gamma and TNF-alpha, which are paracrine inhibitors of melanocytes or initiators of apoptosis, are detected at significantly higher levels in vitiligo patients compared with healthy controls [71, 100,103-105], and IL-17 levels are positively correlated with the extent of body area involvement [106]. In contrast, the level of TGF-beta, required for the maturation of Treg cells, is significantly decreased in vitiligo patients compared with controls [106]. Finally, imbalances of keratinocyte-derived cytokines that affect melanocyte activity and survival are found in vitiligo lesional skin: significantly lower expression of granulocyte-macrophage colony-stimulating factor, stem cell factor and endothelin-1 is detected in depigmented vitiligo lesions compared with normal skin [100].

13. Immuno-regulatory micro RNAs

MicroRNAs (miRNAs) are a class of small non-coding RNAs that negatively regulate gene expression. Abnormal expression of miRNAs which play crucial roles in regulating immunity has been reported in vitiligo. In a mouse model of the disease [107], dysregulated miRNAs included miRNA-146a, which contributes to the regulation of Treg cell function [108] and is implicated in autoimmune disease development in mice [109], as well as miR-191, which mediates in the proliferation and survival of melanocytes [110]. In addition, there is an increase in the expression of immune-regulatory miRNAs miRNA-133b, miRNA-135a, miRNA-9 and miRNA-1 in the lesional skin of vitiligo patients, suggesting an important role for these in vitiligo pathogenesis [111].

14. Treatment modalities

Repigmentation in vitiligo patients receiving treatment with immunosuppressive agents indirectly supports the theory that immune-mediated processes are involved in vitiligo pathogenesis. Topically applied tacrolimus (FK506), a therapeutic agent which exerts a potent immunosuppressive effect on T cells by blocking the action of the cytokine gene-activating cofactor calcineurin [112], has resulted in successful repigmentation responses in vitiligo patients [113,114] Topical corticosteroids, which have anti-inflammatory and immunosuppressive actions, are considered to be an effective first-line treatment in children and adults with segmental or non-segmental vitiligo of recent onset [3,115], and, indeed, following treatment of vitiligo patients with systemic steroids, a reduction in anti-melanocyte antibody levels and in antibody-mediated anti-melanocyte cytotoxicity has been demonstrated [116,117].

Psoralen with ultraviolet radiation (PUVA) is used as a second-line therapy for vitiligo [3,118]. Following PUVA treatment, a reduction in the number of Langerhans cells and a decrease in the expression of vitiligo-associated melanocyte antigens, which could lead to a blocking of antibody-dependent cell-mediated cytotoxicity against melanocytes, have been noted in vitiligo patients [119,120]. In addition, ultraviolet radiation can induce the expression of anti-inflammatory cytokines, modulate the expression of intercellular adhesion molecule-1, and induce apoptosis of skin-infiltrating T lymphocytes [121,122].

Despite the many available therapeutic modalities [115,123], repigmentation in the majority of vitiligo patients is rarely complete or long-lasting, so a better understanding of the precise aetiology and pathogenesis of the disease is crucial to improving the efficacy of treatment regimens.

15. Conclusion

As detailed in this chapter, there is strong evidence for the involvement of autoimmunity in the aetiology and pathogenesis of vitiligo. However, it is most likely that several interacting factors (Figure 1) are responsible for the clinical manifestations of the disease [124]. Indeed, although the evidence for the role of immune-related genes in the aetiology of vitiligo is clear [15], the limited concordance in identical twins [23] indicates that other factors, probably environmental, are also involved in its development, making the disease complex, polygenic, and multi-factorial.

Of note is the finding that oxidative-stress in melanocytes [16-18] results in the secretion of heat-shock protein 70 and chaperoned melanocyte antigens which mediates dendritic cell-activation with the consequential dendritic cell effector functions then playing a role in the destruction of melanocytes [96,125]. This has led to the convergence theory of vitiligo aetiology, which suggests that several factors act synergistically or independently to induce the disappearance of cutaneous melanocytes (Figure 1) [126]. During the elicitation phase of the disease, physical trauma to the skin [126], emotional stresses [12], or imbalances of endogenous neural factors [13], metabolites, cytokines or hormones [87] can lead to oxidative stress within melanocytes, which then respond by actively secreting heat-shock protein 70 and chaperoned melanocyte antigens [125]. In the immune activation stage, these 'danger' signals promote the activation of antigen-presenting dendritic cells with the subsequent activation and recruitment of anti-melanocyte autoreactive cytotoxic T lymphocytes to the skin [19]. Intrinsic damage to melanocytes could, therefore, be the initiating event in vitiligo development followed by a destructive secondary anti-melanocyte immune response from cytotoxic T cells [19,126,127]. Notably, 50% of vitiligo patients experience a Koebner phenomenon, whereby vitiligo develops at a site previously affected by a physical trauma [126]. In addition, different pathogenic mechanisms could account for the various clinical types of vitiligo: pathogenic neural factors are usually related to segmental vitiligo, whereas autoimmunity is most often associated with the non-segmental (generalised) form [2].

As indicated, it is most likely that immune responses in vitiligo are of a secondary nature following melanocyte damage. Indeed, as several vitiligo-associated autoantigens such as tyrosinase and gp100 are located intracellularly, it has been suggested that the formation of neo-antigens due to haptenation, the exposure of cryptic epitopes or the modification of proteins during apoptosis could account for immune responses against these proteins [128,129]. In this scenario, after processing by mature Langerhans cells, antigenic peptides are presented to T cells which have escaped clonal deletion or to naïve T lymphocytes which are not tolerised to cryptic epitopes [128,129]. Activated cytotoxic T cells can then attack directly melanocytes expressing antigenic peptides in the context MHC class I molecules [31,34], and anti-melanocyte autoantibodies can be produced following the stimulation of B lymphocytes by activated helper T cells [128].

In summary, autoimmunity has an important role to play in vitiligo development with key contributions from anti-melanocyte autoreactive cytotoxic T cells [19], T helper 17 cells [74,75], and Treg cells [77-79].

Author details

Mitesh Dwivedi[1,3*], Naresh C. Laddha[2,3], Anthony P. Weetman[4], Rasheedunnisa Begum[3] and Helen Kemp[4]

*Address all correspondence to: mitesh_dwivedi@yahoo.com

1 C. G. Bhakta Institute of Biotechnology, Uka Tarsadia University, Tarsadi, Surat, Gujarat, India

2 Department of Molecular Biology, Unipath Specialty Laboratory Ltd., Ahmedabad, Gujarat, India

3 Department of Biochemistry, The Maharaja Sayajirao University of Baroda, Vadodara, Gujarat, India

4 Department of Human Metabolism, University of Sheffield, Sheffield, United Kingdom

References

[1] Taïeb A, Picardo M. Epidemiology, definitions and classification. In: Taïeb A, Picardo M. (eds) Vitiligo. Berlin: Springer-Verlag; 2010. p13-24.

[2] Taïeb A. Intrinsic and extrinsic pathomechanisms in vitiligo. Pigment Cell Res 2000;13: 41-47.

[3] Gawkrodger DJ, Ormerod AD, Shaw L, Mauri-Sole I, Whitton ME, Watts MJ, Anstey AV, Ingham J, Young K. Vitiligo: concise evidence based guidelines on diagnosis and management. Postgrad Med J 2010;86: 466-471.

[4] Kent G, Al'Abadie M. Psychologic effects of vitiligo: A critical incident analysis. J Am Acad Dermatol 1996;35: 895-898.

[5] Parsad D, Dogra S, Kanwar AJ. Quality of life in patients with vitiligo. Health Qual Life Outcomes 2003;1: 58.

[6] Boisseau-Garsaud AM, Garsaud P, Cales-Quist D, Helenon R, Queneherve C, Claire RC. Epidemiology of vitiligo in the French West Indies (Isle of Martinique). Int J Dermatol 2000;39: 18-20.

[7] Howitz J, Brodthagen H, Schwartz M, Thomsen K. Prevalence of vitiligo: Epidemiological survey on the Isle of Bornholm, Denmark. Arch Dermatol 1977;113: 47-52.

[8] Handa S, Kaur I. Vitiligo: clinical findings in 1436 patients. J Dermatol 1999;10: 653-657.

[9] Sehgal VN, Srivastava G. Vitiligo: compendium of clinico-epidemiological features. Indian J Dermatol Venereol Leprol 2007;73: 149-156.

[10] Kakourou T. Vitiligo in children. World J Pediatr 2009;5: 265-268.

[11] Grimes PE, Sevall JS, Vojdani A. Cytomegalovirus DNA identified in skin biopsy specimens of patients with vitiligo. J Am Acad Dermatol 1996;35: 21-26.

[12] Al'Abadie MS, Kent GG, Gawkrodger DJ. The relationship between stress and the onset and exacerbation of psoriasis and other skin conditions. Br J Dermatol 1994;130: 199-203.

[13] Al'Abadie MS, Senior HJ, Bleehen SS, Gawkrodger DJ. Neuropeptide and neuronal marker studies in vitiligo. Br J Dermatol 1994;131; 160-165.

[14] Gauthier Y, Cario-Andre M, Taieb A. A critical appraisal of vitiligo etiologic theories. Is melanocyte loss a melanocytorrhagy? Pigment Cell Res 2003;16: 322-332.

[15] Spritz RA. Six decades of vitiligo genetics: genome-wide studies provide insights into autoimmune pathogenesis. J Invest Dermatol 2012;132: 268–273.

[16] Dell'Anna ML, Picardo, M. A review and a new hypothesis for non-immunological pathogenetic mechanisms in vitiligo. Pigment Cell Res 2006;19: 406-411.

[17] Schallreuter KU, Moore J, Wood JM, Beazley WD, Peters EMJ, Marles LK, Behrens-Williams SC, Dummer R, Blau N, Thony B. Epidermal H2O2 accumulation alters tetrahydrobiopterin (6BH4) recycling in vitiligo: identification of a general mechanism in regulation of all 6BH4-dependent processes? J Invest Dermatol 2001;116: 167–174.

[18] Schallreuter KU, Wood JM, Berger, J. Low catalase levels in the epidermis of patients with vitiligo. J Invest Dermatol 2001;97: 1081–1085.

[19] Van den Boorn JG, Konijnenberg D, Dellemijn TA, van der Veen JP, Bos JD, Melief CJ, Vyth-Dreese FA, Luiten RM. Autoimmune destruction of skin melanocytes by perilesional T cells from vitiligo patients. J Invest Dermatol 2009;129: 2220-2232.

[20] Kemp EH, Weetman AP, Gawkrodger DJ. Humoral immunity. In: Taïeb A, Picardo M. (eds) Vitiligo. Berlin: Springer-Verlag; 2010. p.248-256.

[21] Boelaert K, Newby PR, Simmonds MJ, Holder RL, Carr-Smith JD, Heward JM, Manji N, Allahabadia A, Armitage M, Chatterjee KV, Lazarus JH, Pearce, S.H., Vaidya B, Gough SC, Franklyn JA. Prevalence and relative risk of other autoimmune diseases in subjects with autoimmune thyroid disease. Am J Med 2010;123: 183.e1-183.e9.

[22] Birlea SA, Fain PR, Spritz RA. A Romanian population isolate with high frequency of vitiligo and associated autoimmune diseases. Arch Dermatol 2008;144: 310-316.

[23] Alkhateeb A, Fain PR, Thody A, Bennett DC, Spritz RA. Epidemiology of vitiligo and associated autoimmune diseases in Caucasian probands and their relatives. Pigment Cell Res 2003;16: 208-214.

[24] Laberge G, Mailloux CM, Gowan K, Holland P, Bennett DC, Fain PR, Spritz RA. Early onset and increased risk of other autoimmune diseases in familial generalized vitiligo. Pigment Cell Res 2005;18: 300-305.

[25] Singh A, Sharma P, Kar HK, Sharma VK, Tembhre MK, Gupta S, Laddha NC, Dwivedi M, Begum R, Indian Genome Variation Consortium, Gokhale RS, Rani R. HLA alleles and amino-acid signatures of the peptide-binding pockets of HLA molecules in vitiligo. J Invest Dermatol 2012;132: 124–134.

[26] Jin Y, Birlea SA, Fain PR, Gowan, K., Riccardi SL, Holland PJ, Mailloux CM, Sufit AJ, Hutton, SM, Amadi-Myers A, Bennett DC, Wallace MR, McCormack WT, Kemp EH, Gawkrodger, D.J., Weetman, A.P., Picardo M, Leone G, Taieb A, Jouary T, Ezzedine K, van Geel N, Lambert J, Overbeck A, Spritz RA. Variant of *TYR* and autoimmunity susceptibility loci in generalized vitiligo. N Engl J Med 2010;362:1686–1697.

[27] Jin Y, Ferrara T, Gowan K, Holcomb C, Rastrou M, Erlich HA, Fain PR, Spritz RA. Next-generation re-sequencing identifies common variants of *TYR* and *HLA-A* that modulate the risk of generalized vitiligo via antigen presentation. J Invest Dermatol 2012;132: 1730–1733.

[28] Liu J1, Tang H, Zuo X, Liang B, Wang P, Sun L, Yang S, Zhang X. A single nucleotide polymorphism rs9468925 of MHC region is associated with clinical features of generalized vitiligo in Chinese Han population. J Eur Acad Dermatol Venereol 2012;26: 1137–1141.

[29] Quan C, Ren YQ, Xiang LH, Sun LD, Xu AE, Gao XH, Chen HD, Pu XM, Wu RN, Liang CZ, Li JB, Gao TW, Zhang JZ, Wang XL, Wang J, Yang RY, Liang L, Yu JB, Zuo XB, Zhang SQ, Zhang, SM, Chen G, Zheng XD, Li P, Zhu J, Li YW, Wei XD, Hong WS, Ye Y, Zhang Y, Wu WS, Cheng H, Dong PL, Hu DY, Li Y, Li M, Zhang X, Tang HY, Tang XF, Xu SX, He SM, Lv YM, Shen M, Jiang HQ, Wang Y, Li K, Kang XJ, Liu YQ, Sun L, Liu ZF, Xie SQ, Zhu CY, Xu Q, Gao JP, Hu, WL, Ni C, Pan TM, Yao S, He CF, Liu YS, Yu ZY, Yin XY, Zhang FY, Yang S, Zhou Y, Zhang XJ. Genome-wide association study for vitiligo identifies susceptibility loci at 6q27 and the MHC. Nat Genet 2010;42: 614–618.

[30] Al Badri AM, Fouli AK, Todd PM, Gariouch JJ, Gudgeon JE, Stewart DG, Gracie JA, Goudie RB. Abnormal expression of MHC class II and ICAM-1 by melanocytes in vitiligo. J Pathol 1993;169: 203-206.

[31] Hedley SJ, Metcalfe R, Gawkrodger DJ, Weetman AP, MacNeil S. Vitiligo melanocytes in long-term culture show normal constitutive and cytokine-induced expression of intercellular adhesion molecule-1 and major histocompatibility complex class I and class II molecules. Br J Dermatol 1998;139: 965-973.

[32] Van den Wijngaard R, Wankowicz-Kalinska A, Le Poole C, Tigges AJ, Westerhof W, Das P. Local immune response in skin of generalised vitiligo patients. Destruction of melanocytes is associated with the prominent presence of CLA+T cells at the perilesional site. Lab Invest 2000;80: 1299-1309.

[33] Ogg GS, Dunbar PR, Romero P, Chen JL, Cerundolo V. High frequency of skin-homing melanocyte-specific cytotoxic T lymphocytes in autoimmune vitiligo. J Exp Med 1998; 188:1203–1208.

[34] Le Poole IC, Mutis T, van den Wijngaard RM, Westerhof W, Ottenhoff T, de Vries RR, Das PK. A novel, antigen-presenting function of melanocytes and its possible relationship to hypopigmentary disorders. J Immunol 1993;151: 7284-7292.

[35] Van den Wijngaard RM, Asghar SS, Pijnenborg AC, Tigges AJ, Westerhof W, Das P. Aberrant expression of complement regulatory proteins, membrane cofactor protein and decay accelerating factor, in the involved epidermis of patients with vitiligo. Br J Dermatol 2002;146: 80-87.

[36] Cui J, Arita Y, Bystryn J-C. Characterisation of vitiligo antigens. Pigment Cell Res 1995;8: 53-59.

[37] Naughton GK, Reggiardo MD, Bystryn J-C. Correlation between vitiligo antibodies and extent of depigmentation in vitiligo. J Am Acad Dermatol 1986;15: 978-981.

[38] Harning R, Cui J, Bystryn, J-C. Relation between the incidence and level of pigment cell antibodies and disease activity in vitiligo. J Invest Dermatol 1991;97: 1078-1080.

[39] Laddha NC, Dwivedi M, Mansuri MS, Singh M, Gani AR, Panchal V, Khan F, Dave D, Patel A, Shajil EM, Gupta R, Marfatia Z, Marfatia YS, Begum R. Role of oxidative stress and autoimmunity in onset and progression of vitiligo. Exp Dermatol 2014;23: 345-368.

[40] Xie P, Geohegan WD, Jordan RE. Vitiligo autoantibodies. Studies of subclass distribution and complement activation. J Invest Dermatol 1991;96: 627.

[41] Aronson PJ, Hashimoto K. Association of IgA anti-melanoma antibodies in the sera of vitiligo patients with active disease. J Invest Dermatol 1987;88: 475.

[42] Kemp EH, Gawkrodger DJ, MacNeil S, Watson PF, Weetman AP. Detection of tyrosinase autoantibodies in patients with vitiligo using 35S-labeled recombinant human tyrosinase in a radioimmunoassay. J Invest Dermatol 1997;109: 69-73.

[43] Baharav E, Merimski O, Shoenfeld Y, Zigelman R, Gilbrud B, Yecheskel G, Youinou P, Fishman P. Tyrosinase as an autoantigen in patients with vitiligo. Clin Exp Immunol 1996;105: 84–88.

[44] Song YH, Connor E, Li Y, Zorovich B, Balducci P, Maclaren N. The role of tyrosinase in autoimmune vitiligo. Lancet 1994;344: 1049-1052.

[45] Kemp EH, Waterman EA, Gawkrodger DJ, Watson PF, Weetman AP. Autoantibodies to tyrosinase-related protein-1 detected in the sera of vitiligo patients using a quantitative radiobinding assay. Br J Dermatol 1998;139: 798-805.

[46] Kemp EH, Gawkrodger DJ, Watson PF, Weetman AP. Immunoprecipitation of melanogenic enzyme autoantigens with vitiligo sera: evidence for cross-reactive autoantibodies to tyrosinase and tyrosinase-related protein-2 (TRP-2). Clin Exp Immunol 1997;109: 495–500.

[47] Okamoto T, Irie RF, Fujii S, Huang S, Nizze AJ, Morton DL, Hoon DS. Anti-tyrosinase-related protein-2 immune response in vitiligo and melanoma patients receiving active-specific immunotherapy. J Invest Dermatol 1998;111: 1034-1039.

[48] Kemp EH, Gawkrodger DJ, Watson PF, Weeman AP. Autoantibodies to human melanocyte-specific protein Pmel17 in the sera of vitiligo patients: a sensitive and quantitative radioimmunoassay (RIA). Clin Exp Immunol 1998;114:333-338.

[49] Waterman EA, Gawkrodger DJ, Watson PF, Weetman AP, Kemp EH. Autoantigens in vitiligo identified by the serological selection of a phage-displayed melanocyte cDNA expression library. J Invest Dermatol 2010;130: 230-240.

[50] Kemp EH, Waterman EA, Hawes BE, O'Neill K, Gottumukkala RV, Gawkrodger DJ, Weetman AP, Watson PF. The melanin-concentrating hormone receptor 1, a novel target of autoantibody responses in vitiligo. J Clin Invest 2002;109: 923-930.

[51] Li Q, Lv Y, Li C, Yi X, Long HA, Qiao H, Lu T, Luan Q, Li K, Wang X, Wang G, Gao, T. Vitiligo autoantigen VIT75 is identified as lamin A in vitiligo by serological proteome analysis based on mass spectrometry. J Invest Dermatol 2010;131: 727-734.

[52] Mandry RC, Ortiz LJ, Lugo-Somolinos A, Sanchez JL. Organ-specific autoantibodies in vitiligo patients and their relatives. Int J Dermatol 1996;35: 18-21.

[53] Farrokhi S, Farsangi-Hojjat M, Noohpisheh MK, Tahmasbi R, Rezaei N. Assessment of the immune system in 55 Iranian patients with vitiligo. J Eur Acad Dermatol Venereol 2005;19: 706-711.

[54] Yu HS, Kao CH, Yu CL.Coexistence and relationship of antikeratinocyte and antimelanocyte antibodies in patients with non-segmental-type vitiligo. J Invest Dermatol 1993:100; 823-828.

[55] Fishman P, Azizi E, Shoenfeld Y, Sredni, B, Yecheskel G, Ferrone S, Zigelman R, Chaitchik S, Floro S, Djaldetti M. Vitiligo autoantibodies are effective against melanoma. Cancer 1993;72: 2365-2369.

[56] Gottumukkala RVSRK, Gavalas NG, Akhtar S, Metcalfe RA, Gawkrodger DJ, Haycock JW, Watson, PF, Weetman AP, Kemp EH. Function blocking autoantibodies to the melanin-concentrating hormone receptor in vitiligo patients. Lab Invest 2006;86: 781-789.

[57] Norris DA, Kissinger RM, Naughton GM, Bystryn J-C. Evidence for immunologic mechanisms in human vitiligo: patients' sera induce damage to human melanocytes in vitro by complement-mediated damage and antibody-dependent cellular cytotoxicity. J Invest Dermatol 1998;90: 783-789.

[58] Gilhar A, Zelickson B, Ulman Y, Etzioni A. In vivo destruction of melanocytes by the IgG fraction of serum from patients with vitiligo. J Invest Dermatol 1995;105: 683-686.

[59] Yi YL, Yu CH, Yu HS. IgG anti-melanocyte antibodies purified from patients with active vitiligo induce HLA-DR and intercellular adhesion molecule-1 expression and an increase in interleukin-8 release by melanocytes. J Invest Dermatol 2000;115: 969-973.

[60] Cario-Andre M, Pain C, Gauthier Y, Taieb A. The melanocytorrhagic hypothesis of vitiligo tested on pigmented, stressed, reconstructed epidermis. Pigment Cell Res 2007;20: 385-393.

[61] Ruiz-Argüelles A, Brito GJ, Reyes-Izquierdo P, Pérez-Romano B, Sánchez-Sosa S. Apoptosis of melanocytes in vitiligo results from antibody penetration. J Autoimmun 2007;29 :281–286.

[62] Michaëlsson G. Vitiligo with raised borders. Report of two cases. Acta Derm Venereol 1968;48: 158-161.

[63] Lang KS, Caroli CC, Muhm D, Wernet D, Moris A, Schittek B, Knauss-Scherwitz E., Stevanovic S, Rammensee H-G, Garbe C. HLA-A2 restricted, melanocyte-specific CD8+T lymphocytes detected in vitiligo patients are related to disease activity and are predominantly directed against MelanA/MART1. J Invest Dermatol 2001;116: 891-897,

[64] Le Gal, FA, Avril M, Bosq J, Lefebvre P, Deschemin JC, Andrieu M, Dore MX, Guillet JG. Direct evidence to support the role of antigen-specific CD8 (+) T-cells in melanoma-associated vitiligo. J Invest Dermatol 2001;117: 1464-1470.

[65] Mandelcorn-Monson RL, Shear NH, Yau E, Sambhara S, Barber BH, Spaner D, DeBenedette MA. Cytotoxic T lymphocyte reactivity to gp100, MelanA/MART-1, and tyrosinase, in HLA-A2-positive vitiligo patients. J Invest Dermatol 2003;121: 550-556.

[66] Palermo B, Campanelli R, Garbelli S, Mantovani S, Lantelme E, Brazzelli V, Ardigó M, Borroni G, Martinetti M, Badulli C, Necker A, Giachino C. Specific cytotoxic T lymphocyte responses against Melan-A/MART1, tyrosinase and gp100 in vitiligo by the use of major histocompatibility complex/peptide tetramers: the role of cellular immunity in the etiopathogenesis of vitiligo. J Invest Dermatol 2001;117: 326–32.

[67] Dwivedi M, Laddha NC, Arora P, Marfatia YS, Begum R. Decreased regulatory T-cells and CD4(+) /CD8(+) ratio correlate with disease onset and progression in patients with generalized vitiligo. Pigment Cell Melanoma Res 2013;26: 586-591.

[68] Al Badri AMT, Todd PM, Garioch JJ, Gudgeon JE, Stewart DG, Goudie RB. An immunohistological study of cutaneous lymphocytes in vitiligo. J Pathol 1993;170: 149-155.

[69] Abdallah M, Lotfi R, Othman W, Galal R. Assessment of tissue FoxP3+, CD4+and CD8+T-cells in active and stable nonsegmental vitiligo. Int J Dermatol 2014;53: 940-946.

[70] Wankowicz-Kalinska A, van den Wijngaard RM, Tigges BJ, Westerhof W, Ogg GS, Cerundolo V, Storkus WJ, Das PK. Immunopolarization of CD4+and CD8+T cells to type-1-like is associated with melanocyte loss in human vitiligo. Lab Invest 2003;83: 683-695.

[71] Dwivedi M, Laddha NC, Shah K, Shah BJ, Begum R. Involvement of interferon-gamma genetic variants and intercellular adhesion molecule-1 in onset and progression of generalized vitiligo. J Interferon Cytokine Res 2013;33: 646-659.

[72] Le Poole IC, Stennett LS, Bonish BK, Dee L, Robinson JK, Hernandez C, Hann SK, Nickoloff BJ. Expansion of vitiligo lesions is associated with reduced epidermal CDw60 expression and increased expression of HLA-DR in perilesional skin. Br J Dermatol 2003;149: 739-748.

[73] Steitz J, Wenzel J, Gaffal E, Tüting T. Initiation and regulation of CD8+T cells recognizing melanocytic antigens in the epidermis: implications for the pathophysiology of vitiligo. Eur J Cell Biol 2004; 83: 797–803.

[74] Kotobuki Y, Tanemura A, Yang L, Itoi S, Wataya-Kaneda M, Murota H, Fujimoto M, Serada S, Naka T, Katayama I. Dysregulation of melanocyte function by Th17-related cytokines: significance of Th17 cell infiltration in autoimmune vitiligo vulgaris. Pigment Cell Melanoma Res 2012;25: 219-230.

[75] Wang CQ, Cruz-Inigo AE, Fuentes-Duculan J, Moussai D, Gulati N, Sullivan-Whalen M, Gilleaudeau P, Cohen JA, Krueger JG. Th17 cells and activated dendritic cells are increased in vitiligo lesions. PLoS One 2011;6: e18907.

[76] Levings MK, Sangregorio R, Roncarolo MG. Human CD25(+)CD4(+) T regulatory cells suppress naive and memory T cell proliferation and can be expanded in vitro without loss of function. J Exp Med 2001;193: 1295-1302.

[77] Lili Y, Yi W, Ji Y, Yue S, Weimin S, Ming L. Global activation of CD8+cytotoxic T lymphocytes correlates with an impairment in regulatory T cells in patients with generalized vitiligo. PLoS One 2012;7: e37513.

[78] Ben Ahmed M, Zaraa I, Rekik R, Elbeldi-Ferchiou A, Kourda N, Belhadj Hmida N, Abdeladhim M, Karoui O, Ben Osman A, Mokni M, Louzir H. Functional defects of peripheral regulatory T lymphocytes in patients with progressive vitiligo. Pigment Cell Melanoma Res 2012;25: 99-109.

[79] Dwivedi M, Kemp EH, Laddha NC, Mansuri MS, Weetman AP, Begum R. Regulatory T cells in vitiligo: Implications for pathogenesis and therapeutics. Autoimmunity Rev 2014;doi: 10.1016/j.autrev.2014.10.002.

[80] Ono S, Tanizaki H, Otsuka A, Endo Y, Koyanagi I, Kataoka TR, Miyachi Y, Kabashima K. Coexistent skin lesions of vitiligo and psoriasis vulgaris. Immunohistochemical analyses for IL-17A-producing cells and regulatory T cells. Acta Derm Venereol 2014;94: 329-330.

[81] Terras S, Gambichler T, Moritz RK, Altmeyer P, Lambert J. Immunohistochemical analysis of FOXP3+regulatory T cells in healthy human skin and autoimmune dermatoses. Int J Dermatol 2014;53: 294-299.

[82] Zhou L, Li K, Shi YL, Hamzavi I, Gao TW, Henderson M, Huggins RH, Agbai O, Mahmoud B, Mi X, Lim HW, Mi QS. Systemic analyses of immunophenotypes of peripheral T cells in non-segmental vitiligo: implication of defective natural killer T cells. Pigment Cell Melanoma Res 2012;25: 602-611.

[83] Klarquist J, Denman CJ, Hernandez C, Wainwright DA, Strickland FM, Overbeck A, Mehrotra S, Nishimura MI, Le Poole IC. Reduced skin homing by functional Treg in vitiligo. Pigment Cell Melanoma Res 2010;23: 276-286.

[84] Abdallah M, Saad A. Evaluation of circulating CD4+CD25highFoxP3+T lymphocytes in active non-segmental vitiligo. J Pan-Arab League Dermatol 2009;20: 1.

[85] Elela MA, Hegazy RA, Fawzy MM, Rashed LA, Rasheed H. Interleukin 17, interleukin 22 and FoxP3 expression in tissue and serum of non-segmental vitiligo: A case-controlled study on eighty-four patients. Eur J Dermatol 2013;23: 350-355.

[86] Dwivedi M, Laddha NC, Imran M, Shah BJ, Begum R. Cytotoxic T-lymphocyte associated antigen-4 (CTLA-4) in isolated vitiligo: a genotype-phenotype correlation. Pigment Cell Melanoma Res 2011;24: 737-740.

[87] Moretti S, Spallanzani A, Amato L, Hautmann G, Gallerani I, Fabiani M, Fabbri P. New insights into the pathogenesis of vitiligo: imbalance of epidermal cytokines at sites of lesions. Pigment Cell Res 2002;15: 87-92.

[88] Tembhre MK, Sharma VK, Sharma A, Chattopadhyay P, Gupta S. T helper and regulatory T cell cytokine profile in active, stable and narrow band ultraviolet B treated generalized vitiligo. Clin Chim Acta 2013;424:27-32.

[89] Tu CX, Jin WW, Lin M, Wang ZH, Man MQ. Levels of TGF-β(1) in serum and culture supernatants of CD4(+)CD25(+) T cells from patients with non-segmental vitiligo. Arch Dermatol Res 2011;303:685-9.

[90] Taher ZA, Lauzon G, Maguiness S, Dytoc MT. Analysis of interleukin-10 levels in lesions of vitiligo following treatment with topical tacrolimus. Br J Dermatol 2009;161: 654-659.

[91] Chatterjee S, Eby JM, Al-Khami AA, Soloshchenko M, Kang HK, Kaur N, Naga OS, Murali A, Nishimura MI, Le Poole IC, Mehrotra S. A quantitative increase in regulatory T cells controls development of vitiligo. J Invest Dermatol 2014;134:1285-1294.

[92] Le Poole IC, van den Wijngaard RMJGJ, Westerhof W, Das, PK. Presence of T cells and macrophages in inflammatory vitiligo skin parallels melanocyte disappearance. Am J Pathol1996;148: 1219-1228.

[93] Oiso N, Tanemura A, Kotobuki Y, Kimura M, Katayama I, Kawada A. Role of macrophage infiltration in successful repigmentation in a new periphery-spreading vitiligo lesion in a male Japanese patient. J Dermatol 2013; 40: 915-918.

[94] Trcka J, Moroi Y, Clynes RA, Goldberg SM, Bergtold A, Perales MA, Ma M, Ferrone CR, Carroll MC, Ravetch JV, Houghton AN. Redundant and alternative roles for activating Fc receptors and complement in an antibody-dependent model of autoimmune vitiligo. Immunity 2002;16: 861-868.

[95] Serarslan G, Yönden Z, Söğüt S, Savaş N, Celik E, Arpaci A. Macrophage migration inhibitory factor in patients with vitiligo and relationship between duration and clinical type of disease. Clin Exp Dermatol 2010;35: 487-490.

[96] Kroll TM, Bommiasamy H, Boissy RE, Hernandez C, Nickoloff BJ, Mestril R, Le Poole IC. 4-tertiary butyl phenol exposure sensitizes human melanocytes to dendritic cell-mediated killing: relevance to vitiligo. J Invest Dermatol 2005;124: 798–806.

[97] Itoi S, Tanemura A, Kotobuki Y, Wataya-Kaneda M, Tsuruta D, Ishii M, Katayama I. Coexistence of Langerhans cells activation and immune cells infiltration in progressive nonsegmental vitiligo. J Dermatol Sci 2014;73: 83-85.

[98] Denman CJ, McCracken J, Hariharan V, Klarquist J, Oyarbide-Valencia K, Guevara-Patiño JA, Le Poole IC. HSP70i accelerates depigmentation in a mouse model of autoimmune vitiligo. J Invest Dermatol 2008;128: 2041-2048.

[99] Basak PY, Adiloglu AK, Koc IG, Tas T, Akkaya VB. Evaluation of activatory and inhibitory natural killer cell receptors in non-segmental vitiligo: a flow cytometric study. J Eur Acad Dermatol Venereol 2008;22: 970-976.

[100] Moretti S, Spallanzani A, Amato L, Hautmann G, Gallerani I, Fabiani M, Fabbri P. New insights into the pathogenesis of vitiligo: imbalance of epidermal cytokines at sites of lesions. Pigment Cell Res 2002;15: 87-92.

[101] Yeo UC, Yang YS, Park KB, Sung HT, Jung SY, Lee ES, Shin MH. Serum concentration of the soluble interleukin-2 receptor in vitiligo patients. J Dermatol Sci 1999;19: 182-188.

[102] Yu HS, Chang KL, Yu CL, Li HF, Wu MT, Wu CS, Wu CS. Alterations in IL-6, IL-8, GM-CSF, TNF-alpha, and IFN-gamma release by peripheral mononuclear cells in patients with active vitiligo J Invest Dermatol 1997;108: 527-529.

[103] Laddha NC, Dwivedi M, Begum R. Increased tumor necrosis factor (TNF)-α and its promoter polymorphisms correlate with disease progression and higher susceptibility towards vitiligo. PLoS One 2012;7:e52298.

[104] Imran M, Laddha NC, Dwivedi M, Mansuri MS, Singh J, Rani R, Gokhale RS, Sharma VK, Marfatia YS, Begum R. Interleukin-4 genetic variants correlate with its transcript and protein levels in patients with vitiligo. Br J Dermatol 2012;167: 314-323.

[105] Birol A, Kisa U, Kurtipek GS, Kara F, Kocak M, Erkek E, Caglayan O. Increased tumor necrosis factor alpha (TNF-alpha) and interleukin 1 alpha (IL1-alpha) levels in the lesional skin of patients with nonsegmental vitiligo. Int J Dermatol 2006;45: 992-993.

[106] Basak PY, Adiloglu AK, Ceyhan AM, Tas T, Akkaya VB. The role of helper and regulatory T cells in the pathogenesis of vitiligo. J Am Acad Dermatol 2009;60: 256-60.

[107] Shi YL, Weiland M, Lim HW, Mi QS, Zhou L. Serum miRNA expression profiles change in autoimmune vitiligo in mice. Exp Dermatol 2014;23:140-142.

[108] Lu LF, Boldin MP, Chaudhry A, Lin LL, Taganov KD, Hanada T, Yoshimura A, Baltimore D, Rudensky AY. Function of miR-146a in controlling Treg cell-mediated regulation of Th1 responses. Cell 2010;142: 914-929.

[109] Boldin MP, Taganov KD, Rao DS, Yang L, Zhao JL, Kalwani M, Garcia-Flores Y, Luong M, Devrekanli A, Xu J, Sun G, Tay J, Linsley PS, Baltimore D. miR-146a is a significant brake on autoimmunity, myeloproliferation, and cancer in mice. J Exp Med 201;208: 1189-1201.

[110] Mueller DW, Rehli M, Bosserhoff AK. miRNA expression profiling in melanocytes and melanoma cell lines reveals miRNAs associated with formation and progression of malignant melanoma. J Invest Dermatol 2009;129: 1740-1751.

[111] Mansuri MS, Singh M, Dwivedi M, Laddha NC, Marfatia YS, Begum R. miRNA profiling revealed differentially expressed miRNA signatures from skin of non-segmental vitiligo patients. Br J Dermatol 2014;doi: 10.1111/bjd.13109.

[112] Homey B, Assmann T, Vohr HW, Ulrich P, Lauerma AI, Ruzicka T, Lehmann P, Schuppe HC. Topical FK506 suppresses cytokine and costimulatory molecule expres-

sion in epidermal and local draining lymph node cells during primary skin immune responses. J Immunol 1998;160: 5331-5340.

[113] Boone B, Ongenae K, Van Geel N, Vernijns S, De Keyser S, Naeyaert JM. Topical pimecrolimus in the treatment of vitiligo. Eur J Dermatol 2007;17: 55-61.

[114] Hartmann A, Brocker EB, Hamm H. Occlusive treatment enhances efficacy of tacrolimus 0.1% ointment in adult patients with vitiligo: results of a placebo-controlled 12-month prospective study. Acta Derm Venereol 2008;88: 474-479.

[115] Abu Tahir M, Pramod K, Ansari SH, Ali J. Current remedies for vitiligo. Autoimmun Rev 2010;9: 516-520.

[116] Hann SK, Kim HI, Im S, Park YK, Cui J, Bystryn JC. The change of melanocyte cytotoxicity after systemic steroid treatment in vitiligo patients. J Dermatol Sci 1993;6: 201-205.

[117] Takei M, Mishima Y, Uda H. Immunopathology of vitiligo vulgaris, Sutton's leukoderma and melanoma-associated vitiligo in relation to steroid effects. I. Circulating antibodies for cultured melanoma cells. J Cutan Pathol 1984;11: 107-113.

[118] Alomar, A. PUVA and related treatment. In: Taïeb A, Picardo M. (eds) Vitiligo. Berlin: Springer-Verlag; 2010. p345-350.

[119] Kao CH, Yu HS. Comparison of the effect of 8-Methoxypsoralen (8-MOP) plus UVA (PUVA) on human melanocytes in vitiligo vulgaris and in vitro. J Invest Dermatol 1992; 98: 734-740.

[120] Viac J, Groujon C, Misery L, Staniek V, Faure M, Schmitt D, Claudy A. Effect of UVB 311 mm irradiation on normal human skin. Photodermatol Photoimmunol Photomed 1997;13: 103-108.

[121] Krutmann J, Morita A. Mechanisms of ultraviolet (UV) B and phototherapy. J Invest Dermatol Symp Proc 1999;4: 70-72.

[122] Duthie MS, Kimber I, Norval M. The effects of ultraviolet radiation on the immune system. Br J Dermatol 1999;140: 995-1009.

[123] Olsson MJ. Surgical therapies. In: Taïeb A, Picardo M. (eds) Vitiligo. Berlin: Springer-Verlag; 2010. p394-406.

[124] Le Poole IC, Das PK, van den Wijngaard RM, Bos JD, Westerhof W. Review of the etiopathomechanism of vitiligo: a convergence theory. Exp Dermatol 1993;2: 145-153.

[125] Hariharan V, Klarquist J, Reust MJ, Koshoffer A, McKee MD, Boissy RE, Le Poole IC. Monobenzyl ether of hydroquinone and 4-tertiary butyl phenol activate markedly different physiological responses in melanocytes: relevance to skin depigmentation. J Invest Dermatol 2010;130: 211-220.

[126] Mosenson JA, Zloza A, Klarquist J, Barfuss AJ, Guevara-Patino JA, Poole IC. HSP70i is a critical component of the immune response leading to vitiligo. Pigment Cell Melanoma Res 2012;25: 88-98.

[127] Le Poole IC, Luiten RM. Autoimmune etiology of generalized vitiligo. Curr Dir Autoimmun 2008;10: 227-243.

[128] Namazi MR Neurogenic dysregulation, oxidative stress, and melanocytorrhagy in vitiligo: can they be interconnected? Pigment Cell Res 2007;20: 360-363.

[129] Westerhof W, d'Ischia M. Vitiligo puzzle: the pieces fall in place. Pigment Cell Res 2007;20: 345-359.

Chapter 8

Will Understanding Methotrexate Modes of Action Teach us About Rheumatoid Arthritis?

Charles F. Spurlock III, Nancy J. Olsen and
Thomas M. Aune

Additional information is available at the end of the chapter

http://dx.doi.org/10.5772/59901

1. Introduction

The traditional paradigm for autoimmunity dates back over a century to the German bacteriologist, and early pioneer of immunology, Paul Ehrlich, who postulated that if the immune system encounters an autoantigen, damaging outcomes ensue. He described the autoimmune phenomenon as "horror autotoxicus" or the horror of self-toxicity. Today, this basic idea persists even in the 'modern era' utilizing biochemical and molecular-based approaches to immunology. We are taught that recognition of self as foreign by the adaptive immune system is the basis for autoimmunity. Thus, the identity of the autoantigen(s) responsible for these illnesses remains the Holy Grail for scientists committed to uncovering the origins of these diseases.

While many are focused on the identity of this antigen, we have opted for a slightly different approach to this centuries-old problem. We would argue that the identity of the autoantigen is not as important as the cell that sees this antigen. Our approach suggests a failure of the responding immune cell, particularly the T helper cell. In fact, recognition of self is essential for T cell survival and immune homeostasis. The immune system must recognize 'self' in order to protect the host.[1, 2] In lieu of traditional approaches that may involve animal models, our work has focused on the patients and their immune cells to investigate the molecular underpinnings of disease. We have also observed that common therapies to treat autoimmune disease, particularly, rheumatoid arthritis (RA), while efficacious, have ill-defined mechanisms elucidating their function. Therefore, a large portion of our investigation of rheumatoid arthritis examines methotrexate (MTX) responses using *in vitro* models and primary cells from RA patients receiving MTX therapy. MTX, which remains the 'gold standard' for the treatment of RA, has become a tool for us to better understand this disease. The resulting body of work reveals novel mechanisms not only for low-dose MTX action but has permitted us to learn a great deal about disease pathogenesis. An important consequence of this MTX-centric approach, has led to us to uncover new understandings for how the human immune system may function, which we will explore in this chapter. In general, many molecular defects are seen in T cells from subjects with RA. MTX alters expression/activity of many of these same targets *in vivo* and in tissue culture models. Studies in tissue culture models have allowed us to unravel some of the phenotypic changes that result from MTX treatment. These are summarized in Table 1.

Gene Target	Status in RA	MTX Target	MTX Function
c-Fos(*FOS*)	UC	+	Increases apoptosis sensitivity
c-Jun (*JUN*)	UC	+	Increases apoptosis sensitivity
CHEK2	UE	-	-
DNA-PKcs (*PRKDC*)	UE	+	Increases lincRNA-p21 transcripts
JNK2 (*MAPK9*)	UE	+	Increases apoptosis sensitivity and p53 protein expression
lincRNA-p21	UE	+	Reduces NF-κB activity
p21 (*CDKN1A*)	UE	+	Activates cell cycle checkpoints
p53 (*TP53*)	UE	+	Activates cell cycle checkpoints and reduces NF-κB activity
NF-κB activity	OE	+	Reduces active NF-κB
RanGAP1 (*RANGAP1*)	UE	-	-

Table 1. Molecular defects in rheumatoid arthritis and methotrexate targets. UC = unchanged, UE = under expressed, OE = over expressed.

2. Body

2.1. Rheumatoid arthritis

Rheumatoid arthritis is a chronic, inflammatory condition of the small and large joints characterized by inflammation of the synovium, or lining of the joint.[3] While the precise etiology of this disease remains unknown, the growing appreciation for the molecular basis of this disease has provided several clues. Particular emphasis has been placed on the cell types found in the joint spaces of patients with active disease.[4, 5] Lymphocytes are the most

http://dx.doi.org/10.5772/59901

common cell infiltrate found in the synovial space. In fact, of these lymphocytes, the majority are T lymphocytes making up approximately 30-50% of all infiltrating cell types in the synovium.[6] Of the T lymphocytes found in the RA synovium, it has been reported that the majority are CD4+CD45RO+ memory cells.[7] B cells constitute about 5% of the sublining synovial cells.[7] Clonal expansion of the B cells in the joint spaces of RA subjects suggests a maturation process driven by an antigen, which still remains unidentified. In normal tissue, the synovial space is only 1 or 2 cells in depth and is comprised of both Type A (macrophage-like) and Type B (fibroblast-like) cells.[7] However, in active RA this number increases ten-fold and is primarily thought to be the consequence of hypercellularlity due to the increase of both Type A and Type B cells.[7, 8] Many studies have suggested that Type A cells in RA display an activated phenotype and via circulation are constantly replenished from the bone marrow. Locally, while in the joint spaces, these Type A, macrophage-like cells produce "pro-inflammatory cytokines, chemokines, and growth factors" that in turn activate fibroblast-like synoviocytes and induce these cells to produce additional pro-inflammatory mediators including "IL-6, prostanoids, and matrix metalloproteinases." [7, 9, 10] This process can create both paracrine and autocrine signaling networks that give rise to the chronic synovitis and recruitment of additional immune cells to the joint, which eventually erodes the extracellular matrix and destroys the joint space. This phenomenon is referred to as the 'pannus', an expansive synovial tissue.[7] Phenotypically, this pannus closely resembles a tumor. Nuclear factor κB (NF-κB), a transcription factor that is ubiquitously expressed and functions as a critical regulator of cell proliferation, differentiation, and inflammation, is also overexpressed in the RA synovium. Briefly, nuclear factor κB consists of five proteins, c-Rel, RelA (p65), RelB, p50/p105, and p52/p100 that form either a homodimer or heterodimer.[7, 9] c-Rel, RelA, and RelB function as the major transactivation subunits. Unless activated, these subunits reside in the cytoplasm along with their inhibitor, IκB.[7] Phosphorylation of IκB causes IκB to be degraded by the proteasome, thus releasing NF-κB dimers to migrate to the nucleus where they localize to promoter regions of target genes.[7] Electromobility shift assays show constitutively high levels of p50 and p65 proteins in the synovium of rheumatoid arthritis subjects and induction of pro-inflammatory cytokines such as IL-1, IL-6, and TNF-α through IKK signaling pathways.[9] Depletion of p65 or the IKK family member, IKKβ, in the synovial tissue with siRNAs or introduction of dominant negative mutants reduces levels of these pro-inflammatory cytokines.[11]

In addition to increased levels of NF-κB, both synoviocytes and T cells in RA exhibit defects in expression and function of the guardian protein p53 leading to inability of these cells to undergo apoptosis and to resulting loss of genomic integrity.[8, 12] p53 is a critical regulator of cell cycle progression and reduced p53 levels or inactivating p53 mutations have also been found in a number of cancers including leukemia. Linking the contribution of these observations to the pervasive, non-resolving inflammation found in RA is a common goal in the management of the disease. Without this understanding, most therapeutics lack the specificity to precisely target the underlying defects contributing to disease progression. As such, most newly developed biologic agents attempt to disrupt the downstream, NF-κB activation-pro-inflammatory cytokine loop, by using drugs like etanercept, which selectively blocks the inflammatory cytokine, TNF-α.[13] These newer biologic therapies have added to the ability of physicians to improve outcomes and decrease disability. However, despite these advances excess mortality observed in patients with RA continues and recent data suggest that the mortality gap between RA patients and the rest of the population continues to widen.[14, 15] How, then, can we design therapies to target these observed defects? In the mid-twentieth century, we witnessed the birth of molecular medicine and the era of intelligent drug design. While most of the drugs developed during this period sought to treat cancer, very few of these early medications remain first in class therapies today and have since been replaced by more targeted therapies. Yet, one drug, MTX, first developed more than a half century ago, remains the standard of care for the treatment of RA.

2.2. Overview and history of MTX

Folates are critical components of cellular division, and DNA and RNA synthesis. The synthetic form of folate, folic acid, was first isolated in the early 1940s and was found to exacerbate acute forms of leukemia when added to a patient's diet.[16-18] Conversely, additional studies found that decreasing dietary amounts of folic acid decreased the leukemia cell counts in patients. From these early observations, work began to design analogues of folic acid, which could be used to treat cancer, particularly leukemia. Aminopterin was designed to reduce proliferation of cancerous cells via the inhibition of folate. Seminal work by Sidney Farber, a pathologist at Harvard Medical School and Boston Children's hospital, demonstrated that aminopterin produced remission in children diagnosed with acute lymphoblastic leukemia (ALL).[18-20] Even though this only produced brief remissions, it was proof of concept that folate antagonism could suppress the proliferation of malignant cells. Thus, the clinical efficacy of aminopterin in the treatment of ALL cemented aminopterin as one of the world's first chemotherapeutics.[18]

Work that followed nearly a decade later by Sidney Futterman, Michael Osborn, and Frank Heunnekens identified dihydrofolate reductase (DHFR) from chicken liver as the enzyme responsible for the reduction of folic acid to metabolically active forms.[18, 21] Thus, blockade of DHFR was implicated as a therapeutic target of chemotherapeutic doses of aminopterin. Isolation of this enzyme allowed for the creation of more potent inhibitors of DHFR. Specifically, another folate analog, MTX, was identified in a study of leukemia-bearing mice and when compared to aminopterin increased survival in these mice.[18] From these initial data in mice, two reports found that MTX at very high doses cured women diagnosed with choriocarcinoma, a malignant trophoblastic cancer of the placenta.[19] This was the first solid tumor to be cured by a drug in humans and stimulated interest in investigating the effects of MTX in additional forms of cancer.[18, 22] Of particular interest was the reduced side effect profile observed in the MTX-treated cohort. Compared to radiation or alkylating agents that can lead to infertility or additional malignancies, MTX monotherapy did not produce these deleterious effects.[18] Today, MTX is currently used in the treatment of large cell or high grade lymphomas, head and neck cancer, breast cancer, bladder cancer, and osteogenic sarcoma.[18] It is often used in combination with other therapies including 6-mercaptopurine (6MP). Studies have shown that the combination of MTX, 6MP, vincristine, and prednisone improve patient outcomes in the treatment of ALL.[18] In particular, a treatment regiment first prescribing MTX and following with 6MP in sequence improves cure rates.[18]

Given the immunosuppressive potential of aminopterin and MTX in the treatment of malignancy, Gubner et al reported in 1951 that proliferative responses of formalin injection in rat paws was abrogated with aminopterin treatment.[18, 23] Further, in a small population of patients with active rheumatoid arthritis, Gubner and colleagues showed that the overwhelming majority of patients treated with aminopterin developed reduced indices of disease activity. When the therapy was stopped, the patients experienced relapse. The toxicities reported included nausea and diarrhea, even at low doses (1-2 mg/day).[18] Due to these discomforts, MTX, which closely resembles aminopterin, was substituted.[18] Patients were able to tolerate MTX reasonably well at low doses. The role of aminopterin, and later MTX, was also investigated in other non-neoplastic diseases including psoriasis, a chronic skin condition producing thick patches of irritated skin that manifest as red or white scales and similar therapeutic benefits were observed.[18] It is interesting to note that this early report describing the therapeutic potential of MTX or other folate analogs was largely ignored for a quarter century. It would not be until the late 1980s that MTX is approved for the treatment of rheumatoid arthritis.[24]

Given the therapeutic potential for MTX in the treatment of these forms of cancer and even autoimmune disease, significant resources have been expended to investigate its mechanism of action. Bertino et al provided significant insight demonstrating that MTX is actively transported into cells through reduced folate transporter 1 (RFT-1).[25] MTX, like naturally occurring folates, is polyglutamated once taken up by the cell. Folates exist in cells as polyglutamates through the addition of 6 glutamyl groups in a gamma peptide linkage to the folate substrate using the enzyme folylpolyglutamate synthase (FPGS).[26] These long-lived MTX polyglutamates remain in the liver of patients for a long period as well as in the bone marrow myeloid precursors.[26] Polyglutamation of MTX occurs within 12-24 hours after treatment and polyglutamates constitute the active form of the drug.[26, 27] Thus, MTX is commonly referred to as a pro-drug, a compound that undergoes a biochemical modification to become its active form. Inhibition of DHFR, at pharmacologically relevant doses of MTX required for the treatment of malignancy, inhibits purine, pyrimidine, and thymidylate biosynthesis through reduced levels of tetrahydrofolate (FH_4) in the cell. Blockade of these enzymes, which are critical for nucleotide generation, halts rapid division of tumor cells through induction of apoptosis. Thus, one goal of MTX therapy is to increase the cellular cytotoxicity profile. Alterations to this pathway in the form of mutated RFT-1 or DHFR can lead to MTX resistance in cancer patients.[19, 26] Interestingly, cancer subjects resistant to MTX often exhibit increased levels of DHFR protein. It is hypothesized that gene amplification events may take place that are long-lived in tumor cells or that amplification occurs through extrachromosomal elements, called amplisomes, that contain DHFR genes.[26] This is currently an area of active exploration and future studies are required to determine the exact mechanisms.

While MTX is still used in the modern treatment of cancer, it is in the treatment of rheumatoid arthritis that physicians have observed MTX's greatest, long-term effectiveness. Often heralded as the drug that revolutionized the field of rheumatology, low-dose, once-weekly MTX differs by approximately three orders of magnitude (milligrams versus grams) compared to dosing schemes required for the treatment of malignancies. When the FDA first approved

MTX in 1988 for the treatment of rheumatoid arthritis, it was assumed that the mechanism of action by which MTX exerts its anti-inflammatory effects in rheumatoid arthritis would closely resemble the mechanism of action found in the treatment of cancer. However, despite considerable experience with MTX in the treatment of RA, we are still uncovering clues as to the exact mechanism or mechanisms MTX employs to produce its anti-inflammatory effects.

2.3. MTX and adenosine

Given the pro-inflammatory, anti-apoptotic phenotype exhibited by both synoviocytes and T cells in RA, and the ability of MTX to mitigate indices of inflammation it is logical to question if MTX may exert its anti-inflammatory properties through modulation of these pathways. For the past 30 years, the precise mechanisms employed by MTX to exert its anti-inflammatory effects in RA have been the focus of thorough investigation.[18, 25, 28-41] In the treatment of cancer, MTX induces apoptosis by blocking the folate-dependent processes involved with DNA and RNA synthesis ultimately leading to cell death. Curiously, however, folic or folinic acid supplementation in RA patients receiving MTX does not reverse its anti-inflammatory effects in randomized, blinded trials.[16, 18, 40, 42] Thus, other mechanisms have been proposed. A prevailing theory is that MTX exerts its mechanism of action through a number of different mechanisms including release of adenosine that function in parallel to blockade of nucleotide synthesis.[16] Reduced levels of methyl donors including tetrahydrofolate (FH_4) and methyltetrahydrofolate through inhibition of DHFR blocks generation of lymphotoxic polyamines through methionine and S-adenosylmethionine (SAM).[17, 27, 36, 40, 42, 43] Polyamine reduction has been posited as one anti-inflammatory mechanism since polyamines can be converted to lymphotoxins.[42] However, use of 3-deazaadensoine, a transmethylation inhibitor, does not demonstrate a significant clinical benefit in RA patients.[42] Yet, low-doses of MTX also inhibit chemotaxis in monocytes through a process reversed by S-adenosylmethionine supporting the contribution of this pathway in RA.[44] The retention of MTX polyglutamates in cells exceeds its half-life in plasma, suggesting that the MTX metabolites persist in tissues. These polyglutamates have also been shown to inhibit aminoimidazolecarboxamidoribonucleotide (AICAR) transformylase resulting in elevated intracellular AICAR levels. RA subjects exhibit high levels of AICAR in their urine during the course of MTX therapy.[16, 42] Increased AICAR levels are strong inhibitors of adenosine monophosphate (AMP) and adenosine deaminases, involved in the consumption of AMP and adenosine to IMP and inosine. Accumulation of adenosine in tissues has anti-inflammatory effects and AICARriboside, which also inhibits adenosine deaminase, is increased in RA.[42, 45] MTX has also been shown to enhance vasodilation leading to increased blood flow through inhibition of adenosine deamination in whole blood in humans.[46] The direct quantification of MTX-mediated adenosine release in humans receiving MTX has been unsuccessful largely because the half life of adenosine in blood and tissue is very brief making these measurements technically challenging.[42, 47] In animal models, however, the anti-inflammatory effects of MTX are mediated by adenosine using the carrageenan-induced air pouch model of inflammation and reversals with A2A adenosine receptor antagonists and supplementation of adenosine deaminase.[42, 48] Thus, one mechanism by which MTX achieves its anti-inflammatory effects is by stimulating increased synthesis and release of adenosine, which in turn, activates adenosine receptors to block various pro-inflammatory paths.

http://dx.doi.org/10.5772/59901

2.4. Novel mechanisms for MTX action

Other studies have also shown that MTX inhibits T cell activation, induces apoptosis, and alters expression of T cell cytokines and adhesion molecules.[28, 32, 49, 50] Additional work by Phillips et al posit that the anti-inflammatory properties of MTX are critically dependent upon the ability to produce reactive oxygen species in both T cells and monocytes, which ultimately lead to apoptosis.[31] Given the pronounced anti-inflammatory properties of low-dose MTX therapy in RA, it is unclear how the known biochemical pathways affected by MTX, e.g. inhibition of DHFR, activation of adenosine synthesis and release, should produce this anti-inflammatory profile. Our work has sought to explore the question of whether either additional biochemical pathways are targeted by MTX or additional biochemical consequences of DHFR inhibition by MTX may produce these anti-inflammatory properties observed in subjects with RA receiving low-dose MTX as therapy.

While initially developed as a chemotherapeutic, MTX (MTX) has been the mainstay for RA treatment for nearly four decades. Once-weekly administration of 7.5 to 25 milligrams yields optimal clinical outcomes, compared to the 5000 mg/week dosage used in the treatment of malignancy.[16, 18] RA patients treated with MTX experience reduced pain, and improved joint score and function typically within three months of initiation of treatment. The tight control and suppression of inflammation in early stages of disease has been advocated as the basis of documented disease modifying effects. Yet, the mechanisms accounting for the anti-inflammatory effects of MTX remain incompletely understood. Questions also remain as to the specific targets necessary to develop new therapeutics beyond MTX for the treatment of RA.

Our initial studies in RA examined differences in expression patterns of genes in healthy control subjects and patients diagnosed with autoimmune disease. The goal of these experiments was to identify a subset of genes that could distinguish between healthy individuals and patients with autoimmune disease.[51-53] Our expectation was that we would identify genes that encode proteins typically involved in pro-inflammatory processes. Instead, we found that patients with RA significantly underexpressed a panel of genes that are typically considered prototypical 'cancer genes' in peripheral blood mononuclear cells that encode proteins required for cell cycle arrest, maintenance of genomic integrity, and induction of apoptosis. Many cancers have inactivating mutations in these genes. Specifically, these studies established that defects in expression of *CHEK2, TP53, CDKN1A,* and *CDKN1B* that encode checkpoint kinase 2, p53, cyclin kinase inhibitor 1A or p21, and cyclin kinase inhibitor 1B or p27, respectively, conferred an inability for RA lymphocytes to undergo apoptosis in response to gamma irradiation.[12] The major obstacle moving forward was how to link these observations to inflammation and RA disease pathogenesis.

Since mechanisms by which low-dose MTX achieve therapeutic benefit in RA are incompletely understood and how the above deficiencies in cell cycle regulation and apoptosis may contribute to RA pathogenesis, we chose to initiate studies to compare RA subjects on MTX to RA subjects not receiving MTX therapy. Initially, we found that RA subjects receiving MTX therapy exhibited increased expression of genes encoding Fos and Jun that form the AP-1 transcription factor. In addition, expression of a number of genes induced by the AP-1 transcription factor is elevated in RA subjects receiving MTX therapy. Further, we were also able to reproduce these findings in tissue culture models via dose-dependent induction of *JUN* and *FOS* expression in T cells treated with sub-micromolar concentrations of MTX.[54]

One signaling pathway that activates the AP-1 transcription factor is via activation of Jun-N-terminal kinase (JNK), a MAP kinase, which phosphorylates Jun resulting in increased transcriptional activity of AP-1. MTX also activates JNK in our tissue culture models and MTX-dependent activation of JNK is responsible for the observed increases in *JUN* and *FOS* transcript levels and increased AP-1 activity. Through JNK activation, MTX increases the sensitivity of T cells to undergo apoptosis by production of reactive oxygen species and alteration of the transcriptional profile in favor of genes whose protein products promote apoptosis including Jun mRNA. Thus the resistance to apoptosis in RA T cells we described previously is reversed by MTX treatment. This process is also mediated by MTX-dependent inhibition of dihydrofolate reductase (DHFR). Besides reduction of folates, DHFR also catalyzes the reduction of dihydrobiopterin (BH_2) to tetrahydrobiopterin (BH_4) and BH_4 is a necessary cofactor of all nitric oxide synthases. MTX also blocks the DHFR catalyzed reduction of BH_2 to BH_4. Loss of BH_4 causes a process called nitric oxide synthase 'uncoupling' that results in production of reactive oxygen species such as hydrogen peroxide by nitric oxide synthases rather than production of nitric oxide. It is this nitric oxide synthase 'uncoupling' that leads to JNK activation and altered sensitivity to apoptosis.

Since our *in vivo* studies of RA patients on low-dose MTX therapy revealed elevated levels of the prototypical JNK-target gene, *JUN*, in response to MTX, our data support the notion that the JNK pathway is also activated by MTX, *in vivo*, and may contribute to the efficacy of MTX in inflammatory disease. Specifically, we now hypothesize that the therapeutic efficacy of MTX may arise at least in part from its ability to deplete BH_4. BH_4 depletion is known to cause a shift in cytokine profiles from a pro-inflammatory profile to an anti-inflammatory profile and our work shows that BH_4 depletion also increases sensitivity of lymphocytes to apoptosis, a process that may improve clearance of self-reactive inflammatory lymphocytes by apoptosis.

We further probed the mechanism by which MTX increases sensitivity of cells to apoptosis by asking if MTX restores the cell cycle checkpoint deficiencies we described previously. Since MTX increases activity of JNK in our tissue culture models, we asked if levels of JNK are decreased in subjects with RA not receiving MTX. We found highly significant deficiencies of *MAPK9* (JNK2) expression in rheumatoid arthritis.[55] This represents the major JNK protein expressed by lymphocytes. Analysis of other MAPK family members including most known ERK and p38 isoforms did not reveal any significant differences in healthy controls versus RA cohorts receiving or not receiving MTX. Following our gene expression studies, we analyzed protein expression in RA lymphocytes and found that these subjects exhibit reduced JNK protein expression. Analysis of additional autoimmune diseases also indicated that this *MAPK9* deficiency observed in RA was not unique to RA, but also extends to multiple sclerosis (MS). It is interesting to note that both RA and MS exhibit similar molecular defects in PBMC specifically through reduced checkpoint kinase 2 (*CHEK2*), p53 and ataxia telangiectasia (AT) mutated (ATM) expression.[56] The contributions of JNK to these defects remains to be explored. We found that MTX increased levels of both p53 and the downstream target p21 in

MTX-treated cells via JNK, which was further confirmed *in vivo* by analyzing transcript levels of *TP53* and *CDKN1A* in subjects receiving and not receiving MTX therapy. These MTX-mediated effects are critically dependent upon MTX depletion of BH_4, generation of ROS, and activation of JNK. Through loss of ATM, RA T cells accumulate a significant amount of DNA damage.[57] One hypothesis is that DNA damage repair deficiencies coupled with depressed levels of p53 and JNK blunt the central pathways of apoptosis resulting in cell survival but loss of genomic integrity. Cell survival comes at a cost and the cost is persistent DNA damage, which may activate NF-κB or alternative pro-inflammatory, pro-survival pathways leading to the 'sterile inflammation' observed in RA pathogenesis.

2.5. The cell cycle checkpoint deficiency-NF-κB activation connection in RA

Our studies outlined above clearly establish that MTX is a strong transcriptional activator, both in tissue culture models as well as in RA patients as part of their therapy. This is achieved in large part via activation of JNK. One of the best-studied proteins induced by MTX is p53, which itself is a strong transcriptional activator and the gene expression program induced by p53 allows p53 to carry out many of its cellular functions such as cell cycle arrest and induction of apoptosis. Further, transcript levels of genes encoding p53 and its transcriptional targets are largely depressed in RA patients. However, whether losses of these gene transcripts and corresponding proteins can contribute to the pro-inflammatory state characteristic of RA or how they might contribute to this pro-inflammatory state is less clear.

The NF-κB transcription factor is probably one of the best-characterized pro-inflammatory transcription factors. Many genes that encode pro-inflammatory cytokines, chemokines, and lymphocyte adhesion molecules possess NF-κB binding sites in their promoters and require activation of NF-κB for their increased expression in response to extracellular inflammatory stimuli. For these reasons, our next series of experiments analyzed the influence of MTX upon transcriptional activity of NF-κB, a central regulator of the inflammatory response, in two cells types: T cells and primary fibroblast-like synoviocytes (FLS) from RA subjects. We also examined NF-κB activity in the PBMC of RA patients receiving and not receiving MTX. In T lymphocytes, we found that MTX is a strong inhibitor of activation of NF-κB in response to various extracellular stimuli. In T cell tissue culture models, MTX inhibits activation of NF-κB via BH_4 depletion and JNK activation. Further, the inhibition of NF-κB activity in T cells by MTX is dependent upon MTX-mediated induction of p53. In patients with RA, NF-κB activity is chronically elevated in T helper cells and this elevation is reversed by MTX therapy. Taken together, we believe these studies provide a direct link between elevated activity of the pro-inflammatory, pro-cell survival transcription factor, NF-κB in RA and depressed levels of the pro-apoptotic, pro-cell cycle control transcription factor, p53, and show how induction of p53 by MTX results in subsequent loss of NF-κB activity in RA T helper cells.

Synovial fibroblast-like cells also activate NF-κB in response to extracellular stimuli and elevated levels of NF-κB activity have been demonstrated in RA synovial tissues. Therefore, we asked if MTX also inhibits activation of NF-κB in response to extracellular stimuli and if this inhibition is achieved via BH_4 depletion and JNK activation. Low concentrations of MTX effectively inhibit NF-κB activation in synovial fibroblasts in tissue culture. However, MTX does not act by depleting BH_4 and activating JNK as it does in T cells. In fact, genes characteristically induced by MTX in T cells, e.g. *TP53, CDKN1A, JUN*, are not induced by MTX in synovial fibroblasts. This appears to be because nitric oxide synthase enzymes are expressed at much lower levels in synovial fibroblasts than in T cells and thus generation of reactive oxygen species via nitric oxide synthase 'uncoupling' is inefficient. Rather, inhibition of NF-κB activation in synoviocytes appears to be mediated by adenosine release and activation of adenosine receptors.[58] This follows earlier work implicating the potential role of adenosine synthesis and activation of adenosine receptors in the anti-inflammatory effects of MTX.[27, 29, 45-47, 59-62] Thus, we conclude that MTX modulates NF-κB through distinct mechanisms and these effects are specific to different cell types (Figure 1).

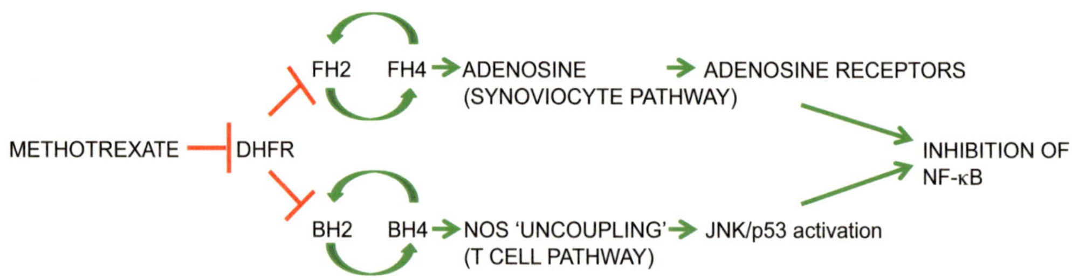

Figure 1. Schematic illustrating alternate pathways of MTX-mediated inhibition of NF-κB activity in T cells and synoviocytes.

We have explored the connection between NF-κB and p53 further, as these transcription factors are two central regulators of the adaptive immune response. NF-κB modulates the response to exogenous stimuli, whereas p53 modulates intrinsic stress responses through initiation of "cell cycle arrest, apoptosis, or senescence, eliminating clones of cells with DNA damage and its resulting mutations".[63] In general terms, NF-κB and p53 are functionally antagonistic. NF-κB is considered a pro-survival, pro-inflammatory transcription factor while p53 is an anti-survival, anti-inflammatory transcription factor. The precise mechanisms explaining the connection between p53 and NF-κB in the context of immune cells remains largely unexplored and is likely to be stimulus-, cell-, and/or disease-specific. The basic understanding in a healthy cell is that DNA damage, hypoxia, or oncogene activation elicit p53 responses that activate cell cycle arrest, senescence or apoptosis, targeting genes that are pro-apoptotic such as *PUMA*, or induce cell cycle arrest proteins such as p21.[63, 64] In the context of DNA damage, ATM is activated which leads to inhibition of MDM-2, an E3 ubiquitin ligase, and subsequent activation of p53.[65-67] While classically thought to be a modulator of cell survival or apoptosis, activation of p53 also creates metabolic consequences via reduced levels of aerobic glycolysis.[63, 68] One example of this regulation is p53-dependent activation of *TIGAR* (*T*P53-*i*nduced *g*lycolysis and *a*poptosis *r*egulator) that decreases fructose-2,6-bisphosphate levels leading to lower rates of cellular glycolysis.[63, 69] Like p53, NF-κB is typically activated via post-translational modifications via degradation of IκB or MDM-2/MDM-4 in response to exogenous signals such as infectious agents, viruses, toll-like receptor agonists, antigen receptors or through inflammatory cytokines, such as TNF-α or interleukin-1β.[63] Thus, NF-κB activation

http://dx.doi.org/10.5772/59901

leads to transcription of mRNAs that encode inflammatory proteins such as: cytokines, IL-6, GM-CSF; cheomokines, IL-8, RANTES, MCP-1; enzymes, COX-2, PLA2; and adhesion molecules VCAM-1 and ICAM-1.(9-11, 70] Interestingly, production of pro-inflammatory cytokines such as IL-1β and TNF-α creates an amplification loop that can lead to constitutive activation of the NF-κB signaling pathway. Therefore, strict regulation of this pathway needs to be employed to avoid persistent NF-κB activity, which could create the basis for chronic inflammatory disease, autoimmunity, and even certain cancers. Metabolically, activation of NF-κB enhances glycolysis and increases glucose transporters (GLUT3) leading to higher amounts of glucose uptake.[63]

Examination of the PBMC and synovium of RA subjects demonstrates that NF-κB is significantly overexpressed. Also present are reduced levels of p53. p53 drives induction of genes that both prevent DNA damage and repair damaged DNA. Together with NF-κB, these master regulators of internal and external stimuli must achieve a careful balance. Each transcription factor responds to a different form of cellular stress, adopting two very different strategies that have evolved into mutually exclusive processes under normal physiologic conditions.[63] It has also recently become appreciated that the metabolic fates of RA T cells are reprogrammed. RA T cells are energy deficient as evidenced by reduced glucose consumption, lactate production, and intracellular stores of ATP.[71, 72] Yang et al identified defects in 6-phosphofructo-2-kinase/fructose-2,6-bisphosphatase 3 (PFKFB3), a critical regulator of glycolysis, as the mediator of the observed defects as constitutive overexpression of PFKFB3 repaired the glycolytic insufficiency. Most interestingly, the study also demonstrated that deficiencies of PFKFB3 reduce ROS levels in cells. Our studies with methotrexate suggest that increased ROS generation is a therapeutic benefit of MTX therapy as apoptotic death of proliferating T cells is essential for T cell homeostasis. Thus, the contribution of metabolic 'rewiring' and the therapeutic potential of targeting these biomarkers represent attractive targets for clinical intervention.

To induce cell cycle arrest or apoptosis, the transcriptional program activated by p53 is mediated, in part, by induction of the long non-coding RNAs (lncRNAs), lincRNA-p21 and PANDA.[73, 74] lncRNAs are relatively newly discovered species of RNA. lncRNAs are transcribed from genes that look like protein-coding genes. Approximately 10,000 lncRNA genes have been discovered in the human genome so they may be as abundant as protein-coding genes.[75] These genes contain exons and introns and lncRNAs are spliced to mature lncRNAs just like mRNAs. The difference between lncRNAs and mRNAs is that lncRNAs are littered with translational stop codons throughout their sequence and thus cannot be translated into proteins and therefore exist as RNA species. As a class, lncRNAs have multiple functions. Major functions are the stimulation or inhibition of transcription of protein-coding genes. These target protein-coding genes are oftentimes, but not always, located in close proximity in the genome to the gene encoding the effector lncRNA. These lncRNAs generally act by recruiting the epigenetic machinery to target gene loci to establish activating or repressive histone marks. lncRNAs also interfere with translation of proteins. Additional mechanisms of action of lncRNAs are to regulate function, stability and activity of proteins. Thus, lncRNAs exhibit a broad spectrum of activities that play key roles in many cellular processes.[76-80]

Further, individual lncRNAs can have multiple modes of action. An example is lincRNA-p21. One function of lncRNA-p21 is to repress transcription of certain genes in response to p53 activation.[73] A second function is to modulate translation of certain mRNAs.[81] A third function is to modulate the stability of the transcription factor HIF-1α, thus regulating its activity.[82] A fourth function is to stimulate transcription of *CDKN1A*, the gene that encodes p21 required for cell cycle arrest.[83] Thus, besides being abundant species of RNAs, individual lncRNAs can possess multiple functions, which increases their cellular phenotypic imprint.

Because both transcript and protein levels of p53 and p21 are depressed in RA and are MTX target genes, we were interested to learn if the lncRNAs, lincRNA-p21 or PANDA, are differentially regulated in RA and/or may be MTX target genes. We have found that lincRNA-p21 transcript levels are depressed in RA T cells and lincRNA-p21 is a MTX target gene in T cells.[84] However, TP53 and lincRNA-p21 levels do not correlate with each other in T cells from subjects with RA or healthy controls suggesting that levels of p53 do not determine levels of lincRNA-p21 in T cells as they do in other cell types. Further, although lincRNA-p21 is strongly induced by MTX in T cells in our tissue culture models and lincRNA-p21 levels are restored to normal in RA patients receiving MTX therapy, induction of lincRNA-p21 does not appear to be dependent upon p53 activation under these conditions in these cell types. In T cells, induction of lincRNA-p21 by MTX is also not mediated by BH_4 depletion, nitric oxide synthase 'uncoupling' and JNK activation or by adenosine release and adenosine receptor activation.[84]

Increased DNA damage is also observed in RA T cells. The two major sentinels of DNA damage responses are the enzymes ATM and DNA-PKcs and these enzymes are also deficient in RA T cells.[57] Thus, these enzyme deficiencies may explain the accumulation of DNA damage observed in RA T cells. In T cells, stimulation with low concentrations of MTX results in activation of DNA-PKcs (phosphorylation) but not activation of ATM. Induction of lincRNA-p21 by MTX requires DNA-PKcs activation. In RA T cells, MTX therapy also restores *PRKDC* (the gene that encodes DNA-PKcs) transcript levels to normal. Mechanistically, we do not understand how MTX activates DNA-PKcs and not ATM in T cells. We also do not understand how activation of DNA-PKcs leads to induction of lincRNA-p21. One obvious mechanism would be via induction of p53 but this appears not to be the case. It may be that p21 contributes to this process but that remains to be investigated. Further studies will be necessary to more fully understand this mechanism.

We also asked if activation of DNA-PKcs and induction of lincRNA-p21 by MTX contributes to MTX-dependent activation of NF-κB in response to extracellular stimuli, such as TNF-α. This is clearly the case. Inhibition of DNA-PKcs, but not ATM, reverses MTX-dependent inhibition of TNF-α mediated NF-κB activation. Further, use of siRNAs to deplete either p53 mRNA or lincRNA-p21 reverses the ability of MTX to inhibit TNF-α mediated NF-κB activation. Thus, we conclude from these studies that multiple pathways are activated in T cells by methotrexate to achieve its anti-inflammatory effects. A graphic summary of the pathways we have discovered as a result of these studies is summarized in Figure 2.

http://dx.doi.org/10.5772/59901

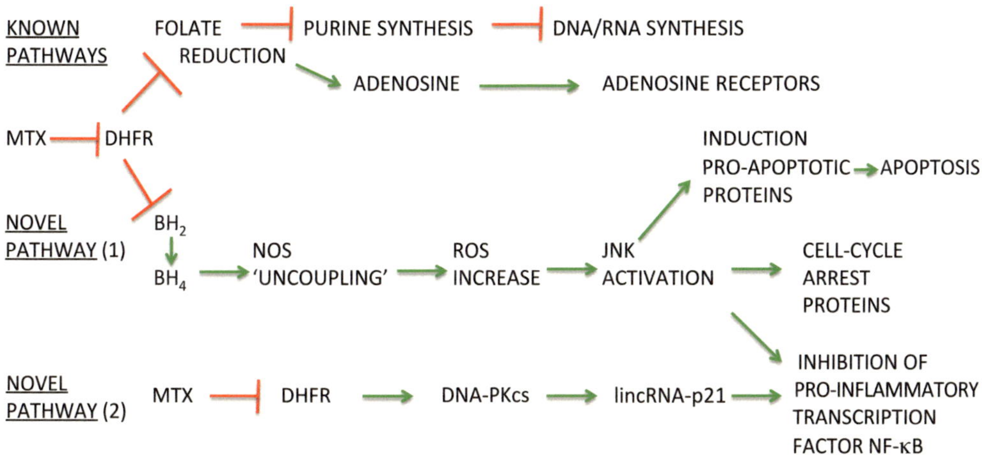

Figure 2. Summary of previously known and new mechanisms of methotrexate action

2.6. Other considerations

It has also been shown that telomeres of CD4+ cells are shortened in subjects with rheumatoid arthritis. On average, the telomeres of lymphocytes and even progenitor cells, such as CD34+ hematopoietic stem cells, are 1.5kb shorter compared to control resulting in accelerated immune system aging. [85, 86] Given that the immune system divides on average once a year and the average telomeric base pair (bp) loss is approximately 50bp, the immune system of RA subjects is approximately 25-30 years older than that of an unaffected individual. This phenotype is present in early disease and in untreated patients. So a question to ask is how are these traits conferred? Genetic studies have informed our knowledge of this disease by revealing the association of human leukocyte antigen (HLA) serotypes with autoimmune disease susceptibility. In the case of rheumatoid arthritis, susceptibility is associated with the HLA-DR4 allele. The relative risk for RA is four times greater in carriers compared to unaffected individuals with current female to male ratios suggesting an approximate 3:1 distribution.[87-89] Specifically, HLA-DRB1*04 remains the most important genetic risk factor for rheumatoid arthritis. If you examine healthy donors, and track the telomeric length of HLA-DRB1*04 +/- individuals as they age, donors with a positive HLA-DRB1*04 haplotypes exhibit premature aging in their CD4+ T cells with average telomeric length approximately 1.0-1.5kb shorter than HLA-DRB1*04 negative individuals.[64-66] It was further observed that this phenomenon of early immune aging was also found in the neutrophils of HLA-DRB1*04 positive individuals with concomitant accumulation of pre-senescent CD4+ T cells in healthy HLA-DRB1*04+ individuals measured by accumulation of CD28 null T cells in the total CD4+ lymphocyte population.[90-92]

In general, telomere loss is a measure of what is termed cellular senescence. Cellular senescence can arise by a number of mechanisms that include DNA damage, deficiencies of DNA damage response and repair pathways, as well as elevated NF-κB activity. It has also been argued that cellular senescence is a pathogenic mechanism in RA. Further, in experimental models, loss of p21, p27 or p53 can produce cellular senescence as well as pro-inflammatory or autoimmune phenotypes. Similarly, increased NF-κB activation can produce pro-inflammatory or autoimmune phenotypes. These same defects are seen in RA. Thus, one can imagine a continuous pathogenic loop of deficiencies in proteins involved in DNA damage responses and cell cycle control and increased NF-κB activity culminating in RA pathogenesis (Figure 3). MTX-dependent restoration of these deficiencies in DNA damage response and cell cycle control proteins that culminate in inhibition of chronic NF-κB activation reinforces this point. What is unclear is if there are dominant 'drivers' in this pathway or will any of the aforementioned defects that arise produce this pathogenic loop? This model raises the question of whether these defects arise via genetic or environmental mechanisms and understanding this question may improve our understandings of the origins of this disease. There may be other methods to interfere with this pathogenic loop. If developed, these methodologies may aid in the treatment of RA.

3. Conclusions

One hundred years ago, the only drug in the physician armamentarium to manage RA was aspirin.[93] Soon after, gold salts were commonly prescribed from approximately 1930-1980. Penicillamine, anti-malarial drugs, and sulfasalazine were subsequently introduced from in the 1970s and 1980s.[24] However, despite introduction of these pharmacologics, the disease course of most RA patients progressed and was not adequately controlled. It wasn't until the introduction of disease-modifying anti-rheumatic drugs, such as MTX, that physicians saw significant improvement in long-term outcomes, especially when MTX was combined with other therapies. When we initiated our studies to examine the anti-inflammatory properties of MTX, we thought that there would be a single biomarker we could target to achieve the same outcome with less toxicity, as subjects taking MTX have reported hair loss, nausea, and fatigue. However, as we examine the molecular basis for this drug in RA, we find that not only does it stimulate the adenosine pathway, which results in reduced NF-κB activation in FLS, but it also activates the BH_4 pathway and induces lincRNA-p21 in T cells. Both of these pathways lower NF-κB transcriptional activity and function *in vivo* in RA.

Targeted therapies that have been approved over the past decade have resulted in many first-in-class drugs. However, the majority of these first in class drugs were the result of phenotypic assay screening, and not through targeted approaches.[94] Interestingly, most targeted approaches result in follow-on drugs that are prescribed in combination with other 'anchor' therapies in human disease. An interesting area of future investigation would be to design small molecules that selectively target BH_2 reduction to BH_4 and alternatively induce lincRNA-p21 expression. Given the diverse effects we see both *in vitro* and *in vivo* in RA patients receiving MTX, it would be difficult to envision a single therapy that could supplant the multi-faceted pathway MTX employs in the management of RA. While these new therapeutics could be of utility, an important future direction of this work is setting the stage for a better understanding the origins of the cellular defects we have observed. We would argue that treatment of the

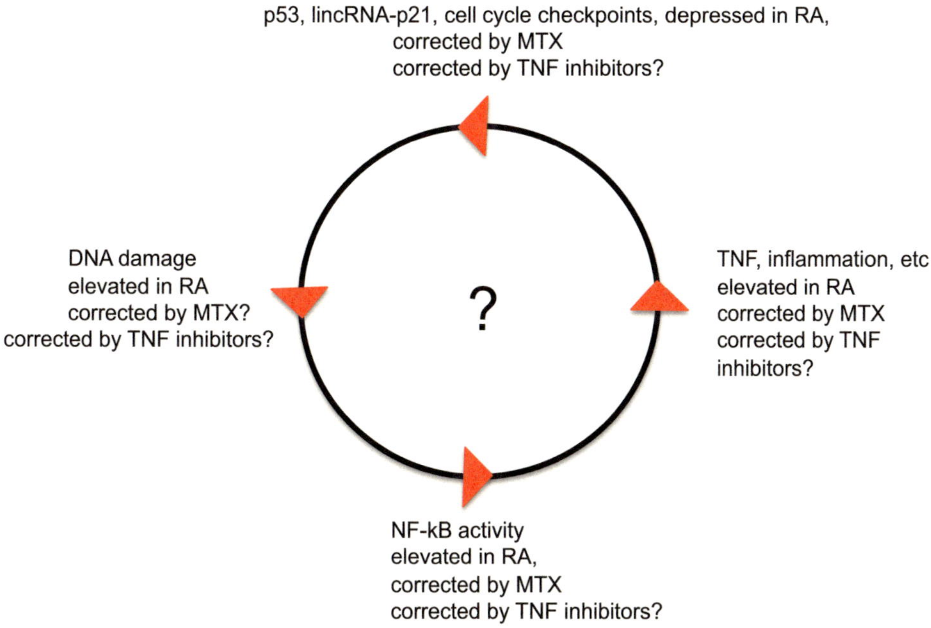

Figure 3. Hypothetical mechanistic loop that connects known molecular defects in RA to pathogenesis.

most proximal events in disease pathogenesis lead to more effective therapeutic strategies and improved clinical outcomes. Most newly developed therapies attempt to disrupt the downstream NF-κB activation-pro-inflammatory cytokine loop, such as etanercept through blockade of TNF-α. We argue that interfering with the upstream pathways of deficiency cell cycle arrest and DNA repair will produce improved therapeutic outcomes for subjects with RA. To this end, we have considered prevailing theories of immunity and autoimmunity. The general view is that initiation of adaptive immune responses to pathogens is divided into two parts, the recognition of 'danger' via the innate immune system and the recognition of foreign antigen by the adaptive immune system.[95, 96] It is widely accepted that a breach in tolerance in the adaptive immune response leads to recognition of self-antigen contributing to autoimmunity. In this model, the source of 'danger' to initiate the immune response to self has never been completely identified.[95] We would propose a new model whereby the source of 'danger' is actually internal or intracellular and not external, which we plan to explore.

In our model, DNA damage accumulates every day in individuals as a result of environmental exposures, UV or ionizing radiation, oxidative stress, chemical exposures, cell replication, inflammatory stress in response to infection, normal metabolic activities produce oxidants, or smoking.[97-104] Smoking is well established as a significant environmental risk factor for RA. Normally, activation of cell cycle checkpoints and the DNA damage response machinery repair DNA damage. However, in RA, via intrinsic mechanisms regulated by the presence of HLA-DRB1*04 alleles or other pathways, these repair mechanisms, DNA-PKcs, ATM, and cell cycle checkpoints, JNK2, p53, p21, p27, CHEK2, RANGAP1 are defective, resulting in failure to repair DNA and loss of genomic integrity.[53, 105-108] Failure to repair DNA and/or cell cycle checkpoint defects results in chronic NF-κB activation and induction of pro-inflammatory cytokines, producing a continuous cycle of events causing chronic inflammation, which underlies the pathogenesis of RA. Future studies are planned to examine the contribution of these defects to the pathogenesis of RA.

4. Nomenclature

Gene symbol-Protein names

ATM – Atm, Ataxia Telangiectasia Mutated

Functions: senses DNA damage and initiates DNA repair pathways and pathways to induce cell cycle arrest or apoptosis, also involved in telomere maintenance

PRKDC – DNA-PKcs, DNA-dependent protein kinase catalytic subunit

Functions: senses DNA damage and initiates similar pathways as Atm, also involved in non-homologous recombination, necessary for successful formation of T and B cell receptors

CHEK2 – Chek2, Chk2, checkpoint kinase 2

Functions: activated by Atm in response to DNA damage, phosphorylates and activates p53

TP53 – p53, tumor protein p53,

Functions: transcription factor, participates in an array of stress responses inducing cell cycle arrest, apoptosis, senescence, DNA repair, or changes in metabolism.

CDKN1A – Cdkn1a, p21, cyclin-dependent kinase inhibitor 1a

Functions: Inhibits activity of cyclin-CDK2 or –CDK4 complexes to inhibit cell cycle progression at G1, p53 target gene

CDKN1B – Cdkn1b, p27, kip1, cyclin-dependent kinase inhibitor 1b

Functions: Inhibits activity of cyclin E-CDK2 or cyclin D-CDK4 complexes to inhibit cell cycle progression at G1, p53 target gene

MAPK9 – Mapk9, Jnk2, c-Jun N-terminal kinase

Functions: Phosphorylates a number of transcription factors including c-Jun to activate the AP-1 transcription factor and regulate stress responses and apoptosis, also pro-inflammatory as many genes that encode cytokines and chemokines have AP-1 binding sites in their promoter

JUN – c-Jun, Jun proto-oncogene

Functions: along with Fos, forms the AP-1 transcription factor

FOS – Fos, c-Fos

Functions: along with Jun, forms the AP-1 transcription factor

http://dx.doi.org/10.5772/59901

RANGAP1 – RanGAP1, Ran GTPase activation protein 1

Functions: GTPase activator for the nuclear Ras-related protein, Ran, and converts it from the active state to the GDP-bound inactive state

RelA – NF-κB p65 subunit, nuclear factor-kappa B

Functions: transcription factor involved in many cellular processes commonly categorized as a pro-survival, pro-inflammatory transcription factor

Telomeresregions of repetitive DNA sequences at the ends of each chromosome, telomere ends shorten after each cell division, cellular senescence occurs when the telomeres become too short and this inhibits further cell division

Acknowledgements

Supported by grants from the National Institutes of Health (R21 AR063846, R01 AI044924, R42 AI53948), the National Center for Advancing Translation Sciences (UL1TR000445), the American College of Rheumatology Within Our Reach grant program (ACR124405) and the National Science Foundation Graduate Research Fellowship Program (DGE0909667).

Author details

Charles F. Spurlock III[1], Nancy J. Olsen[2] and Thomas M. Aune[1,3*]

*Address all correspondence to: tom.aune@vanderbilt.edu

1 Department of Medicine, Vanderbilt University School of Medicine, Nashville, TN, USA

2 Division of Rheumatology, Department of Medicine, Penn State M.S. Hershey Medical Center, Hershey, Pennsylvania, USA

3 Department of Pathology, Microbiology and Immunology, Vanderbilt University School of Medicine, Nashville, Tennessee, USA

References

[1] Stefanova I, Dorfman JR, Tsukamoto M, Germain RN. On the role of self-recognition in T cell responses to foreign antigen. Immunol Rev. 2003;191:97-106.

[2] Stefanova I, Dorfman JR, Germain RN. Self-recognition promotes the foreign antigen sensitivity of naive T lymphocytes. Nature. 2002;420(6914):429-34.

[3] Olsen NJ, Spurlock CF, Aune TM. Methotrexate induces production of IL-1 and IL-6 in the monocytic cell line U937. Arthritis Res Ther. 2014;16(1).

[4] St. Clair EW, Pisetsky DS, Haynes BF. Rheumatoid arthritis. Philadelphia: Lippincott Williams & Wilkins; 2004. xiv, 555 p. p.

[5] Goronzy JJ, Weyand CM. Developments in the scientific understanding of rheumatoid arthritis. Arthritis Res Ther. 2009;11(5):249.

[6] Lundy SK, Sarkar S, Tesmer LA, Fox DA. Cells of the synovium in rheumatoid arthritis. T lymphocytes. Arthritis Res Ther. 2007;9(1):202.

[7] Bartok B, Firestein GS. Fibroblast-like synoviocytes: key effector cells in rheumatoid arthritis. Immunological Reviews. 2010;233(1):233-55.

[8] Firestein GS, Echeverri F, Yeo M, Zvaifler NJ, Green DR. Somatic mutations in the p53 tumor suppressor gene in rheumatoid arthritis synovium. Proc Natl Acad Sci U S A. 1997;94(20):10895-900.

[9] Firestein GS. NF-kappaB: Holy Grail for rheumatoid arthritis? Arthritis and Rheumatism. 2004;50(8):2381-6.

[10] Tak PP, Firestein GS. NF-kappaB: a key role in inflammatory diseases. J Clin Invest. 2001;107(1):7-11.

[11] Simmonds RE, Foxwell BM. Signalling, inflammation and arthritis: NF-kappaB and its relevance to arthritis and inflammation. Rheumatology (Oxford). 2008;47(5): 584-90.

[12] Maas K, Westfall M, Pietenpol J, Olsen NJ, Aune T. Reduced p53 in Peripheral Blood Mononuclear Cells From Patients With Rheumatoid Arthritis Is Associated With Loss of Radiation-Induced Apoptosis. Arthritis and Rheumatism. 2005;52(4):1047-57.

[13] Dichamp I, Bourgeois A, Dirand C, Herbein G, Wendling D. Increased nuclear factor-kappaB activation in peripheral blood monocytes of patients with rheumatoid arthritis is mediated primarily by tumor necrosis factor-alpha. J Rheumatol. 2007;34(10): 1976-83.

[14] Gabriel SE. Why do people with rheumatoid arthritis still die prematurely? Ann Rheum Dis. 2008;67:30-4.

[15] Gabriel SE, Crowson CS, Kremers HM, Doran MF, Turesson C, O'Fallon WM, et al. Survival in rheumatoid arthritis: a population-based analysis of trends over 40 years. Arthritis and Rheumatism. 2003;48(1):54-8.

[16] Cronstein BN. Low-Dose Methotrexate: A Mainstay in the Treatment of Rheumatoid Arthritis. Pharmacological Reviews. 2005;57(2):163-72.

[17] Cronstein BN. Molecular therapeutics. Methotrexate and its mechanism of action. Arthritis and Rheumatism. 1996;39(12):1951-60.

[18] Cronstein BN, Bertino JR. Methotrexate: Springer; 2000.

[19] Chabner BA, Roberts TG, Jr. Timeline: Chemotherapy and the war on cancer. Nat Rev Cancer. 2005;5(1):65-72.

[20] Farber S, Diamond L, Mercer RD, Sylvester RF, Wolff JA. Temporary remissions in acute leukemia in children produced by folic antagonist, 4-aminopteroylglutamic acid (aminopterin).. N Engl J Med. 1948;238:787–93.

[21] Huennekens FM. In search of dihydrofolate reductase. Protein Sci. 1996;5(6):1201-8.

[22] Bertino JR. Karnofsky memorial lecture. Ode to methotrexate. J Clin Oncol. 1993;11(1):5-14.

[23] Gubner R, August S, Ginsberg V. Therapeutic suppression of tissue reactivity: II. Effect of aminopterin in rheumatoid arthritis and psoriasis. Am J Med Sci. 1951;221:176–82.

[24] Pincus T, Yazici Y, Sokka T, Aletaha D, Smolen JS. Methotrexate as the "anchor drug" for the treatment of early rheumatoid arthritis. Clin Exp Rheumatol. 2003;21(5 Suppl 31):S179-85.

[25] Jolivet J, Cowan KH, Curt GA, Clendeninn NJ, Chabner BA. The pharmacology and clinical use of methotrexate. N Engl J Med. 1983;309:1094-104.

[26] Kremer JM. Toward a better understanding of methotrexate. Arthritis and Rheumatism. 2004;50(5):1370-82.

[27] Chan ES, Cronstein BN. Molecular action of methotrexate in inflammatory diseases. Arthritis research. 2002;4(4):266-73.

[28] Paillot R, Genestier L, Fournel S, Ferraro C, Miossec P, Revillard JP. Activation-dependent lymphocyte apoptosis induced by methotrexate. Transplant Proc. 1998;30(5): 2348-50.

[29] Montesinos MC, Desai A, Delano D, Chen JF, Fink JS, Jacobson MA, et al. Adenosine A2A or A3 receptors are required for inhibition of inflammation by methotrexate and its analog MX-68. Arthritis Rheum 2003;48:240-7.

[30] Johnston A, Gudjonsson JE, Sigmundsdotti H, Ludviksson BJ, Valdimarrsson H. The anti-inflammatory action of methotrexate is not mediated by lymphocyte apoptosis, but by the suppression of activation and adhesion molecules. Clinical Immunology. 2005(114):154-63.

[31] Phillips DC, Woollard KJ, Griffiths HR. The anti-inflammatory actions of methotrexate are critically dependent upon the production of reactive oxygen species. Br J Pharmacol. 2003;138:501-11.

[32] Constantin A, Loubet-Lescoulié P, Lambert N, Yassine-Diab B, Abbal M M, B., de Préval C, et al. Antiinflammatory and immunoregulatory action of methotrexate in the treatment of rheumatoid arthritis: evidence of increased interleukin-4 and inter-

leukin-10 gene expression demonstrated in vitro by competitive reverse transcriptase-polymerase chain reaction. Arthritis Rheum 1998;41:48-57.

[33] Olsen NJ, Murray LM. Antiproliferative effects of methotrexate on peripheral blood mononuclear cells. Arthritis Rheum. 1989;32:378-85.

[34] Williams HJ, Willkens RF, Samuelson COJ, Alarcón GS, Guttadauria M, Yarboro C, et al. Comparison of low-dose oral pulse methotrexate and placebo in the treatment of rheumatoid arthritis. A controlled clinical trial. Arthritis Rheum. 1985;28:721-30.

[35] Braun J, Kastner P, Flaxenberg P, Wahrisch J, Hanke P, Demary W, et al. Comparison of the clinical efficacy and safety of subcutaneous versus oral administration of methotrexate in patients with active rheumatoid arthritis: results of a six-month, multicenter, randomized, double-blind, controlled, phase IV trial. Arthritis Rheum. 2008;58:73-81.

[36] Cronstein BN. The mechanism of action of methotrexate. Rheum Dis Clin North Am. 1997;23(4):739-55.

[37] Dervieux T, Furst D, Lein DO, Capps R, Smith K, Caldwell J, et al. Pharmacogenetic and metabolite measurements are associated with clinical status in patients with rheumatoid arthritis treated with methotrexate: results of a multicentred cross sectional observational study. Ann Rheum Dis 2005;64:1180-5.

[38] Dalrymple JM, Stamp LK, O'Donnell JL, Chapman PT, Zhang M, Barclay ML. Pharmacokinetics of oral methotrexate in patients with rheumatoid arthritis. Arthritis Rheum 2008;58:3299-308.

[39] van Dieren JM, Kuipers EJ, Samsom JN, Nieuwenhuis EE, van der Woude CJ. Revisiting the immunomodulators tacrolimus, methotrexate, and mycophenolate mofetil: their mechanisms of action and role in the treatment of IBD. Inflamm Bowel Dis. 2006;12:311-27.

[40] Tian H, Cronstein BN. Understanding the mechanisms of action of methotrexate: implications for the treatment of rheumatoid arthritis. Bull NYU Hosp Jt Dis. 2007;65:168-73.

[41] Braun J, Rau R. An update on methotrexate. Curr Opin Rheumatol. 2009;21:216-23.

[42] Chan SLC, Cronstein BN. Methotrexate-how does it really work? Nature Reviews/ Rheumatology. 2010;6:175-8.

[43] Cronstein BN. Molecular mechanism of methotrexate action in inflammation. Inflammation. 1992;16(5):411-23.

[44] Nesher G, Moore TL, Dorner RW. In vitro effects of methotrexate on peripheral blood monocytes: modulation by folinic acid and S-adenosylmethionine. Ann Rheum Dis. 1991;50(9):637-41.

[45] Morabito L, Montesinos MC, Schreibman DM, Balter L, Thompson LF, Resta R, et al. Methotrexate and sulfasalazine promote adenosine release by a mechanism that re-

http://dx.doi.org/10.5772/59901

quires ecto-5'-nucleotidase-mediated conversion of adenine nucleotides. J Clin Invest. 1998;101(2):295-300.

[46] Riksen NP, Barrera P, van den Broek PH, van Riel PL, Smits P, Rongen GA. Methotrexate modulates the kinetics of adenosine in humans in vivo. Ann Rheum Dis. 2006;65(4):465-70.

[47] Dolezalová P, Krijt J, Chládek J, Nemcová D, Hoza J. Adenosine and methotrexate polyglutamate concentrations in patients with juvenile arthritis. Rheumatology (Oxford). 2005;44:74-9.

[48] Cronstein BN, Naime D, Ostad E. The antiinflammatory mechanism of methotrexate. Increased adenosine release at inflamed sites diminishes leukocyte accumulation in an in vivo model of inflammation. J Clin Invest. 1993;92(6):2675-82.

[49] Wessels JAM, Huizinga TWJ, Guchelaar H-J. Recent insights in the pharmacological actions of methotrexate in the treatment of rheumatoid arthritis. Rheumatology (Oxford). 2008;47:249-55.

[50] Genestier L, Paillot R, Fournel S, Ferraro C, Miossec P, Revillard JP. Immunosuppressive properties of methotrexate: apoptosis and clonal deletion of activated peripheral T cells. J Clin Invest 1998;102:322-8.

[51] Maas K, Chan S, Parker J, Slater A, Moore J, Olsen NJ, et al. Cutting edge: molecular portrait of human autoimmune disease. J Immunol. 2002;169:5-9.

[52] Olsen N, Sokka T, Seehorn CL, Kraft B, Maas K, Moore J, et al. A gene expression signature for recent onset rheumatoid arthritis in peripheral blood mononuclear cells. Ann Rheum Dis. 2004;63:1387-92.

[53] Liu Z, Maas K, Aune TM. Identification of gene expression signatures in autoimmune disease without the influence of familial resemblance. Hum Mol Genet. 2006;15(3):501-9.

[54] Spurlock CF, 3rd, Aune ZT, Tossberg JT, Collins PL, Aune JP, Huston JW, 3rd, et al. Increased sensitivity to apoptosis induced by methotrexate is mediated by JNK. Arthritis and Rheumatism. 2011;63(9):2606-16.

[55] Spurlock CF, 3rd, Tossberg JT, Fuchs HA, Olsen NJ, Aune TM. Methotrexate increases expression of cell cycle checkpoint genes via JNK activation. Arthritis and Rheumatism. 2012;64(6):1780-9.

[56] Deng X, Ljunggren-Rose A, Maas K, Sriram S. Defective ATM-p53-mediated apoptotic pathway in multiple sclerosis. Annals of neurology. 2005;58(4):577-84.

[57] Shao L, Fukii H, Ines C, Oishi H, Goronzy JJ, Weyand CM. Deficiency of the DNA repair enzyme ATM in rheumatoid arthritis. J Exp Med. 2009;206(6):1435-49.

[58] Spurlock CF, 3rd, Gass HMt, Bryant CJ, Wells BC, Olsen NJ, Aune TM. Methotrexate-mediated inhibition of nuclear factor kappaB activation by distinct pathways in T cells and fibroblast-like synoviocytes. Rheumatology. 2015; 54:178-187

[59] Cristalli G, Lambertucci C, Marucci G, Volpini R, Dal Ben D. A2A adenosine receptor and its modulators: overview on a druggable GPCR and on structure-activity relationship analysis and binding requirements of agonists and antagonists. Current pharmaceutical design. 2008;14:1525–52.

[60] Jacobson KA, Gao ZG. Adenosine receptors as therapeutic targets. Nature reviews Drug discovery. 2006;5:247–64.

[61] Montesinos MC, Yap JS, Desai A, Posadas I, McCrary CT, Cronstein BN. Reversal of the antiinflammatory effects of methotrexate by the nonselective adenosine receptor antagonists theophylline and caffeine: evidence that the antiinflammatory effects of methotrexate are mediated via multiple adenosine receptors in rat adjuvant arthritis. Arthritis and Rheumatism. 2000;43(3):656-63.

[62] Majumdar S, Aggarwal BB. Methotrexate suppresses NF-kappaB activation through inhibition of IkappaBalpha phosphorylation and degradation. J Immunol. 2001;167:2911-20.

[63] Ak P, Levine AJ. p53 and NF-κB: different strategies for responding to stress lead to a functional antagonism. FASEB. 2010;24:3643-52.

[64] Zhang XP, Liu F, Wang W. Two-phase dynamics of p53 in the DNA damage response. Proc Natl Acad Sci U S A. 2011;108(22):8990-5.

[65] Lee J-H, Paull TT. ATM Activation by DNA Double-Strand Breaks Through the Mre11-Rad50-Nbs1 Complex. Science. 2005;308(5721):551-4.

[66] Liu S, Opiyo SO, Manthey K, Glanzer JG, Ashley AK, Amerin C, et al. Distinct roles for DNA-PK, ATM and ATR in RPA phosphorylation and checkpoint activation in response to replication stress. Nucleic Acids Res. 2012;40(21):10780-94.

[67] Maya R, Balass M, Kim ST, Shkedy D, Leal JF, Shifman O, et al. ATM-dependent phosphorylation of Mdm2 on serine 395: role in p53 activation by DNA damage. Genes Dev. 2001;15(9):1067-77.

[68] Matoba S, Kang JG, Patino WD, Wragg A, Boehm M, Gavrilova O, et al. p53 regulates mitochondrial respiration. Science. 2006;312(5780):1650-3.

[69] Bensaad K, Tsuruta A, Selak MA, Vidal MN, Nakano K, Bartrons R, et al. TIGAR, a p53-inducible regulator of glycolysis and apoptosis. Cell. 2006;126(1):107-20.

[70] McInnes IB, Schett G. Cytokines in the pathogenesis of rheumatoid arthritis. Nature Reviews Immunology. 2007;7(6):429-42.

[71] Yang Z, Goronzy JJ, Weyand CM. The glycolytic enzyme PFKFB3/phosphofructokinase regulates autophagy. Autophagy. 2014;10(2):382-3.

[72] Yang Z, Fujii H, Mohan SV, Goronzy JJ, Weyand CM. Phosphofructokinase deficiency impairs ATP generation, autophagy, and redox balance in rheumatoid arthritis T cells. J Exp Med. 2013;210(10):2119-34.

[73] Huarte M, Guttman M, Feldser D, Garber M, Koziol MJ, Kenzelmann-Broz D, et al. A large intergenic noncoding RNA induced by p53 mediates global gene repression in the p53 response. Cell. 2010;142(3):409-19.

[74] Hung T, Wang Y, Lin MF, Koegel AK, Kotake Y, Grant GD, et al. Extensive and coordinated transcription of noncoding RNAs within cell-cycle promoters. Nat Genet. 2011;43(7):621-9.

[75] Rinn JL, Chang HY. Genome regulation by long noncoding RNAs. Annu Rev Biochem. 2012;81:145-66.

[76] Wang KC, Yang YW, Liu B, Sanyal A, Corces-Zimmerman R, Chen Y, et al. A long noncoding RNA maintains active chromatin to coordinate homeotic gene expression. Nature. 2011.

[77] Gupta RA, Shah N, Wang KC, Kim J, Horlings HM, Wong DJ, et al. Long non-coding RNA HOTAIR reprograms chromatin state to promote cancer metastasis. Nature. 2010;464(7291):1071-6.

[78] Tsai MC, Manor O, Wan Y, Mosammaparast N, Wang JK, Lan F, et al. Long noncoding RNA as modular scaffold of histone modification complexes. Science. 2010;329(5992):689-93.

[79] Guttman M, Amit I, Garber M, French C, Lin MF, Feldser D, et al. Chromatin signature reveals over a thousand highly conserved large non-coding RNAs in mammals. Nature. 2009;458(7235):223-7.

[80] Khalil AM, Guttman M, Huarte M, Garber M, Raj A, Rivea Morales D, et al. Many human large intergenic noncoding RNAs associate with chromatin-modifying complexes and affect gene expression. Proc Natl Acad Sci U S A. 2009;106(28):11667-72.

[81] Yoon JH, Abdelmohsen K, Srikantan S, Yang X, Martindale JL, De S, et al. LincRNA-p21 suppresses target mRNA translation. Molecular Cell. 2012;47(4):648-55.

[82] Yang F, Zhang H, Mei Y, Wu M. Reciprocal regulation of HIF-1alpha and lincRNA-p21 modulates the Warburg effect. Molecular Cell. 2014;53(1):88-100.

[83] Dimitrova N, Zamudio JR, Jong RM, Soukup D, Resnick R, Sarma K, et al. LincRNA-p21 activates p21 in cis to promote Polycomb target gene expression and to enforce the G1/S checkpoint. Mol Cell. 2014;54(5):777-90.

[84] Spurlock CF, 3rd, Tossberg JT, Matlock BK, Olsen NJ, Aune TM. Methotrexate Inhibits NF-kappaB Activity Via Long Intergenic (Noncoding) RNA-p21 Induction. Arthritis & Rheumatology. 2014;66(11):2947-57.

[85] Koetz K, Bryl E, Spickschen K, O'Fallon WM, Goronzy JJ, Weyand CM. T cell homeostasis in patients with rheumatoid arthritis. Proc Natl Acad Sci U S A. 2000;97(16): 9203-8.

[86] Colmegna I, Diaz-Borjon A, Fujii H, Schaefer L, Goronzy JJ, Weyand CM. Defective proliferative capacity and accelerated telomeric loss of hematopoietic progenitor cells in rheumatoid arthritis. Arthritis Rheum. 2008;58(4):990-1000.

[87] Ritchie MD, Denny JC, Crawford DC, Ramirez AH, Weiner JB, Pulley JM, et al. Robust replication of genotype-phenotype associations across multiple diseases in an electronic medical record. Am J Hum Genet. 2010;86(4):560-72.

[88] Weyand CM, Goronzy JJ. Association of MHC and rheumatoid arthritis. HLA polymorphisms in phenotypic variants of rheumatoid arthritis. Arthritis research. 2000;2(3):212-6.

[89] Weyand CM, Goronzy JJ. HLA polymorphisms and T cells in rheumatoid arthritis. International reviews of immunology. 1999;18(1-2):37-59.

[90] Hohensinner PJ, Goronzy JJ, Weyand CM. Targets of immune regeneration in rheumatoid arthritis. Mayo Clin Proc. 2014;89(4):563-75.

[91] Weyand CM, Yang Z, Goronzy JJ. T-cell aging in rheumatoid arthritis. Curr Opin Rheumatol. 2014;26(1):93-100.

[92] Schonland SO, Lopez C, Widmann T, Zimmer J, Bryl E, Goronzy JJ, et al. Premature telomeric loss in rheumatoid arthritis is genetically determined and involves both myeloid and lymphoid cell lineages. Proc Natl Acad Sci U S A. 2003;100(23):13471-6.

[93] Ragan C. Rheumatoid arthritis; the natural history of the disease and its management. Bull N Y Acad Med. 1951;27(2):63-74.

[94] Swinney DC, Anthony J. How were new medicines discovered? Nat Rev Drug Discov. 2011;10(7):507-19.

[95] Matzinger P. Friendly and dangerous signals: is the tissue in control? Nat Immunol. 2007;8(1):11-3.

[96] Gallucci S, Matzinger P. Danger signals: SOS to the immune system. Curr Opin Immunol. 2001;13(1):114-9.

[97] Kaarniranta K, Salminen A. Control of p53 and NF-KB signaling by WIP1 and MIF: Role in cellular senescence and organismal aging. Cellular Signaling. 2010;23:747-52.

[98] Perry JJP, Tainer JA. All Stressed Out Without ATM Kinase. Sci Signal. 2011;4(167).

[99] Hadian K, Krappmann D. Signals from the Nucleus: Activation of NF-kappa B by Cytosolic ATM in the DNA Damage Response. Sci Signal. 2011;4(156).

[100] Bredemeyer AL, Helmink BA, Innes CL, Calderon B, McGinnis LM, Mahowald GK, et al. DNA double-strand breaks activate a multi-functional genetic program in developing lymphocytes. Nature. 2008;456(7223):819-23.

[101] Matsuoka S, Ballif BA, Smogorzewska A, McDonald ER, Hurov KE, Luo J, et al. ATM and ATR substrate analysis reveals extensive protein networks responsive to DNA damage. Science. 2007;316(5828):1160-6.

[102] Wu ZH, Shi Y, Tibbetts RS, Miyamoto S. Molecular linkage between the kinase ATM and NF-kappaB signaling in response to genotoxic stimuli. Science. 2006;311(5764): 1141-6.

[103] Parker A, Izmailova ES, Narang J, Badola S, Le T, Roubenoff R, et al. Peripheral blood expression of nuclear factor-kappab-regulated genes is associated with rheumatoid arthritis disease activity and responds differentially to anti-tumor necrosis factor-alpha versus methotrexate. J Rheumatol. 2007;34:1817-22.

[104] Oleinik NV, Krupenko NI, Krupenko SA. Cooperation between JNK1 and JNK2 in activation of p53 apoptotic pathway. Oncogene. 2007;26:7222-30.

[105] Gutierrez GJ, Tsuji T, Cross JV, Davis RJ, Templeton DJ, Jiang W, et al. JNK-mediated Phosphorylation of Cdc25C Regulates Cell Cycle Entry and G(2)/M DNA Damage Checkpoint. Journal of Biological Chemistry. 2010;285(19):14217-28.

[106] Quimby BB, Dasso M. The small GTPase Ran: interpreting the signs. Curr Opin Cell Biol. 2003;15(3):338-44.

[107] Weyand CM, Fujii H, Shao L, Goronzy JJ. Rejuvenating the immune system in rheumatoid arthritis. Nat Rev Rheumatol. 2009;5(10):583-8.

[108] Fujii H, Shao L, Colmegna I, Goronzy JJ, Weyand CM. Telomerase insufficiency in rheumatoid arthritis. Proc Natl Acad Sci U S A. 2009;106(11):4360-5.